Textbook of
Applied Psychology

Textbook of Applied Psychology

As per the Revised INC Syllabus for BSc Nursing

Sukhbir Kaur
BSN RN (PGI, Chandigarh) PGDHM MSN (CMC, Ludhiana) PhD (N)
Associate Professor
Department of Psychiatric Nursing
College of Nursing, Sri Guru Ram Das University of Health Sciences
Amritsar, Punjab, India

Co-author
Onkardeep Kaur
BSN RN MSN (SGRDUHS, Amritsar) PhD (N) Scholar
Lecturer
Department of Obstetric and Gynecological Nursing
College of Nursing, Sri Guru Ram Das University of Health Sciences
Amritsar, Punjab, India

Forewords
Triza Jiwan
Parvesh Saini

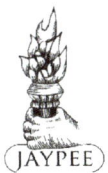

JAYPEE BROTHERS MEDICAL PUBLISHERS
The Health Sciences Publisher
New Delhi | London

Jaypee Brothers Medical Publishers (P) Ltd

Headquarters
Jaypee Brothers Medical Publishers (P) Ltd
EMCA House, 23/23-B
Ansari Road, Daryaganj
New Delhi 110 002, India
Landline: +91-11-23272143, +91-11-23272703
+91-11-23282021, +91-11-23245672
Email: jaypee@jaypeebrothers.com

Corporate Office
Jaypee Brothers Medical Publishers (P) Ltd
4838/24, Ansari Road, Daryaganj
New Delhi 110 002, India
Phone: +91-11-43574357
Fax: +91-11-43574314
Email: jaypee@jaypeebrothers.com

Overseas Office
J.P. Medical Ltd
83 Victoria Street, London
SW1H 0HW (UK)
Phone: +44 20 3170 8910
Fax: +44 (0)20 3008 6180
Email: info@jpmedpub.com

Website: www.jaypeebrothers.com
Website: www.jaypeedigital.com

© 2022, Jaypee Brothers Medical Publishers

The views and opinions expressed in this book are solely those of the original contributor(s)/author(s) and do not necessarily represent those of editor(s) and publisher of the book.

All rights reserved. No part of this publication may be reproduced, stored or transmitted in any form or by any means, electronic, mechanical, photocopying, recording or otherwise, without the prior permission in writing of the publishers.

All brand names and product names used in this book are trade names, service marks, trademarks or registered trademarks of their respective owners. the publisher is not associated with any product or vendor mentioned in this book.

Medical knowledge and practice change constantly. This book is designed to provide accurate, authoritative information about the subject matter in question. However, readers are advised to check the most current information available on procedures included and check information from the manufacturer of each product to be administered, to verify the recommended dose, formula, method and duration of administration, adverse effects and contraindications. It is the responsibility of the practitioner to take all appropriate safety precautions. Neither the publisher nor the author(s)/editor(s) assume any liability for any injury and/or damage to persons or property arising from or related to use of material in this book.

This book is sold on the understanding that the publisher is not engaged in providing professional medical services. If such advice or services are required, the services of a competent medical professional should be sought.

Every effort has been made where necessary to contact holders of copyright to obtain permission to reproduce copyright material. If any have been inadvertently overlooked, the publisher will be pleased to make the necessary arrangements at the first opportunity.

Inquiries for bulk sales may be solicited at: jaypee@jaypeebrothers.com

Textbook of Applied Psychology

First Edition: **2022**

ISBN: 978-93-5465-933-1

Reviewers

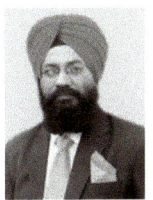

Amandeep Singh PhD (Clinical Psychology)
Assistant Professor-cum Clinical Psychologist
SGRD University of Health Sciences
Vallah, Punjab, India

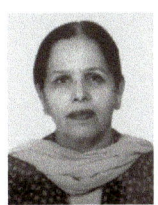

Avinash Kaur Rana
Ex-Lecturer
Postgraduate Institute of Medical Education and Research
Chandigarh, India
Ex-Professor-cum Principal
Swami Devi Dyal College of Nursing
Panchkula, Haryana, India

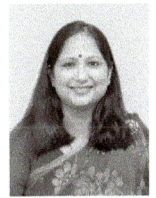

Bandana Bisht BSN MSN PhD (N)
Assistant Professor
Faculty
Department of Psychiatry
Government Medical College and Hospital
Chandigarh, India

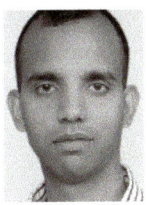

Bhartendra Sharma BSN MSN PhD (N)
Professor
Mahatma Gandhi Nursing College
Jaipur, Rajasthan, India

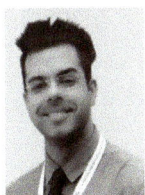

Deepak Sethi BSN MSN PhD (N)
Professor
Sharda University
Greater Noida, Uttar Pradesh, India

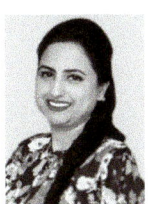

Kanika Sharma PhD Scholar
Associate Professor
University Institute of Nursing
Chandigarh University
Chandigarh, India

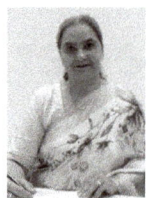

Kirandeep Dhaliwal BSN MSN PhD (N)
Professor-cum Vice-Principal
MM College of Nursing
Maharishi Markandeshwar University
Mullana, Haryana, India

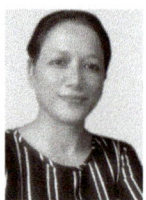

Monika Dogra BSN MSN PhD (N)
Professor
Department of Mental Health Nursing
Khalsa College of Nursing
Amritsar, Punjab, India

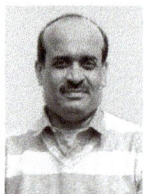

Rajesh Konnur MPhil (N) PhD MBA PGDGC PGDCA
Professor
College of Nursing
Kurji Holy Family Hospital
Patna, Bihar, India

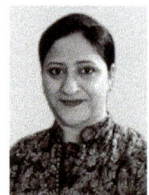

Rupinder Kaur Oberoi MBBS MD Psychiatry (IGMC, Shimla)
Specialist Medical Officer
Gurdaspur, Punjab, India

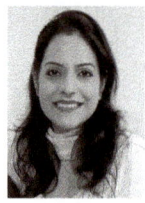

Shailza Sharma BSN MSN (Mental Health Nursing)
Associate Professor
Dayanand Medical College and Hospital, College of Nursing
Ludhiana, Punjab, India

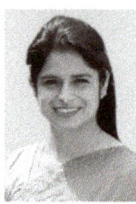

Suman Vashist BSN MSN PhD (N) Scholar
Associate Professor
Faculty of Nursing
SGT University
Gurugram, Haryana, India

Foreword

I am delighted to pen down this foreword for *Textbook of Applied Psychology* for nurses by Dr Sukhbir Kaur and Ms Onkardeep Kaur as I believe in educative values of teaching and applying comprehensive approach to imparting knowledge as reflected in this book. I am sure the readers will be benefited with the simple and comprehensive information in this book. I congratulate the authors of this book for compilation of the content matter in well-organized manner.

This book widely covers the basic concepts of psychology as per the needs of the nursing students. It is written in simple, understandable language and formatted as per the convenience of students. This book covers all the chapters as per the latest Indian Nursing Council (INC) syllabus for BSc Nursing students and also ready references and covers the topics related to GNM and Post Basic Nursing courses. The author has used diagrams, flowcharts, figures to extensively elaborate the difficult concepts which students can easily grasp. Application of each aspect of psychology is highlighted at the end of each chapter. For self-evaluation action summary is laid down at the end of each chapter.

I am confident enough that this book will provide adequate knowledge to the students and enhance teacher knowledge as well.

Triza Jiwan BSN MSN (Mental Health Nursing), PhD (N)
Professor-cum-Principal
College of Nursing
Dayanand Medical College and Hospital
Ludhiana, Punjab, India

Foreword

Nursing is a profession within the healthcare sector focused on the care of individuals, families and communities by understanding about their behavior and implementing care accordingly, so they may attain, maintain or recover optimal health and quality of life. Nurses must have extended knowledge into the psychology of their clients so that they can give holistic care.

It gives me an immense happiness to write foreword for Textbook of Applied Psychology written by Dr Sukhbir Kaur and Ms Onkardeep Kaur. The text is written in simple English to ensure that the students are able to grasp the fundamental concepts and theories in psychology easily. The content of this book is structured and organized according to the syllabus of Indian Nursing Council with particular aim to provide a systematic knowledge to the nursing students and professionals, i.e., Post Basic BSc Nursing and BSc Nursing as per their academic curriculum.

The book contains ample number of tables, figures, flowcharts and in the end of each chapter the multiple choice questions are also included keeping in view the examination prospective of undergraduates. I am sure that this book will be widely used and will make a worthy contribution to the nursing profession. I wish all the best to the author for such a contribution in the field of nursing.

Parvesh Saini PhD MSc (N) MCH
Principal
College of Nursing
Sri Guru Ram Das University of Health Sciences
Amritsar, Punjab, India

Preface

Nursing profession is based on the core of understanding patient behavior and then responding appropriately based on sound professional knowledge and evidences. Therefore, psychology being the study of human behavior is of utmost relevance to the profession and should be thoroughly emphasized through a structured curriculum as provided by Indian Nursing Council (INC) in various nursing programs.

The current *Textbook of Applied Psychology* attempts to emphasize the core concepts of psychology which help in understanding behavior of patients and significant others. Students will get enlightened their knowledge regarding psychological aspects by reading various units which are organized as per INC syllabus for BSc Nursing and also beneficial for Post Basic Nursing and GNM nursing as well.

This 1st edition of book contains the general concepts of psychology and their application in nursing. The book exclusively and extensively covers the topics like scope of psychology, relevance of learning, perception and attention in nursing, emotion regulation by nurses, thinking and intelligence, motivation, conflict and frustration and various other mental processes. New topics added in the curriculum like communication skills, interpersonal relationship, soft skills, empowerment, professional etiquettes, time management topics are comprehensively covered with their application.

This book can be used as a reference source for PG nursing students and nurse educators. This book is termed with illustrations, flowcharts, tables for better understanding of topics. Each chapter contains multiple choice questions, short answers questions, long answer questions and learning activities. Each chapter is summarized under the heading review which provides the basic understanding of each chapter.

We hope that this book will be of immense utility for all those for whom it is intended. We will always appreciate the comment and suggestion for improving the book.

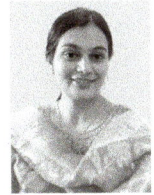

Sukhbir Kaur

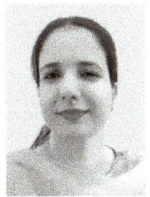

Onkardeep Kaur

Acknowledgments

"Let no man in the world live in delusion, without Guru none can cross over to the other shore"
— ***Guru Nanak Dev ji***

No one walks alone on the journey of life. Just where do you start to thank those that joined you, walked beside you, and helped you along the way continuously urged us to write a book, to put our thoughts down on over the years, those that we have met and worked with have paper, and to share our insights together with the secrets to our continual, positive approach to life and all that life throws at us.

Special acknowledgement should be made for the invaluable assistance given by many people during the preparation of this book. Among them Dr (Mrs) Triza Jiwan, Principal and Professor, Dayanand Medical College, College of Nursing, Ludhiana, Punjab, India, for forwarding content of this book. We are also privileged to Dr Parvesh Saini, Principal and Professor, Sri Guru Ram Das College of Nursing, Vallah, Amritsar, Punjab, for forwarding content and unending support.

We can never complete this book without encouragement of our family members and relatives who gave us inspiration and everlasting support.

We are also very grateful to Vice-Chancellor Dr Daljeet Singh, Sri Guru Ram Das University of Health Sciences, for continuous motivation.

A word of gratitude to M/s Jaypee Brothers Medical Publishers (P) Ltd, New Delhi, India, who helped and guided me, especially Shri Jitendar P Vij (Group Chairman), Mr Ankit Vij (Managing Director), and Mr MS Mani (Group President). A Special thanks to Mr Gurdeep Singh (Executive-Key Accounts), for compiling this content beautifully and making it more presentable for the users of this book.

Last but not the least, we thanks to almighty God, who showered immense blessings.

Contents

Unit I: Introduction ... 1
- Nature and Meaning of Psychology *1*
- Relationship with Other Subject *6*
- Methods of Psychology *7*
- Relevance of Psychology to Nursing *10*
- Importance of Psychology in Nursing Profession *11*
- Applications of Psychology to Everyday Situations *11*

Unit II: Biological and Behavior ... 15
- Mind–Body Relationship *16*
- Brain and Behavior *19*
- Association Cortex *27*
- Muscular Control of Behavior *27*
- Glandular Controls of Behavior *29*
- Genetics and Behavior *31*
- Psychology of Sensation *34*

Unit III: Mental Health and Mental Hygiene ... 38
- Concept of Mental Health and Mental Hygiene *38*
- Characteristics of Mentally Healthy Individual *40*
- Warning Signs of Poor Mental Health *42*
- Mental Hygiene *43*
- Promotive and Preventive Mental Health Services *46*
- Defense Mechanism *50*
- Dealing with Ego *55*
- Frustration and Conflict—Types of Conflicts and Measurements to Overcome *55*
- Nurses as a Facilitator of Conflict Resolution *62*

Unit IV: Developmental Psychology ... 65
- Developmental Theory *65*
- Development of Individual Across Life Span *68*
- Death and Dying *74*
- Psychology of Vulnerable Groups *75*
- Psychology of Groups *80*
- Development of Groups *81*

Unit V: Personality ... 84
- Meaning and Definition of Personality *84*
- Traits or Constituents of Personality *84*
- Factors/Determinants Affecting Personality *86*
- Theories and Classification of Personality *87*
- Measurement and Evaluation of Personality *94*
- Alterations in Personality *97*
- Role of Nurse in Identification of Individual Personality *98*

Unit VI: Coginitive Psychology ... 101
- Attention *101*
- Distraction *105*

- Perception *106*
- Learning *111*
- Habit Formation *121*
- Memory and Forgetting *124*
- Thinking *130*
- Intelligence *134*
- Aptitude *139*
- Types of Aptitude Test *141*

Unit VII: Motivation and Emotional Processes — 146
- Motives *153*
- Emotions *156*
- Stress and Adaptation *165*
- Attitude *172*

Unit VIII: Psychological Assessment and Tests — 182
- Methods Used for Psychosocial Assessment *182*
- Role of Nurse in Psychological Testing *194*

Unit IX: Application of Soft Skills — 196
- Types of Soft Skill/Communication *197*
- How to Develop Soft Skills? *198*
- Communication and Interpersonal Relationships *206*
- Resilience *208*
- Stress Management *211*
- Time Management *214*
- Work-Life Balance *215*
- Applying Soft Skills to Workplace and Society *216*
- Application of Soft Skills in Nursing *218*

Unit X: Self-empowerment — 220
- Self-empowerment *220*
- Personal Empowerment *220*
- Nursing Empowerment *220*
- Dimensions of Self-empowerment *220*
- Steps of Self-empowerment Development *221*
- Techniques to Build Personal Empowerment *222*
- Example of Self-empowerment *222*
- Women's Empowerment *222*
- Professional Etiquette and Personal Grooming *224*
- Personal Grooming *225*
- Role of Nurse in Empowering Others *226*

Bibliography — 229
Index — 233

INC Syllabus

Description: This course is designed to enable the students to develop understanding about basic concepts of sociology and psychology and its application in personal and community life, health, illness and nursing. It further provides students opportunity to recognize the significance and application of soft skills and self-empowerment in the practice of nursing.

Competencies: On completion of the course, the students will be able to:
1. Identify the scope and significance of sociology in nursing.
2. Apply the knowledge of social structure and different culture in a society in identifying social needs of sick clients.
3. Identify the impact of culture on health and illness.
4. Develop understanding about types of family, marriage and its legislation.
5. Identify different types of caste, class, social change and its influence on health and health practices.
6. Develop understanding about social organization and disorganization and social problems in India.
7. Integrate the knowledge of clinical sociology and its uses in crisis intervention.
8. Identify the importance of psychology in individual and professional life.
9. Develop understanding of the biological and psychological basis of human behavior.
10. Identify the role of nurse in promoting mental health and dealing with altered personality.
11. Perform the role of nurses applicable to the psychology of different age groups.
12. Identify the cognitive and affective needs of clients.
13. Integrate the principles of motivation and emotion in performing the role of nurse in caring for emotionally sick client.
14. Demonstrate basic understanding of psychological assessment and nurse's role.
15. Apply the knowledge of soft skills in workplace and society.
16. Apply the knowledge of self-empowerment in workplace, society and personal life.

COURSE OUTLINE

Unit 1	Describe scope, branches and significance of psychology in nursing	• Introduction • Meaning of psychology • Development of psychology—scope, branches and methods of psychology • Relationship with other subjects • Significance of psychology in nursing • Applied psychology to solve everyday issues
Unit II	• Describe biology of human behavior • Biological basis of behavior	• Introduction • Body–mind relationship • Genetics and behavior • Inheritance of behavior • Brain and behavior • Psychology and sensation—sensory process—normal and abnormal
Unit III	• Explain mentally healthy person and defence mechanisms • Mental health and mental hygiene	• Concept of mental health and mental hygiene • Characteristic of mentally healthy person • Warning signs of poor mental health • Promotive and preventive mental health strategies and services • Defense mechanism and its implication • Frustration and conflict—types of conflicts and measurements to overcome • Role of nurse in reducing frustration and conflict and enhancing coping
Unit IV	Describe psychology of people in different age groups and role of nurse	**Developmental psychology** • Psychological needs of various groups in health and sickness—infancy, childhood, adolescence, adulthood and old age • Introduction to child psychology and role of nurse in meeting the psychological needs of children • Psychology of vulnerable individuals challenged, women, sick, etc. • Role of nurse with vulnerable group
Unit V	Explain personality and role of nurse in identification and improvement in altered personality	**Personality** • Meaning, definition of personality • Classification of personality • Measurement and evaluation of personality—introduction • Alteration in personality • Role of nurse in identification of individual personality and improvement in altered personality
Unit VI	Explain cognitive process and their applications	**Cognitive process** • Attention—definition, types, determinants, duration, degree and alteration in attention • Perception—meaning of perception, principles, factor affecting perception • Intelligence—meaning of intelligence—effect of heredity and environment in intelligence, classification, introduction to measurement of intelligence tests—mental deficiencies

- Learning—definition of learning, types of learning, factors influencing learning—learning process, habit formation
- Memory—meaning and nature of memory, factors influencing memory, methods to improve memory, forgetting
- Thinking—types, level, reasoning and problem solving
- Aptitude—concept, types, individual differences and variability
- Psychometric assessment of cognitive processes—introduction
- Alteration in cognitive processes

Unit VII	Describe motivation, emotion, attitude and role of nurse in emotionally sick client	**Motivation and emotional processes** • Motivation—meaning, concept, types, theories of motivation, motivation cycle, biological and special motives • Emotions—meaning of emotions, development of emotions, alteration of emotion, emotions in sickness—handling emotions in self and other • Stress and adaptation—stress, stressor, cycle, effect, adaptation and coping • Attitudes—meaning of attitudes, nature, factor affecting attitude, attitudinal change, role of attitude in health and sickness • Psychometric assessment of emotions and attitude—introduction • Role of nurse in caring for emotionally sick client
Unit VIII	Explain psychological assessment and tests and role of nurse	• Psychological assessment and tests—introduction • Types, development, characteristics, principles, uses, interpretation • Role of nurse in psychological assessment
Unit IX	• Explain concept of soft skill and its application in work place and society • Application of soft skill	• Concept of soft skill • Types of soft skill—visual, aural and communication skill • The way of communication • Building relationship with client and society • Interpersonal relationships (IPR)—definition, types, and purposes, interpersonal skills, barriers, strategies to overcome barriers • Survival strategies—managing time, coping stress, resilience, work-life balance applying soft skill to workplace and society • Use of soft skill in nursing
Unit X	Explain self-empowerment	**Self-empowerment** • Dimensions of self-empowerment • Self-empowerment development • Importance of women's empowerment in society • Professional etiquette and personal grooming • Role of nurse in empowering others

UNIT 1

Introduction

OUTLINE

- ❏ Introduction
- ❏ Nature, Meaning, Definition of Psychology
- ❏ Development of Psychology
- ❏ Scope, Branches and Methods of Psychology
- ❏ Relationship with other Subjects
- ❏ Significance of Psychology in Nursing
- ❏ Applied Psychology to Solve Everyday Issues

■ INTRODUCTION

Psychology is fairly a new science. Until 19th century, this was recognized as a separate field of study. The birth of formal psychology can be traced back to 1879. It was founded by Wilhelm Wundt in Leipzig, Germany (Father of Psychology). The word "Psychology" is derived from two Greek words—"psyche" (spirit or soul, mind) and "logos" (study). The word "soul" means spiritual or immortal elements in a person.

■ NATURE AND MEANING OF PSYCHOLOGY

The nature of psychology is scientific which has been emphasized by various psychologists and thinkers as it is the scientific study of human behavior. Therefore, its nature can be explained as follows:

- ❖ It is positive or natural science since we describe behavior as we discover or find it without evaluating.
- ❖ It discovers and explains the underlying laws and principles of behavior and forms well-organized theory of human behavior.
- ❖ Psychology deals with the mind and its working, and the knowledge of psychology helps in reading other people's mind.
- ❖ Psychology has its applied aspects in the form of various branches of applied psychology such as industrial, legal, clinical, and educational psychology.
- ❖ Psychology is factual as it is objective based on observation and experiments.
- ❖ Laws of psychology are universal and at all times and places the laws are same and are verifiable.
- ❖ Psychology describes the cause and effect relationship in human behavior.

The subject matter of psychology is affect, behavior, and cognition. The affect for psychology is the actual mental processes that make up moods, feeling, and emotional state. An example of affect would be feeling sad about something happening. Behavior includes the actual actions and responses of organisms. Behavior can include the way we act in any given situation, for example, when we get up in the morning. The order in the way we prepare ourselves for going out into public can be categorized as our behavior. Cognition is the actual mental events and the processes that result from them. Memories of an event are great examples of an organism's cognition.

Before discussing about concept of psychology which is considered as study of behavior let us focus on what is behavior.

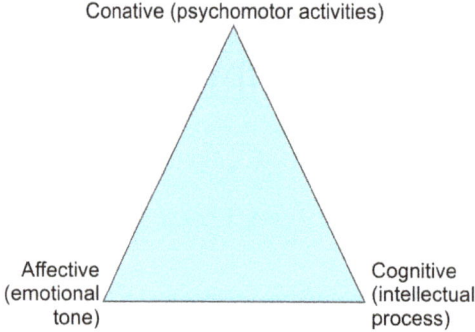

Fig. 1: Components of behavior.

In broad sense, behavior includes conative (motor activities), cognitive (thinking), and affective (feelings) components **(Fig. 1)**.

According to Woodworth, behavior can be defined as any manifestation of life activities. It is also defined as a process in which an animal or a person behaves in response to a particular situation or stimulus.

Brief History

- Word "psychology" used by Rudolf Gockle—1590
- In 19th century psychology was recognized as separate field of study. The birth of formal psychology can be tracked back to 1879.
- William James used the word "mind" instead of "soul" in 1890. Mind is abstract and cannot be seen but behavior is what mind does. Mind is a stream of consciousness.
- According to Aristotle, psychology is the study of soul. (not accepted).
- Later on, Philosopher Plato said Psychology is the study of mind. (incomplete).
- According to Sigmund Freud "mind" is divided into three parts—conscious, subconscious, and unconscious. This was also rejected.
- Later on in the 18th century, experimental psychology or scientific psychology came into being—founder was William Wundt (1832-1920); first psychology laboratory in Leipzig, Germany, 1879.
- Definition of psychology changed to: "Psychology is the systematic study of behavior".
- By this definition psychology became a subject of science and it comes under behavioral sciences.
- Scientific study of behavior by measuring tools or tests called psychological tests.
- Modern era of Indian psychology began in 1915 and first syllabus of psychology was introduced and first psychology laboratory was established at Calcutta University.
- Department of applied psychology in Calcutta University was started in 1938.
- Indian psychoanalytical association was established by Professor Bose in 1922.

Definition

Psychology is the scientific study of mental processes and behavior. It is study of mind and how it works.

—Oxford Dictionary

Psychology is the science of human and animal behavior which includes the application of this science to solve human behavior.

—W Hamilton

Psychology is the scientific study of the human mind and its functions, especially that affecting behavior in given context.

Psychology is the scientific study of behavior and mental processes and how they are affected by an organism's physical state, mental state, and external environment.

Subfields/Areas/Scope of Psychology

There are few areas of psychology. Areas of psychology and its scope are widespread as the spares of human life. Some such areas of study in psychology are as follows **(Fig. 2)**:

i. **General psychology:** It is that branch of psychology that deals with the study of behavior of a normal person in normal life conditions. It includes learning,

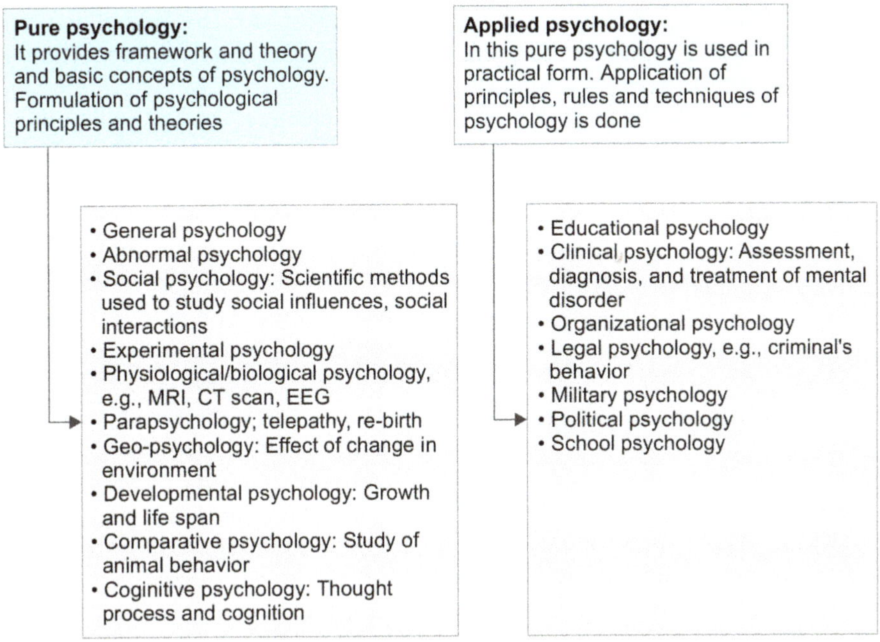

UNIT I: Introduction

```
┌─────────────────────────────────┐    ┌─────────────────────────────────┐
│ Pure psychology:                │    │ Applied psychology:             │
│ It provides framework and theory│    │ In this pure psychology is used │
│ and basic concepts of psychology│    │ in practical form. Application  │
│ Formulation of psychological    │    │ of principles, rules and        │
│ principles and theories         │    │ techniques of psychology is done│
└─────────────────────────────────┘    └─────────────────────────────────┘
```

- General psychology
- Abnormal psychology
- Social psychology: Scientific methods used to study social influences, social interactions
- Experimental psychology
- Physiological/biological psychology, e.g., MRI, CT scan, EEG
- Parapsychology; telepathy, re-birth
- Geo-psychology: Effect of change in environment
- Developmental psychology: Growth and life span
- Comparative psychology: Study of animal behavior
- Coginitive psychology: Thought process and cognition

- Educational psychology
- Clinical psychology: Assessment, diagnosis, and treatment of mental disorder
- Organizational psychology
- Legal psychology, e.g., criminal's behavior
- Military psychology
- Political psychology
- School psychology

Fig. 2: Subfields/areas/scope of psychology.

intelligence, sensation, perception, and memory.

ii. **Abnormal psychology:** Study of behavior of an abnormal person. Abnormal persons are those who are suffering from psychological disorders, personality disorder, and drug addiction. It includes the clinical picture and treatment of abnormalities.

iii. **Childhood psychology:** It is the study of behavior of the children. It studies the physical, emotional, and moral development of children. It includes characteristics behavior as how they think, feel, preserve, and react to different situations of life.

iv. **Developmental psychology:** It deals with the study of behavior of an individual in the different development stages of life from birth to death. These developmental stages are prenatal, infancy, childhood, adolescence, adulthood, and late-adulthood.

v. **Educational psychology:** Study of behavior of an individual in educational settings. It studies the classroom behavior of student and teacher and relationship between student and teacher.

vi. **Industrial psychology:** Behavior is studied in industrial setting. It deals with the relationship between man and machine, productivity of individual in behavior in industrial setting, job satisfaction, etc. It tends to deal with human problems in industries so as to make the condition suitable.

vii. **Comparative psychology:** It studies the animal behavior. Theories and principles obtained working on animal enhance understanding the nature. As behavior of animal and human are compared, it is called comparative psychology.

viii. **Clinical psychology:** It studies the mentally sick person with references to symptoms and treatment of their sickness.

ix. **Experimental psychology:** It deals with those theories and principles and studies which are obtained using experimental method. This branch raises the status of psychology to other scientists.

UNIT I: Introduction

x. **Social psychology:** Behavior of an individual in social situation and social groups is studied. It studies how the behavior of an individual is related to social situation and how it is influenced with social groups.

xi. **Parapsychology:** This is the field of psychology that investigates all psychological phenomena that apparently cannot be explained in scientific law like telepathy.

Schools of Thought in Psychology (Fig. 3)

1. **Structuralism**: This early school of psychology grew upon the ideas of Wilhelm Wundt in Germany and founded by the follower of Wundt, Edward B Titchener (1867–1927). The goal of the structuralist was to find out the units or elements which make up the mind. The main method used to discover these elementary units of mind was introspection.

2. **Behaviorism**: This school of thought was founded by John B. Watson. It emphasized the need to study what is observable. Its objective was to predict and control behavior. It focuses on observable behavior and modification of behavior.

3. **Functionalism**: Various psychologists do not follow the structuralism and thought of more functional process influencing psychology. The main influencers were William James, John Dewey, Harvey Carr, Thorndike, and Woodworth. In 1890, William James criticized the study of structure of mind and gave the concept of study of mental activities. Perception, emotions, memory, attention, and concentration were considered as important mental activities. It was considered that the conscious experience is organized to help in adjustment with the environment.

4. **Gestalt psychology:** The pioneer of this school of thought was Max Wertheimer in 1912 who termed the word "gestalt"

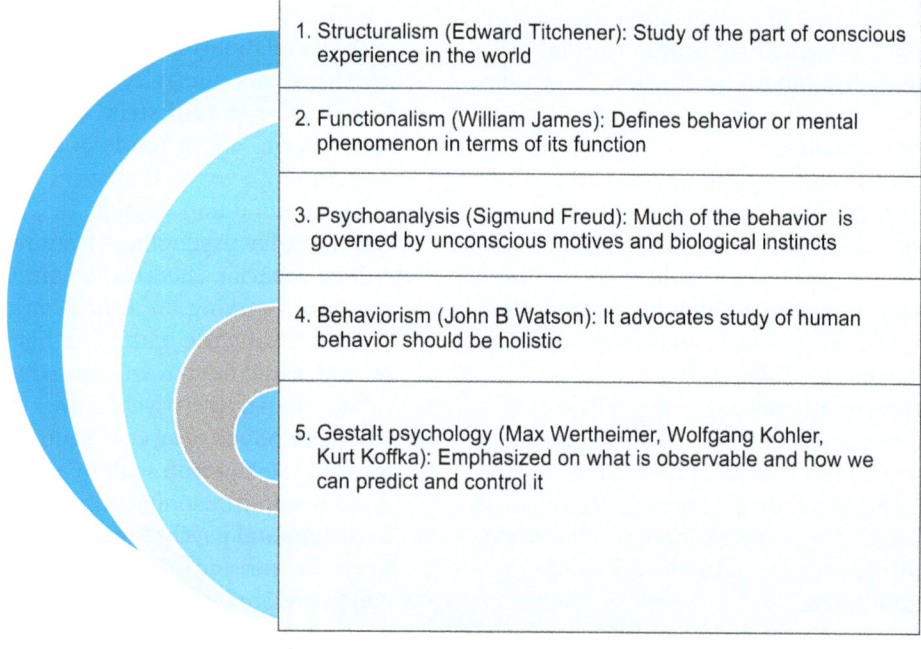

Fig. 3: Schools of thought in psychology.

which means whole in German. This school emphasizes on whole rather than parts. Rather than analyzing conscious experience or behavior in its parts, it must be studied as a whole in relation to each other. It will give better understanding about organization of mental activities such as perception, thinking, learning, etc. Gestalt school has provided different laws of organization in perception. Insight theory of learning by Kohler is another contribution of this school.

5. **Psychoanalysis:** Sigmund Freud considered as the "Father of Modern Psychology" was the father of this school of thought. While experiencing with patients Freud developed the concept of psychoanalysis which emphasized on components of personality as id, ego and superego, and topography of mind, that is, conscious, unconscious, and subconscious parts. The iceberg of mind plays an important role in deciding and resolving upon daily life issues and regulation of wanted and unwanted thoughts. He not only gave concept of normal and abnormal behavior but also developed therapeutic techniques based on psychoanalysis such as free association, dream analysis, analysis of resistance, etc. Various other contributors of this school of thought were Carl Jung, Adler, etc.

Contemporary Approaches to Psychology

Each contemporary perspective represents a different point of view about human behavior and mental processes. Each perspective has its own assumptions, questions, and explanations of behavior and mental processes which are as follows:

- **Psychodynamic approach:** It is a systematic study of psychological forces. Freud believes that behavior is motivated by inner unconscious force over which a person has little control. The psychology which is developed at early childhood later on affects the behavior and mental states of individual. It also helps individual to understand about their emotions and unconscious patterns of behavior and it also emphasizes that any behavior has underlying cause.
- **Cognitive approach:** This examines how people understand and think about the world. Psychologists such as Edward Tolman and Jean Piaget are associated with the further propagation of the ideas of their psychology. They believe that there is more to the human nature than a series of stimulus–response connections; they concentrate on mental processes such as thinking, reasoning, and self-awareness.
- **Humanistic approach:** It contends that people can control their behavior and they naturally try to reach their full potential. Advocated by the contemporary psychologists such as Maslow, Rogers Arthur Combs, Gordon Allport and reflects the recent human trends in psychology. A school called humanistic psychology was developed as an alternative to behaviorism and psychoanalysis. They believe that individuals are controlled by their own values and choices and not entirely by the environment.
- **Evolutionary approach:** This is an approach to psychology centered on evolutionary ideas such as adaptation, reproduction, and natural selection as the basis for explaining specific human behaviors.
- **Sociocultural approach:** This is an approach to psychology that examines the ways in which social and cultural environments influence behavior. It is an emerging approach which emphasizes on the contribution of society to the individual development. It focuses on the interaction between various societies, cultures, ethnic groups, religion, and particular behavior influence pertaining to the sociocultural changes.

- **Positive psychology**: It is a new form or modern version of psychology. It emphasizes on the importance of positivity in individual life. This theory is based on the belief that happiness is derived from both emotional and mental factors. It is also considered as a branch of psychology which focuses on building positive life skills which flourish an individual's strengths and behavior.
- **Biological**: This focuses on the biological influences on behavior and mental processes including the brain and the rest of the nervous system. All of our thoughts, feelings, and behaviors are associated with underlying bodily activities and processes, for example, when you think specific areas of your brain are activated to trigger the appropriate muscle and tendons into action and to coordinate all the required movements. Brain works through the actions of chemicals called neurotransmitters. Neurotransmitters communicate messages between nerve cells (called neurons) within the brain. The neurotransmitter called dopamine is involved in complex bodily movements and in regulating emotional responses, particularly our experience to pleasure and excitement. Dopamine is used in medication to help people with Parkinson's disease. Neurotransmitter called serotonin is involved in the onset of sleep and the moods we experience. Serotonin is used in medication to help people with severe depression.
- **Behavioral**: This focuses on how behavior is acquired or modified by environmental consequences such as rewards and punishments. It explains how rewards and punishments in an individual's environment shape, maintain, and change his behavior through a type of learning that he called operant conditioning. In Skinner's view, this was evidence of an operant conditioning principle called reinforcement. Reinforcement states that the consequences of a behavior determine whether the behavior will be more or less likely to be repeated.

Different Types of Reinforcement

- Positive reinforcement increases the likelihood of doing something by providing a desirable consequence, such as pressing the lever to get food.
- Negative reinforcement also increases the likelihood of doing something for a desired consequence, but it involves the removal or avoidance of something that is unpleasant.

▌RELATIONSHIP WITH OTHER SUBJECT

Psychology is derived from various other fields such as philosophy and physiology. Roots of psychology can be traced back 2000 years ago to the early philosophers, biologists, and physiologists of ancient Greece. Relationship of the subject with other sciences provides its relevance, credibility, and authenticity. Psychological aspect is almost present in every field of study.

1. **Philosophy and psychology:** The roots of psychology are derived from philosophy as it was considered as study of soul. The nature of humans was understood and invested often with the philosophers at that time. Even the term "psychology" was composed by philosopher Aristotle. Later on, psychology was separated from philosophy by various schools of thoughts and they started to consider it as soft science. Philosophy emphasizes on studying the pattern of life and psychology studies about how this pattern can be achieved. Various branches of philosophy such as epistemology, ethics, logics, and esthetics are based on psychological perspective.
2. **Sociology and psychology:** They both are considered as positive sciences. Sociology is a social science and is a study based on

society and the individuals of the society. It involves family, community, social institutions, origin and development of psychology, cultures, traditions, social customs, social problems, and interrelationship between individuals. The society is formed by individuals.

3. **Anthropology and psychology:** Anthropology is the scientific study of human species. It studies the fact that how human being lives, what their culture is, what they think, what they do, and how they interact with their environments. Anthropology emphasizes on studying full range of human diversity as well as what people share in common. Therefore, social psychology and cultural psychology are the branches of psychology included in anthropology. The knowledge of anthropology is of great importance in understanding various topics of cross cultural psychology and social psychology. Anthropology also relies on various contents from historical evolution of psychology to know about early life and behavior of human beings.

4. **Physiology and psychology**: Physiology is the study of structure and functions of the human organs and body and how these functions alter during the motor activities or during performing certain behavior. There is a connection associated with psychology that what bodily changes takes place when individual perform particular behavior. Various psychologists have done lot of work on mind–body relationship. Therefore, psychology has one of its branches as physiological psychology. Psychology also contributes to physiology in certain aspects as understanding its significance in human behavior.

5. **Physics and psychology**: Physics is the study of constituents and materials of universe. Human being also lives in this universe and these constituents of the universe do influence human behavior. Environmental changes such as temperature, sound waves, and chemicals affect the physiological mechanism and sensory processes. Therefore, psychophysics is the branch of psychology which studies the relationship between physical dimensions of the world and sensory dimensions of human.

6. **Psychiatry and psychology**: Psychiatry is the branch of medicine which treats the patient with psychological problems. It is derived from the branch of abnormal psychology which is the study of maladaptive behavior of individuals in particular situations. It also studies about the clinical description, diagnosis, and treatment of mental illnesses. Various treatment modalities in psychiatry are based on psychological approaches known as psychotherapy.

7. **Biochemistry and psychology:** Biochemistry is the study of various biochemical changes taking place in the body of human being. The biochemical changes taking place in brain and body are related to behavior of the individuals. It is seen in various experiments that different types of behavioral reactions are associated with certain biochemical changes and therefore by altering these biochemical reactions behavior modification can be done in an individual.

■ METHODS OF PSYCHOLOGY

Introspection Method

Introspection or self-observation is the oldest method for the study of behavior, which was introduced by Wilhelm Wundt, Father of Psychology. It was formerly used in philosophy and then in psychology to collect data about the conscious experience of the subject. It means to see within oneself or self-observation, to understand one's own mental health and the state of mind. This method was developed by the structuralisms in psychology who defined psychology as the study of conscious experiences of the individual.

Merits
- It gives information about one's own self which is difficult by other methods.
- It is an easy method and needs no equipment.
- It makes a base for other methods such as experimental and observation method.

Demerits
- This method is subjective in nature and lacks scientific objectivity. The observer and the observed are the same; the mind is both the field and the instrument of observation.
- Introspection cannot be employed on children and insane people.

Observation Method

With the development of psychology as an objective science of behavior, the method of introspection was replaced by careful observation of human and animal behavior. Observation literally means looking outside oneself. It is a very important method for collecting data in almost all types of research studies. Different types of observation used in research are direct or indirect, scheduled or unscheduled, natural or artificial, and participant and non-participant. But there are two basic types of observation.

- **Natural observation:** In natural observation, the observer observes the specific behavior and characteristics of subjects in natural settings and the subjects are not aware of the fact that their behavior is being observed by someone.
- Participant observation: In participant observation, the observer becomes a part of the group which he wants to observe. There is no doubt that observation is a scientific technique of collecting data, whose results can be verified and relied upon to locate behavioral problems.

Merits
- This type of observation is a natural and normal way of knowing not only the external world but also the mind of the subject.
- This method is objective in nature and free from personal bias and prejudice.
- Through this method, we can observe as many children as we like.
- This method is quite suitable for children and abnormal persons who cannot be examined through introspection. This can be used anytime and anywhere.

Demerits
- Observation is useful only for collecting data about overt behavior which is manifested in a number of activities. This overt behavior does not provide reliable information regarding the internal mental process. It becomes very difficult to draw any conclusion in case of adults who can hide their actual behavior in the presence of the observer.
- Subjectivity of interpretation is another limitation of this method.

Scientific Method

It is a form of critical thinking based on careful measurement and controlled observation.

Six basic slements involved in scientific method are as follows:
1. Observation
2. Defining a problem
3. Proposing a hypothesis (an educated guess that can be tested)
4. Gathering evidence/testing the hypothesis
5. Publishing results
6. Building a theory

It is also called experimental method. This approach is used by psychologists to systematically acquire knowledge and understanding about behavior and other phenomena of interest.

UNIT I: Introduction

Merits

- This method is the most systematic procedure for solving problems. It provides reliable information.
- It is a revisable method and makes psychology a scientific study.
- It provides objective and precise information about the problems.
- It gives observer an easy approach to the mind of an individual.
- It provides innovative ideas for the further experimentation.
- It enables us to control and direct human behavior
- It is applicable in educational, individual, and social problems.

Demerits

- It is arranged in an artificial laboratory-like situation.
- Behavior is a natural phenomenon and it may change under artificial environment.
- It is time-consuming and costly requiring specialized knowledge and skills.
- Psychologists have criticized the fact that mostly the experiments have been conducted on rats, cats, and dogs. The results are analyzed and then applied on human beings.
- It sometimes interferes with the very thing that we are trying to observe.

Clinical Method

This method is primarily used to collect detailed information on the behavior problems of maladjusted and deviant cases. The main objective of this method is to study individual case or cases of group to detect and diagnose their specific problems and to suggest therapeutic measures to rehabilitate them in their environment.

It involves the following steps:
1. Interview
2. Information gathering
3. A hypothesis formulated
4. Diagnoses made
5. Planned treatment program

Case Study

Case study is in-depth study of the subject. It is the in-depth analysis of a person, group, or phenomenon. A variety of techniques are employed including personal interviews, psychometric tests, direct observation, and archival records. Case studies are most often used in psychology in clinical research to describe the rare events and conditions of the subject; case study is especially used in education psychology. It deals with education for the following problems:

- Lack of interest in students
- Aggressive behavior in student
- Daydreaming
- Poor academic performance
- Emotional problems
- Social problems
- Empathetic understanding
- Find the problem
- Establish rapport
- Treatment

Correlation Method

The correlation method involves systematically measuring the relationship between two or more variables. Correlation coefficient: +1.00 to –1.00

- Positive Correlation
- Negative Correlation
  Example—assessing relationship between adjustment and academic achievement of students.

Interview Method

Only recently, however, interview has been used systematically for scientific purposes, both in the laboratory and in the field. According to PV. Young, "Interviewing is not a simple way to conversation between an interrogator and informant. Gestures, glances, facial expressions and pauses often reveal subtle feelings."

Types of Interview Method

There are different types of interview—focused interview, repeated interview, clinical interview, diagnostic interview, research interview, personal interview, etc.

Merits

- High participation of the subject or respondent
- This method is very flexible.
- The subject's emotions can be studied well.
- Through the interview method, the investigator may get to know the cause of any behavior pattern of the subject and the historical background of each incident.
- The data collected through the interview method is reliable.
- The interview method can be applied on all types of people—literate or illiterate children and adults and at times also on mentally unbalanced persons since it provides proper in-depth information as compared to the other methods.
- In the interview method, the subject and investigator are face to face with each other.

Demerits

- It is a costly method.
- It is also time-consuming as the interviewer has to physically locate a subject.
- It requires lot of planning.
- The subject may not reveal his true feelings and emotions.
- The investigator must be very proficient and must have proper insight into human nature.
- There can be difficulty in persuading the subject to be interviewed.

■ RELEVANCE OF PSYCHOLOGY TO NURSING

1. **Development and maturation**: By understanding developmental stage, nurses will not misidentify normal process as diseases.
2. **Learning and motivation**: When nurses need to give education, they know when, where, and what to do.
3. **Personality and behavior:**
   - Expand nurse's perception
   - Understanding patient's reaction. Change negative behavior to positive
   - Practice effective interaction.
   - Help nurses to deal with their own emotion when dealing with the patient
4. **Adaptation:**
   - Nurses help patients to adapt with their diseases, anxiety, and disability.
   - This helps nurses to understand and deal with the patient's reaction.
5. **Counseling:**
   - Preventing illness—psychologist changes behavior to prevent illness.
   - Psychologist counsels regarding healthy behavior and how to get rid of stress.
6. **Research:**
   - To explore more about human behavior
   - To improve quality of care
   - Critical analysis of health policy: Scope of health psychology
7. **Others:**
   - Understanding behavioral factors—behavior which promotes health
   - Effects of disease—disease affects psychological well-being
   - Improves relationship between health team members
   - Managing pain
   - Improving adherence to medical advice

IMPORTANCE OF PSYCHOLOGY IN NURSING PROFESSION

Psychology has become necessary in every profession including nursing today. This is because of increasing emphasis being laid on the interplay of body, mind, and spirit in the health status of every individual. The learning of psychology helps a nurse in the following ways:

- **Understand the mind–body relationships:** The understanding of psychology helps nurses to realize the relationship between the physiological and mental processes. This understanding will help nurses to deal with patients and understand how well the physiological process disturbed the psychological functions.
- **Enable to understand one's own self:** The knowledge of psychology helps nurses to understand their own behavior and know their strengths and weaknesses. This insight makes them control and attain self-discipline.
- **Understand individual differences:** The knowledge of psychology helps the nurses to understand the individual differences among the human behavior and enable them to provide effective services to different patients.
- **Deal with mentally-disturbed patients:** The understanding of abnormal psychology helps the nurses to know the behavior pattern of abnormal patients and handle them more effectively by applying the principles of psychology to modify their behavior.
- **Enable nurses to make better judgments:** The knowledge of psychology helps nurses to make effective adjustments in the environment as it makes them happier and to develop harmonious relationship with others such as doctors and other nurses.
- **Provide effective counseling:** Nurses also play the role of a counselor. The knowledge of psychology helps them to provide effective counseling for emotionally disturbed patients.

APPLICATIONS OF PSYCHOLOGY TO EVERYDAY SITUATIONS

Psychology is the study of people's behavior, performance, and mental operations. It also refers to the application of the knowledge, which can be used to understand events, treat mental health issues, and improve education, employment, and relationships. Psychology is very important especially because it deals with the study of the mental processes and behavior at the same time. It is also applied in our daily life and in many things.

1. **Understanding mental processes:** How we behave, how we react to situations, and how we perform are all associated with psychology. That is because psychology studies our nature, how we think and how it is related to what we do, and why we think and act the way we do. It is actually very complicated because unlike the study of disease processes and the physical body, studying the human mind is very complicated and it is hard to study in an unbiased way.
2. **Explaining the disease conditions:** Its importance in the society has grown significantly over the years. Psychology is used to study various kinds of mental and life-threatening diseases such as Alzheimer's, Parkinson's, and many other types of neurological disorders. Psychology is also used to better understand and help those with pervasive developmental disorders such as autism. The study of psychology in these disorders and diseases has helped the medical professionals in developing cure and treatment for certain diseases.
3. **Knowing oneself:** With psychology, we are able to learn about ourselves.

To fully understand ourselves we have to know about the causes of our own behavior and our perspectives in life. By knowing ourselves and learning our own personality, we can develop goals for ourselves. Also, by learning about ourselves, we are able to learn about other people and their differences. Gaining understanding of oneself and of others can help improve the way relationships and communications work.

4. **Making interpersonal relationships:** In addition to learning about oneself, the field of psychology allows us to learn about others. For example, we may gain insight into personality traits that are different from our own personality traits. It is important to gain an understanding of others to improve social relationships. We may wish to build rapport and communicate more effectively.

5. **Problem-solving:** Ideas and findings in psychology may help to think of practical ideas and possible solutions to important problems. We may gain insight concerning possible applications of psychology and solutions to certain important problems.

6. **Adjustment to life:** Knowledge about Psychology helps to provide guidance and counseling to persons with problems of adjustment, in the field of education, employment, and private life.

7. **Professional education:** Psychology has large scope as a teaching subject in college and universities. Background knowledge of human behavior is essential in every professional field.

8. **Therapeutic modalities:** Psychology has contributed various valuable therapeutic measures which help to modify the abnormal behavior or psychiatric disorders, e.g., behavior therapy, group therapy etc.

QUESTION BANK

MULTIPLE CHOICE QUESTIONS

1. Which subfield is most directly concerned with studying how marketing effects human behavior?
    a. Clinical
    b. Personality
    c. Engineering psychology
    d. Industrial-organizational
    e. Counseling
2. Which of the following individuals is also a physician?
    a. Clinical psychologist
    b. Psychologist
    c. Experimental psychologist
    d. Psychiatrist
    e. Developmental psychologist
3. A person working within this subfield of psychology might work closely with his local police department to explain the behavior of a suspect:
    a. Health psychologist
    b. Criminal psychologist
    c. Clinical psychologist
    d. Forensic psychologist
    e. Counseling psychologist
4. Two historical roots of psychology are the disciplines of:
    a. Philosophy and chemistry
    b. Physiology and chemistry
    c. Philosophy and physiology
    d. Philosophy and physics
5. The 17th century philosopher who believed that the mind is blank at birth and that most knowledge comes through sensory experience is:
    a. Plato
    b. Aristotle
    c. Descartes
    d. Locke

UNIT I: Introduction

6. The Greek philosopher who believed that intelligence was inherited was:
   a. Aristotle
   b. Plato
   c. Descartes
   d. Simonides
7. This German philosopher and psychologist was the first to set up a laboratory to gather empirical data related to psychology?
   a. Wundt, 1879
   b. James, 1890
   c. Freud, 1900
   d. Watson, 1913
8. Which of the following schools of thought would be most likely to reject the method of introspection to study human experience?
   a. Behaviorism
   b. Psychoanalysis
   c. Structuralism
   d. Functionalism
   e. None of the above
9. Which of the following deals with the study of how a person's action, feelings, or thoughts are influenced by others?
   a. Social psychology
   b. Clinical psychology
   c. Educational psychology
   d. Health psychology
10. Behavior includes which of the following activities?
    a. Motor
    b. Cognitive
    c. Affective
    d. All of the above
11. Understanding of psychology is relevant for nurses because:
    a. It helps a nurse to understand herself
    b. It helps a nurse to understand others
    c. It helps a nurse to solve the problems according to situations
    d. All of the above
12. Which of the following is scientific method of psychology?
    a. Introspection
    b. Observation
    c. Interview
    d. Experimental
13. Who is considered the founder of psychodynamic perspective in psychology?
    a. Jean Piaget
    b. Ivan Pavlov
    c. Sigmund Freud
    d. William James
14. The psychology school of thought that emphasized on whole or complete view of situation was:
    a. Structuralism
    b. Behaviorism
    c. Gestalt
    d. Functionalism
15. According to which school of thought to understand human behavior one must focus on unconscious mind and early life experiences?
    a. Psychoanalysis
    b. Functionalism
    c. Behaviorism
    d. Gestalt
16. Who established the first psychology laboratory in the US?
    a. Mary Whiton Calkins
    b. G Stanley Hall
    c. William James
    d. William Wundt
17. The Greek philosopher who believed that intelligence is inherited was:
    a. Aristotle
    b. Plato
    c. Descartes
    d. Simonides
18. By 1920s, the definition of psychology was said to be a study of science of _____.
    a. Consciousness
    b. Mind
    c. Philosophy
    d. Behavior

UNIT I: Introduction

19. **Educational psychology attempts to apply knowledge of psychology in:**
    a. Medicine
    b. Education
    c. Social sciences
    d. Industries
20. **The oldest method of study of behavior is:**
    a. Introspection
    b. Observation
    c. Experimental
    d. Intelligence tests
21. **Functionalist emphasizes that only those things should be taught to children:**
    a. Which they could apply in everyday life
    b. Which they can remember only
    c. Which they can use on special events
    d. Which are related to their self only
22. **Introspection means:**
    a. Looking outward
    b. Looking inward
    c. Observing events
    d. None of these
23. **Psychologist does experiments to study behavior related to:**
    a. Teaching
    b. Learning
    c. Changing cognitions
    d. None of these
24. **Who is recognized as the father of modern scientific psychology?**
    a. John B Watson
    b. Wilhelm Wundt
    c. William James
    d. BF Skinner

ANSWER KEY

1. d	2. c	3. b	4. c	5. d	6. b	7. a	8. a
9. a	10. d	11. d	12. d	13. c	14. c	15. a	16. b
17. b	18. d	19. b	20. a	21. a	22. b	23. b	24. b

SHORT ANSWER TYPE QUESTIONS

1. What is behavior?
2. What is experimental method?
3. What is behaviorism?
4. What is Gestalt psychology?
5. What is clinical method?
6. Discuss scope of psychology.
7. Discuss advantages and limitations of introspection method.
8. Discuss similarities and differences between observation and introspection method.
9. Discuss relationship of psychology to sociology.
10. How will you define term "behavior" in psychology?
11. Explain clinical method of psychology.

LONG ANSWER TYPE QUESTIONS

1. Define psychology. How does psychology help in good nurse–patient relationship?
2. Describe the scope of psychology.
3. Explain various methods of psychology.
4. Discuss implications of psychology to nursing students.
5. Discuss the importance of psychology in everyday life situations with example.
6. Explain in detail nature and importance of psychology.
7. List the different methods of psychology and discuss any one method.

UNIT II

Biological and Behavior

OUTLINE

- Introduction
- Body–Mind Relationship
- Brain and Behavior
- Genetics and Behavior, Inheritance of Behavior
- Psychology and sensation—sensory process—normal and abnormal

■ INTRODUCTION

Understanding human behavior is incomplete without an analysis of the biological process. It includes both mental and bodily reactions which may be external or internal. The behavior of an individual is based on certain physiological and psychological processes, the way in which one acts or conducts oneself, especially toward others. Various parts of the body form the basis of all behaviors such as how people talk, how they walk, read, or do all the actions. Psychologists nowadays, are widely focusing on the role of bodily process on behavior and also the effect of psychological process on the body. The behavior is closely related to both physical and mental activity. Behavior means all the covert and overt activities of human beings that can be observed.

Definition

Behavior can be broadly defined as any reaction, response, or action of any individual.

It can also be defined as the way in which an animal or a person behaves in response to a particular situation or stimulus, person, or environment **(Fig. 1)**.

Cognitive (thinking): It is related to the intellectual process—how the individual thinks as he gets the information through

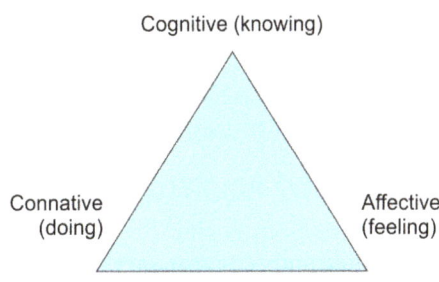

Fig. 1: Constituents of behavior.

various sensory processes, how it is interpreted by our brain to produce a particular kind of response in the form of behavior. For example, a hardworking student hears the news of failing in the examination and starts thinking of the reason for the failure.

Affective (mood): It is the emotional tone associated with the information interpreted and will be shown in the form of actions or behavior of an individual. For example, on hearing news about failure in examination, the student becomes sad.

Connative (psychomotor activity): These are the actions or reactions shown after interpreting the information and can be seen in the form of a person's behavior toward a particular situation. For example, a student after hearing the news of failure felt sad and started crying and wanted to be alone for some time.

A process is called cognitive, affective, or connative depending on the element that predominates in it.

Biological explanations of behavior fall into four categories:
1. Physiological—relates a behavior to the activity of the brain and other organs
2. Ontogenetic—describes the development of a structure or behavior
3. Evolutionary—reconstructs evolutionary history of a behavior or structure
4. Functional—describes *why* a structure or behavior evolved as it did

Therefore, human behavior is a result of both the psychological and physiological processes taking place in the body which depend on each other. Early philosophers, therefore, focused more attention on understanding this relationship which they called as mind-body relationship.

MIND–BODY RELATIONSHIP

Modern psychologists view the relationship between mind and body as interrelated. Mind-body relationship dated back to several years ago and is being studied since ancient times.

History of Mind-Body Relationship

From the earliest times, the mind and body were generally thought of as one unit and was widely explored by the pioneers such as Plato, Aristotle, Buddha, and ancient Greek and eastern thinkers. They have solved the question in many ways—how the mind or soul is related to the body.

Disease was understood as resulting from some type of divine (supernatural) cause or possession, punishment from God(s), etc. Greeks and Arabs were among the first to suggest natural causes of illness, e.g., Hippocrates' humoral theory. Galen was the first to attribute disease to a specific pathogen.

This emphasis on natural causation was lost with the fall of the Roman Empire and the subsequent rise in power of the Church. This view became less tenable; however, with the contributions of Sigmund Freud, hysterical patients had obvious, profound physical symptoms, with no apparent organic cause.

Later in the 1920s, Psychosomatic Medicine concept came up which led to an emphasis on the autonomic nervous system. In the Middle Ages, the Church was the guardian of medical knowledge—the functions of the priest and physician merged. This began to change during the Renaissance, however, especially due to the influence of René Descartes who theorized Cartesian Dualism. Descartes proposed that mind and body be considered as two separate entities.

A different explanation can be given about mind-body relationship and mind refers to all the mental processes of the brain.

Concept of Mind and Body (Fig. 2)

Mind is used synonymously with terms such as soul, brain, or consciousness. Mind is a common term used casually and is considered an abstract component.

It is the element of a person that enables him/her to be aware of the world and his/her experiences, to think, and to feel; the faculty of consciousness and thought; the element or complex of elements in an individual that feels, perceives, thinks, wills, and especially reasons.

Mind is the sum total of various mental processes such as observing, knowing, thinking, reasoning, feeling, wishing, imagining, remembering, and judging.

Mind the 'psyche' by which one is aware of surroundings and able to experience emotions, reasons and make decisions
—*Miller and Keane*

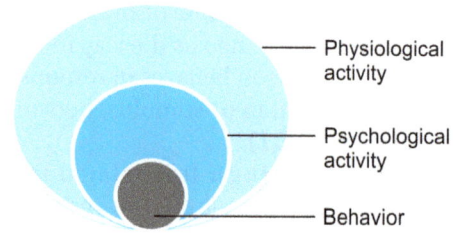

Fig. 2: Mind–body interaction.

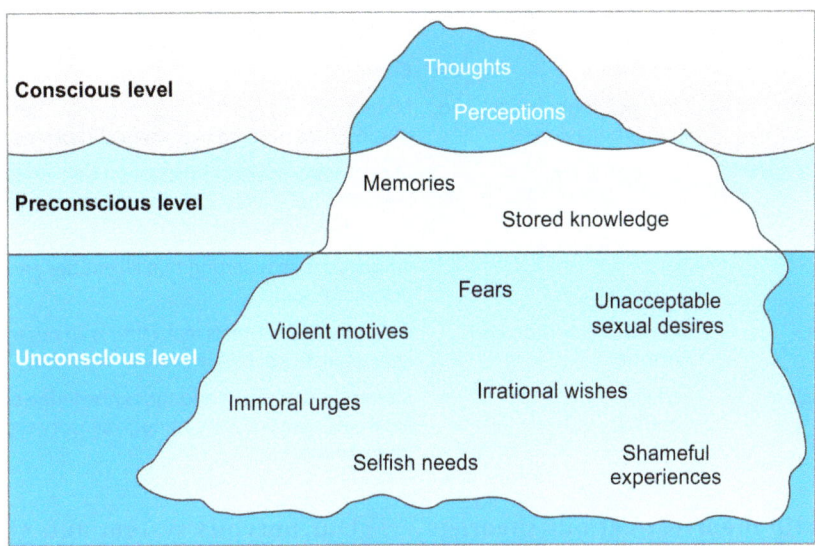

Fig. 3: Freud's iceberg of mind.

The mind arises out of central nervous system (CNS) and it develops along with other body parts. Therefore, it has two components, i.e., organic or physiological component which is made of tissues and cells and the psychological components, i.e., emotions and perception. The brain is a body component.

Body works mechanistically and, thus, can be understood scientifically.

It is defined as the physical structure, including the bones, flesh, and organs of a person or an animal; the entire material or physical structure of an organism, especially of human or animal.

Biological psychology is the study of the physiological, evolutionary, and developmental mechanisms of behavior and experience. For the next 200 years, physicians looked exclusively at organic and cellular changes and pathology to understand and treat illness, until physical evidence became the only basis for diagnosis and treatment of disease.

Mind or mental process is always connected to a body and more intimately connected with the brain or cortical processes. According to earlier psychologists, mind was regarded as a conscious part or the processes which one is aware of at times. It was the sum total of conscious mental processes only. But later on, it was hypothesized by Sigmund Freud in his work "Iceberg of Mind" that it consists of three parts—conscious, preconscious or subconscious and unconscious part (**Fig. 3**).

At the conscious level, we are aware of our mental activities; at the unconscious level, we are not aware of mental processes; and the subconscious level acts like a filter that selects which processes to bring into awareness.

Theories of Mind–Body Relationship (Table 1)

Broadly, theories of mind-body relationship are categorized into two:
1. **Monistic theories:** This theory emphasizes that mind and body are not separate substances. Aristotle, Hobbs, Hegel, and various behaviorists stated that mind is not separate. It is one of the bodily functions and involves mental processes just like other physiological processes. It is generally thought to be a substance other than physical substance and body is just a mental representation.

Table 1: Theories of mind–body relationship.

Name	Proponents	Concepts
Monism	Aristotle, Hobbs, Hegel, and various behaviorists	Mind is a bodily function and generally thought to be of substance other than a physical substance
Dualism (Cartesian)	René Descartes	Mind is not a physical substance. Mind affects the body and body affects the mind. They are separate and they affect each other.
Idealism	Plato	Emphasizes on asserting that all entities are composed of mind or spirit.
Materialism	Greeks, Democritus, and Aristotle	Only physical matter is real. Mind is an organic process, characteristics of highly evolved organisms.
Phenomenalism	Berkely, Hume, and Condillac	Matter does not exist and thus knowledge of the external world is always through sensory experience of phenomena.

2. **Dualistic theories:** Various theorists such as Descartes, Locke, and James who belong to the school of thought known as interactionism theorized that mind is a different substance from other physical substances. Sometimes, the mind affects the body and sometimes body affects the mind. We are physical as we extended in space and mental beings because we can think. Mind is not a physical thing; it exists separately from the body.

The arguments between psychologists and various thinkers are still controversial whether the mind governs body or body governs mind.

Psychosomatic medicine and mind–body interactions also emphasize the intimate relationship that exists between the body and mind. Both neural and chemical processes are important to our understanding of the relationship between the brain and behavior.

Effect of Body on Mind

Mind and body interact with each other. Our nervous system and various glands are responsible to a great extent for our ways of thinking, feeling, and wishing. Various bodily functions affect mental functioning which we can analyze through various identifiable changes in the body.

Our nervous system and glands are responsible, to a great extent, for our ways of thinking, feeling, and wishing. Below are few examples depicting the effect of body on mind:

❖ Increase in blood pressure or heart rate increases the mental activity or mental alertness.
❖ When we feel tired or fatigued we are not able to concentrate on particular work.
❖ Any bodily discomfort or illness causes irritability and feelings of sadness which can lead to certain mental illnesses such as depression.
❖ Certain bodily glands such as thyroid overactivity lead to mental restlessness and overexcitability whereas decreased inactivity of thyroid gland leads to fatigue and lethargy.
❖ Drugs that effect our mood or behavior are used to treat various psychological symptoms like relieving from anxiety, etc.; study of drugs' effects is widely researched to study about mind–body interaction.

Certain drugs such as stimulants (nicotine, cocaine) increase central nervous system activity by increasing dopamine activity. Anti-anxiety drugs such as benzodiazepines, diazepam, and lorazepam cause depression of central nervous system by reducing serotonin and norepinephrine secretions and increasing gamma-aminobutyric acid (GABA) activity.

Effect of Mind on Body

Our mind also affects our bodily function or physical states. Mind activates all the physical and motor activity. Our behavior can affect our health. Psychosomatic medicine is the branch that deals with the effect of mind on body. It can be traced back 2000 years ago as there were traditional healers and Ayurveda. Psychosomatic medicine focuses on the study and treatment of diseases believed to be caused by emotional conflicts, e.g., asthma, peptic ulcers, and hypertension. Certain examples are given below showing the effect of mind on body.

- ❖ Unpleasant emotions like fear, anger, and worry cause headaches, insomnia, indigestion, etc.
- ❖ Emotional conflicts are responsible for various neurotic illnesses such as hysteria, neurasthenic and gastrointestinal troubles such as peptic ulcer, ulcerative colitis, or flatulence.
- ❖ Overthinking or negative thoughts cause physical fatigue.
- ❖ Meditation or relaxation techniques have been found to be more effective in concentration and attention and also increase in overall productivity as confirmed by functional magnetic resonance imaging (fMRI).
- ❖ Chronic stress affects both neural and hormonal pathways and also affects the immune system and makes our body prone to physical illness. This also leads us to a new area of research and study that is "**Psychoneuroimmunology**" (**Fig. 4**)
- ❖ Stress is the result of various factors which can be physical, psychological, or environmental and in turn there is secretion of stress hormone cortisol as a result of bodily response to stress. These stress hormones suppress the immune cells and natural antibodies making the body at risk of getting various diseases

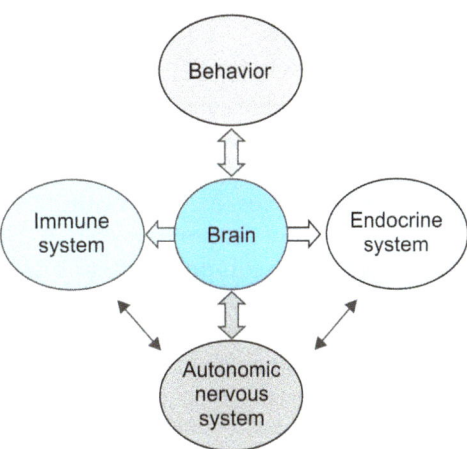

Fig. 4: Concept of psychoneuroimmunology.

such as rheumatoid arthritis, asthma, and various types of infections.

Mind–Body Interventions

There is huge amount of data that reveal that there is relationship between mind and body. Therefore, various techniques or modalities have been developed based on this fact and that is called mind–body interventions. Various relaxation therapies, guided imagery, and hypnosis have been found to have profound effect in treating coronary artery disease, reducing pain in cancer patients, and these can be used pre- and postsurgery to reduce anxiety symptoms. Psychological intervention has been found to be very effective in reducing distress in daily life, improving mood, quality of life, and certain physical disease-related symptoms such as chemotherapy-induced nausea, vomiting, pain, etc.

Therefore, psychosomatic medicine and mind–body interventions emphasized the intimate relationship between mind and body.

▌BRAIN AND BEHAVIOR

Behavior of an individual involves the interaction between mind and body. As already discussed mind–body interaction has two aspects, physical or bodily and mental or psychological. The physical aspect involves the nervous system.

UNIT II: Biological and Behavior

Nervous System

The behavior of an individual is regulated and formulated by the nervous system. Nervous system interprets and regulates our thoughts, emotions, perception, learning, and various other mental processes. The brain is the central processor of the nervous system. The nervous system is composed of a network of nerves which transmits messages and the nervous system is classified as follows:
- Central nervous system
- Peripheral nervous system

Central Nervous System (Flowchart 1)

The central nervous system is composed of brain and the spinal cord. Both brain and the spinal cord are composed of neurons and glial cells that control various bodily functions. The brain is the central processing unit of nervous system as it collects information via sense organs and interprets it and then sends information through various muscles and body parts.

Brain

The brain is the highest nerve center in the nervous system where a large amount of nerves meet each other. The brain is situated in the cavity of skull. Its average weight is 1.3 kg and volume is approximately 1.3 L. It is composed of 180 million nerve cells, 50 million of which are processing the information. It is divided into four lobes, i.e., frontal lobe, parietal lobe, temporal lobe, and occipital lobe. The brain is divided into three main parts—forebrain, midbrain, and hindbrain (**Figs. 5 and 6**).

Forebrain: It consists of cerebrum, thalamus, hypothalamus, and diencephalon.

Midbrain: It consists of mesencephalon, tectum, and tegmentum.

Hindbrain: It consists of pons, medulla, and cerebellum (together known as the brainstem).

Cerebrum

It is composed of two hemispheres—the left hemisphere and the right hemisphere separated by a deep groove that houses a band of 200 million neurons called the corpus callosum which attaches the two hemispheres. The outer part of the cerebrum is called cortex and the inner part is the medulla part. The left hemisphere controls the right part of the body and is dominant in most of the population. It controls various mental functions such as speech, comprehension, rationality, and cognition. The right hemisphere controls the left part of the body and is non-dominant in most population. Each hemisphere is divided into four lobes.

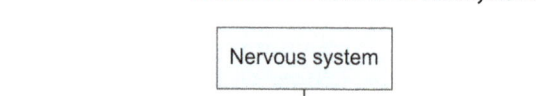
Flowchart 1: Central nervous system.

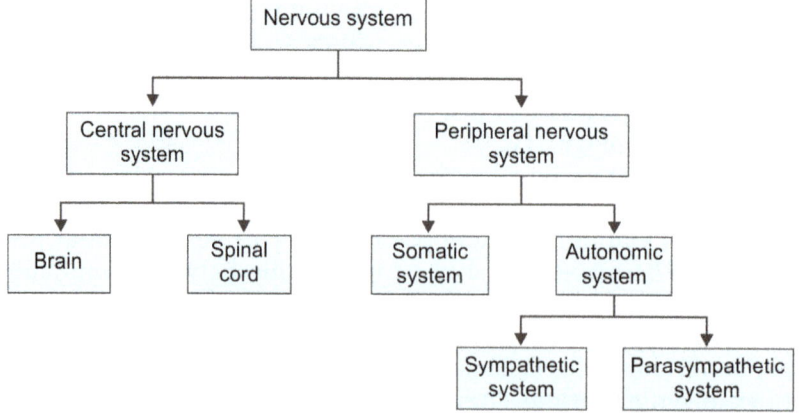

UNIT II: Biological and Behavior

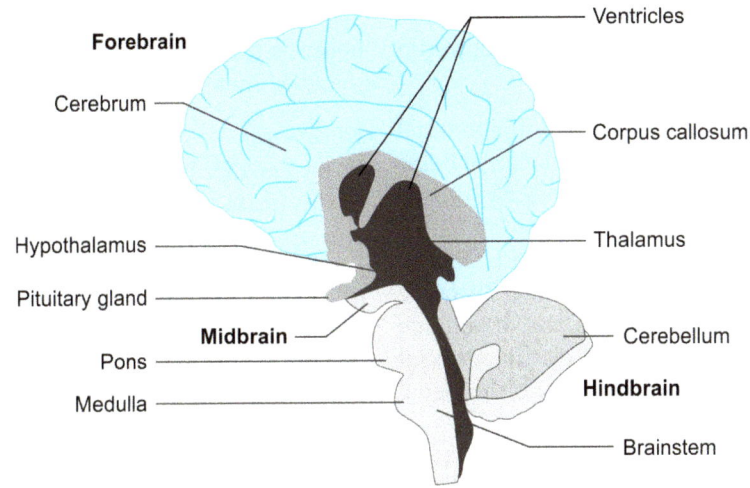

Fig. 5: Parts of brain.

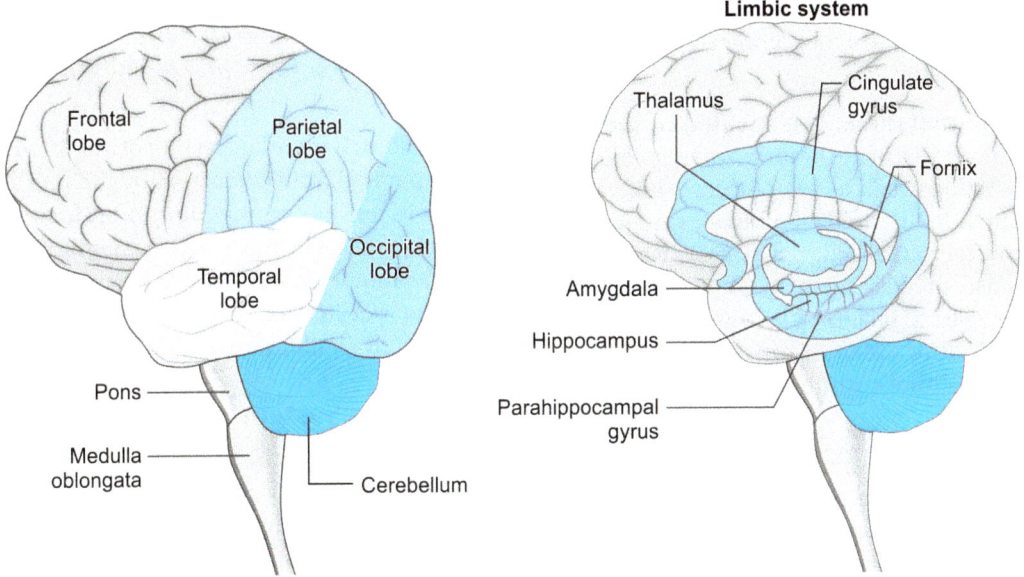

Fig. 6: Anatomy of the brain.

Frontal lobe: It controls voluntary body movement including that permits speaking, thinking, and judgment formation. The frontal lobe may also play a role in the emotional experience. The alteration includes fear, aggressiveness, depression, rage, euphoria, irritability, and apathy and is probably related to a frontal lobe in connection with the limbic system.

Parietal lobe: It controls perception and interpretation of most sensory information including touch, pain, taste, body position; language interpretation is associated with the left hemisphere of the parietal lobe.

Temporal lobe: The upper anterior temporal lobe is concerned with the auditory functions while the lower part is dedicated to short-term memory. It also plays a role in the expression of emotions through an interconnection with the limbic system.

Occipital lobe: It is located in the cerebral hemisphere in the back of the hat and it helps to control vision. It is the primary area of visual perception and language interpretation. Visual perception gives individuals the ability to judge special relationships such as distance and to see in three dimensions. Language interpretation is influenced by the occipital lobes through an association with the visual experience.

Thalamus: It is a small structure located just above the brainstem between the cerebral cortex and the midbrain. It mainly receives sensory impulses. It also regulates the actions of many of the higher centers of sensation and movement.

Hypothalamus: It is located in the lower central area of the brain which regulates body functions such as temperature, hunger, and thirst. It also holds the higher centers which control mental behavior, consciousness, moral sense, intellect, speech, language, etc. It also receives all incoming sensory nerve impulses including those of touch, pain, pressure, temperature, texture, shape, size, etc.

Diencephalon: It is situated between the telencephalon and the midbrain and it acts as a primary relay and processing center for secondary information and autonomic control and it is functionally a diverse area.

Midbrain
Mesencephalon: It is located above the pons and adjoined rostrally to the thalamus. Its functions include particular movement of the eyes, important functions in motor movement, and also in auditory and visual processing. It is the connection point between the forebrain and the hindbrain.

Tectum and tegmentum: These are the dorsal and the ventral parts of the midbrain respectively. It is a network of multisynaptic neurons that are involved in many subconscious homeostatic and reflexive pathways.

Hindbrain
Pons Varolii: It forms the middle portion of the brainstem and contains ascending and descending pathways. It acts as a relay center between the cerebellum and cerebral hemispheres. It helps in regulating breathing and sleeping [REM (rapid eye movement) sleep cycle].

Medulla oblongata: It is the lower portion of the brainstem which connects to the spinal cord. It provides a pathway for all ascending and descending pathways. It contains vital centers of control which regulate heart rate, blood pressure, respiration, and reflex centers for swallowing, sneezing, coughing, and vomiting.

Cerebellum: It is the largest part of hindbrain. It is separated from brainstem by the fourth ventricle but has connection to brainstem through bundles of fiber tracts. It is concerned with involuntary movements such as muscular tone and coordination and the maintenance of posture and equilibrium.

The Limbic System

This is not a specific area but the most important area which influences human behavior. It is a circuit covering many areas and their interconnections. It includes the hypothalamus, the amygdala, portions of the cerebral cortex such as the hippocampus, and a number of other nuclei and pathways. The amygdala is also called "emotional brain" and is associated with feelings of fear and anxiety, anger and aggression, love, joy, happiness, sexuality, and social behavior. The limbic system has been implicated in a number of functions including motivation and emotion. Stimulation of certain parts of the limbic system may produce eating, drinking, or emotions. Damage to certain areas may produce docility and other emotional changes.

Stimulation of certain areas of the limbic system and some areas connected with it can produce an extremely pleasurable sensation. Recent theories postulated that certain types of abnormal behavior, particularly depressive states, may result from the functional abnormalities in these pleasure centers.

The Extrapyramidal System

It is a biological neural network that is part of the motor system causing involuntary movements. Extrapyramidal tract can be distinguished from tracts of motor cortex that reach their targets by traveling through the pyramids of the medulla. The pyramidal pathways (corticospinal and corticobulbar tracts) may directly innervate motor neurons of the spinal cord or brainstem, whereas the extrapyramidal system centers on the modulation and regulation (indirect control) of anterior (ventral) horn cells.

Neurons

The human brain is estimated to contain at least 150 billion nerve cells called neurons. Neurons are linked to one another in a long chain. Each neuron receives messages from other neurons and sends its own messages to others. There are different types of neurons for different functions, such as motor neuron, sensory neuron, and interneuron. Cell division, a feature common to most other kinds of cells, does not occur in most adult cells. Nerve cells lost are never replaced. Speculation is that an average of 10,000 neurons die each day.

Parts of Neuron

On the basis of its structure, it can be divided into three parts (**Fig. 7**):
1. **Cell body:** It is the topmost part of neuron which is filled with a fluid called cytoplasm. In the center of cell body, a dense substance is present called nucleus. It controls all the cellular activities of nerve cells such as oxygen utilization and energy production. For example, energy synthesis occurs in

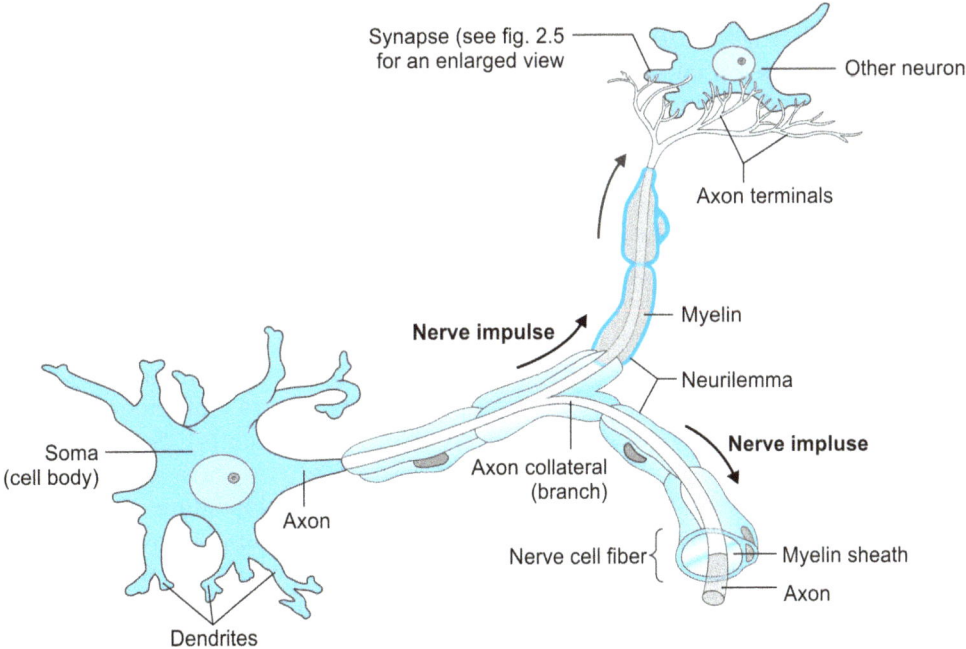

Fig. 7: Structure of neuron.

organelles that are known as mitochondria and protein synthesis on structure known as ribosomes. Certain short fibers or processes extend from the cell body called dendrites. These dendrites are the receiving centers which pick up the signals from other neurons.

2. **Axons:** Each neuron has a single long fiber that extends away from the cell body. Its length varies in different neurons. These axons construct nerve fibers and nerve pathways in association with the axons of other neurons. Axon is covered with a white membrane called myelin sheath. This membrane is not continuous on axon; some gaps are present in between at regular intervals called nodes of Ranvier. It helps the conductance of nerve impulse received from cell body across the axon. Myelin sheath increases the cell's rate of conduction and its action potential.

3. **Terminal:** The axon at the end is divided into various small branches called telodendria that are connected with dendrites of other neurons. These telodendria terminate in small swellings which are termed synaptic terminals. The terminal of one neuron is attached with the dendrite of another neuron at a gap observed microscopically called synapse.

Therefore, synapse contains a physical space that separates two cells which is referred to as synaptic space or cleft. The synaptic membrane toward the terminal of neuron is called presynaptic membrane and the other toward the dendrite of the other cell is called postsynaptic membrane.

Information transfer along the neurons is a chemical process. It involves the release of chemical neurotransmitter molecules by the presynaptic membrane which fills the space of synapse to help in nerve impulse transmission from one neuron to another neuron. These neurotransmitter molecules are stored in synaptic vesicles. Synaptic transmission is a process that requires energy and for this transmission, energy is supplied with mitochondria.

Therefore, the connection between nerve cells is known as synapse and the chemicals that pass information from one neuron to another are known as neurotransmitters.

Nerve Impulse Conduction (Fig. 8)

When stimulation is received by a neural cell, the right end of the top axon is at rest. Thus, it has a negative charge inside. An action potential begins when ion channels open and sodium ions (Na^+) rush into the axon. The action potential would travel from left to right along the axon. In the lower axon, the action potential has moved to the right. After it passes, potassium ions (K^+) flow out of the axon. This quickly renews the negative charge inside the axon, so it can fire again. Sodium ions that enter the axon during an action potential are pumped out more slowly. Removing them restores the original resting potential.

Neurotransmitters

Neurotransmitters are chemicals located and released in the brain to allow an impulse from one nerve cell to pass to another nerve cell **(Table 2)**.

Description

There are approximately 50 neurotransmitters identified. There are billions of nerve cells located in the brain, which do not directly touch each other. Nerve cells communicate messages by secreting neurotransmitters. Neurotransmitters can excite or inhibit neurons (nerve cells). Some common neurotransmitters are acetylcholine, norepinephrine, dopamine, serotonin, and GABA. Acetylcholine and norepinephrine are excitatory neurotransmitters while dopamine, serotonin, and GABA are inhibitory. Each neurotransmitter can directly or indirectly influence neurons in a specific portion of the brain, thereby affecting behavior.

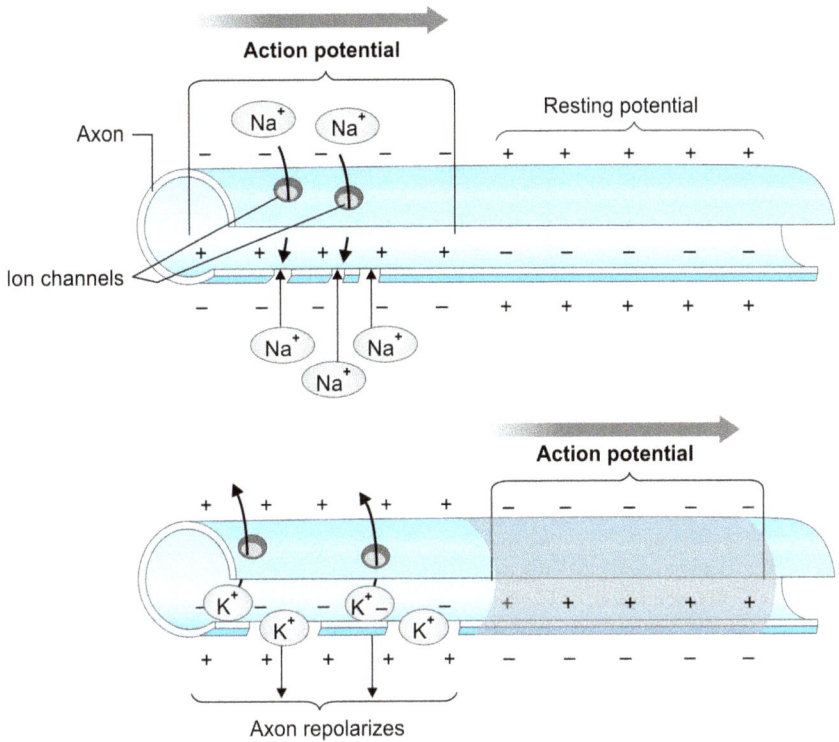

Fig. 8: The nerve impulse.

Mechanism of Impulse Transmission

A nerve impulse travels through a nerve in a long, slender cellular structure called an axon, and it eventually reaches a structure called the presynaptic membrane, which contains neurotransmitters to be released in a free space called the synaptic cleft. Freely flowing neurotransmitter molecules are picked up by receptors (structures that appear on cellular surfaces that pick up molecules that fit into them like a "lock and key") located.

Neurotransmitters are chemicals that transmit messages from one nerve cell (neuron) to another. The nerve impulse travels from the first nerve cell through the axon—a single smooth body arising from the nerve cell—to the axon terminal and the synaptic knobs. Each synaptic knob communicates with a dendrite or cell body of another neuron, and the synaptic knobs contain neurovesicles that store and release neurotransmitters. The synapse lies between the synaptic knob and the next cell. For the impulse to continue traveling across the synapse to reach the next cell, the synaptic knobs release the neurotransmitter into that space, and the next nerve cell is stimulated to pick up the impulse and continue it in a structure called the postsynaptic membrane of another nearby neuron. Once the neurotransmitter is picked up by receptors in the postsynaptic membrane, the molecule is internalized in the neuron and the impulse continues. This process of nerve cell communication is extremely rapid.

Once the neurotransmitter is released from the neurotransmitter vesicles of the presynaptic membrane, the normal movement of molecules should be directed to receptor sites located on the postsynaptic membrane. However, in certain disease states, the flow of the neurotransmitter is defective. For example, in depression, the flow of the inhibitory neurotransmitter serotonin is defective, and

Table 2: Various types of neurotransmitter and their description.

Neurotransmitter	Type	Location	Effect	Variations
Acetylcholine	Both excitatory and inhibitory	Brain and peripheral neuromuscular junctions	Contracts smooth muscles, dilates blood vessels, increases bodily secretions, and slows heart rate, thinking and comprehension motivation, arousal, attention, learning and memory	Decreased levels cause dementia, Alzheimer's disease. Increased level causes cramps, paralysis, muscarinic, and nicotinic toxicity
Norepinephrine (noradrenaline)	Both excitatory and inhibitory Acts as both stress hormone and neurotransmitter	Cell bodies in the pons and medulla, whole body, produced by adrenal medulla	Alert, motivated, controls appetite, energy, sexual arousal, increases heart rate, blood pressure, and glucose levels	Decreased level causes depression and sleep disorders. Increased level causes schizophrenia and mania
Dopamine	Excitatory Both hormone (feel good) and neurotransmitter	Produced in the substantia nigra, ventral tegmentum, and hypothalamus of brain	Pleasure, increased heart rate, thinking and planning, executive function, motor control, arousal, and reinforcement	Increased level causes anxiety, sleep disturbance, increased energy, mania, schizophrenia. Decreased level causes depression, Parkinson's disease, psychosis
Serotonin	Inhibitory	Produced by neurons originating in the raphe nuclei located in the midline of brainstem	Modulates mood, cognition, reward, learning, memory Also aids in sleeping, eating, and digestion	Increased level leads to confusion, restlessness, headaches, high blood pressure, unconsciousness. Decreased levels cause depression, anxiety, and sleep trouble
GABA (gamma-aminobutyric acid)	Inhibitory	Synthesized in cytoplasm of presynaptic neuron	Essential in normal brain function, information processing, calmness. Relieves anxiety, stress	Increased level causes decreased brain activity, hypersomnia, daytime sleepiness. Decreased level causes ADHD, anxiety, panic disorders, Parkinson's disease, and insomnia

(ADHD: attention deficit hyperactivity disorder)

molecules flow back to their originating site (the presynaptic membrane) instead to the receptors on the postsynaptic membrane that will transmit the impulse to a nearby neuron.

The mechanism of action and localization of neurotransmitters in the brain has provided valuable information concerning the cause of many mental disorders, including clinical depression and chemical dependency, and in researching medications that allow normal flow and movement of neurotransmitter molecules.

Neurotransmitter Disease Variability: Example

Drug addictions

Cocaine and crack cocaine are psychostimulants that affect neurons containing dopamine in the areas of the brain known as the limbic and frontal cortex. When cocaine is used, it generates a feeling of confidence and power. However, when large amounts are taken, people "crash" and suffer from physical and emotional exhaustion as well as depression.

Attempts to counteract the effects of the drugs involve using medications that mimic them, such as nalorphine, naloxone, and naltrexone.

Alcohol is one of the depressant drugs in the widest use and is believed to cause its effects by interacting with the GABA receptor. Initially, anxiety is controlled, but greater amounts reduce muscle control and delay reaction time due to impaired thinking.

ASSOCIATION CORTEX (FIGS. 9A AND B)

Most of the cerebral cortex lies outside the primary sensory areas and principal motor areas. These regions in the frontal, parietal, temporal, and occipital lobes are called association areas. The two hemispheres of the cortex are connected by a bundle of nerves called corpus callosum.

Frontal Lobe Association Cortex

It is interconnected with visual, auditory, and somatosensory cortical areas, with other association cortex in the parietal and temporal lobes. In case of frontal damage, changes in personality, general behavior, and intellectual ability are seen.

Parietal Lobe Association Cortex

It lies behind the somatosensory cortex and receives inputs from the visual cortex, auditory cortex, and thalamus. Major output goes to the frontal and temporal association cortex, to the thalamus, and to subcortical structures involved in the control of movements. Its damage leads to difficulty in recognizing common objects, say a pencil. The patients would know they are touching something but not able to identify what they are handling.

A circle is flashed to the left brain of a split-brain patient, and he is asked what he saw. He easily replies, "A circle." He can also pick out the circle by merely touching shapes with his right hand, out of sight behind a screen. However, his left hand cannot identify the circle. If a triangle is flashed to the patient's right brain, he cannot say what he saw (speech is controlled by the left hemisphere). He also cannot identify the triangle by touch with the right hand. Now, however, the left hand has no difficulty picking out the triangle. In other tests, the hemispheres reveal distinct skills, as listed in **Figures 9A and B**.

Temporal Lobe Association Cortex and Related Structures

The temporal lobe of each hemisphere lies below the lateral fissure. The upper portions of each temporal lobe contain the primary sensory cortex and related cortex involved in hearing. Below the hearing or involved areas is the association cortex of the temporal lobes. Buried within each temporal lobe are two limbic system structures in the formation of memories. These are the hippocampus and amygdala.

MUSCULAR CONTROL OF BEHAVIOR

Whether we engage our diaphragm muscle to improve oxygenation and immune function, move our limbs when we take bath, eat, dress, run or walk, or practice yoga while lying in bed, our ability to move is an essential aspect of our well-being. Thus, our muscles with bones are responsible for bodily movements, internal and external.

The term "muscle tissue" refers to all the contractile tissues of the body—skeletal,

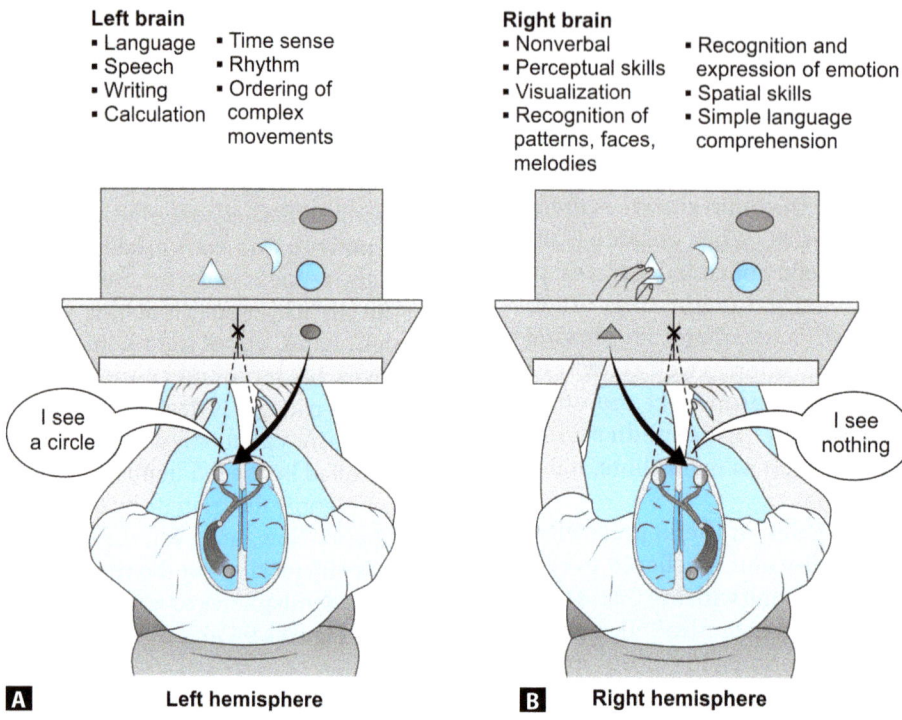

Figs. 9A and B: Association of cortex.

cardiac, and smooth muscle. The skeletal muscle tissues and connective tissue make up individual muscle organs, such as the biceps brachia muscle. Cardiac muscle is located in the heart and is therefore considered part of the cardiovascular system. Smooth muscle of intestines is a part of the digestive system, whereas smooth muscle tissue of the urinary bladder is a part of the urinary system and so on.

Integration of sensory input and motor output: Sensory systems provide the input that keeps the central nervous system informed of changes in the external and internal environment. Output from the central nervous system (CNS) is then conveyed to motor systems, which enables us to move about, alter glandular secretions, and change our relationship to the world around us. As the sensory information reaches the CNS, it becomes part of a large pool of sensory input. Every bit of input the CNS receives does not elicit a response. Rather, the incoming information is integrated with other information arriving from all other operating sensory receptors. The integration process occurs not just once but at many stations along the pathways of the CNS and at both conscious and subconscious levels. It occurs within the spinal cord, brainstem, cerebellum, basal ganglia, and cerebral cortex. As a result, a muscle contracts or a gland secretes with a motor response. Motor portions of cerebral cortex play a major role in initiating and controlling precise, discrete, and muscular movements. The basal ganglia largely integrate semivoluntary, automatic movements such as walking, swimming, and laughing. The cerebellum assists the motor cortex and basal ganglia by making body movements smooth and coordinated and by contributing significantly in maintaining normal posture and balance.

Motor Pathways in Brain

Most motor pathways extend from the cortex of the brain to the skeletal muscles.

- **Direct (pyramidal) pathways:** Voluntary motor impulses are propagated from the motor cortex to somatic efferent neurons that innervate skeletal muscles via the direct (pyramidal) pathways. The simplest pathways consist of upper and lower motor neurons.
- **Indirect (extrapyramidal) pathways:** These involve the motor cortex, basal ganglia, thalamus, cerebellum, reticular formation, and nuclei in the brainstem.

The muscle control is lost when the nerve centers or fibers are injured or diseased. General muscular tension causes flaccid paralysis and spastic paralysis, respectively.

■ GLANDULAR CONTROLS OF BEHAVIOR (FIG. 10)

The endocrine glands secrete products called hormones which are chemical messengers that deliver stimulatory or inhibitory signals to the target cells.

Pituitary gland: The pituitary gland is a body 1.2 cm (1/2 inch) in diameter extending downward from the floor of the brain's third ventricle by a stalk (infundibulum). It is composed of an anterior lobe (adenohypophysis) and a posterior lobe (neurohypophysis). Many of the hormones respond due to hypothalamus. Pituitary regulation may have implication for behavioral functioning. The action of pituitary hormones is summarized in **Table 3**.

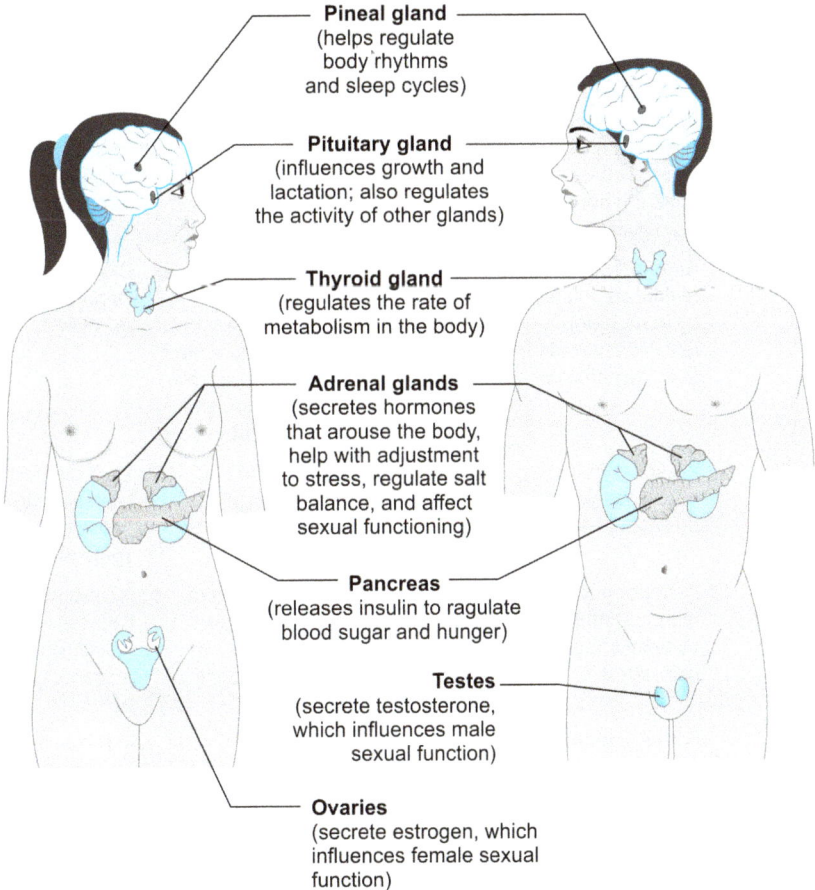

Fig. 10: Endocrine glands and their functions.

Table 3: Hormones and the behavior.

Hormone	Location and stimulation	Target organ	Function	Possible behavioral correlation to altered secretion
Growth hormone (GH)	Anterior pituitary; release stimulated by a thyrotropin-releasing hormone from hypothalamus	Bones and tissues	Growth in children and protein synthesis in adults	Anorexia nervosa
Thyroid-stimulating hormone (TSH)	Pituitary; release stimulated by thyrotropin-releasing hormone from hypothalamus	Thyroid gland	Stimulation of secretion of thyroid hormones needed for metabolism of food and regulation of temperature	Increased levels: Insomnia, anxiety, emotional lability, apprehension Decreased levels: depression, fatigue, dull mental processes, apathy
Adrenocorticotropic hormone (ACTH)	Anterior pituitary; release stimulated by corticotrophin-releasing hormone from hypothalamus	Adrenal cortex	Stimulation of secretion of cortisol, which plays a role in response to stress.	Increased level: Mood Disorders, psychosis, increased libido Decreased levels: depression, apathy, fatigue
Prolactin	Anterior pituitary; release stimulated by prolactin-releasing hormone from hypothalamus	Breasts	Stimulation of milk production	Increased levels: depression, anxiety, decreased libido, irritability
Gonadotropic hormone	Anterior pituitary; release stimulated by gonadotropin-releasing hormone from hypothalamus	Ovaries and testes	Stimulation of secretion of estrogen, progesterone, and testosterone; role in ovulation and sperm production	Decreased levels: Depression and anorexia nervosa
Melanocyte-stimulating hormone (MSH)	Anterior pituitary; release stimulated by onset of darkness	Pineal gland	Stimulation of secretion of melatonin	Increased testosterone: Increased sexual behavior and aggressiveness
Antidiuretic hormone (ADH)	Posterior pituitary; release stimulated by dehydration, pain, stress	Kidney	Conservation of body water and maintenance of blood pressure	Increased levels: Depression Polydipsia, altered pain response modified sleep patterns
Oxytocin	Posterior pituitary; release stimulated by end of pregnancy, stress during sexual arousal	Uterus, breasts	Contraction of the uterus for labor; release of breast milk	May play in stress response by stimulation of ACTH

The adenohypophysis: The hypothalamus produces releasing hormones that pass through capillaries and veins of the hypophyseal portal system to the capillaries in the anterior pituitary, where they stimulate the secretion of specialized hormones. It includes growth hormone, thyroid-stimulating hormone, adrenocorticotropic hormone, prolactin, gonadotropic hormone, and melanocyte-stimulating hormone.

The neurohypophysis: The hypothalamus has direct control over the posterior pituitary through efferent neural pathways. Two hormones are found in the posterior pituitary, i.e., vasopressin or antidiuretic hormone (ADH) and oxytocin.

GENETICS AND BEHAVIOR

Both genes and the environment interact to shape human behavior. The fundamental issue is how much role genetics play in shaping human behaviors. Brain function involves thousands of genes. 30% of the genetic disorders are due to neural tube defects during embryonic life. Various psychological disorders, weight gain, personality, and sexual orientation all involve genetics as one of the common etiological factors.

Various genes affect the behavior of a person through influence on the structure and pattern of genes and their anatomical configuration. Therefore, genetics is the study of how traits are inherited from parents to offsprings. In the 19th century monk Gregor Mendel first studied genetics scientifically and demonstrated that inheritance occurs through genes.

Genes

Genes are basic units of heredity that maintain their structural identity from one generation to another. Genes are aligned along chromosomes (strands of genes) and come in pairs. A gene is a portion of a chromosome and is composed of deoxyribonucleic acid (DNA). DNA serves as a model for the synthesis of ribonucleic acid (RNA). RNA is a single-strand chemical that can serve as a template/model for the synthesis of proteins. Living organisms are made up of proteins. Proteins determine the development of the body by:

❖ Forming part of the structure of the body
❖ Serving as enzymes and biological catalysts that regulate chemical reactions in the body
❖ Types of genes include:
  ▪ Homozygous for a gene means that a person has an identical pair of genes on the two chromosomes.
  ▪ Heterozygous for a gene means that a person has an unmatched pair of genes on the two chromosomes.
  ▪ Genes are either dominant, recessive, or intermediate.
  ▪ Examples: Eye color, ability to taste PTC
  ▪ A dominant gene shows a strong effect in either the homozygous or heterozygous condition.
  ▪ A recessive gene shows its effect only in the homozygous condition.
  ▪ Autosomal genes—all other genes except for sex-linked genes
  ▪ Sex-linked genes—genes located on the sex chromosomes
❖ In mammals, the sex chromosomes are designated X and Y.
  ▪ Females have two X chromosomes (XX).
  ▪ Males have an X and a Y chromosome (XY).

The human Y chromosome has genes for 27 proteins. The human X chromosome has genes for approximately 1,500 proteins. Thus, sex-linked genes usually refer to X-linked genes (e.g., red–green color deficiency). Sex-limited genes are genes that are present in both sexes but mainly have an effect on one sex (chest hair, breast size, etc.).

Almost all behaviors have both a genetic component and an environmental component. Researchers study monozygotic ("from one egg") and fraternal ("from two eggs") twins to infer contributions of heredity and environment. Researchers also study adopted children and their resemblance to their biological parents to infer hereditary influences **(Fig. 11)**. Heritability refers to how much characteristics depend on genetic differences. Estimates of hereditary influences are often difficult to infer and are prone to error.

Sources of error include the following:
❖ The inability to distinguish between the effects of genes and prenatal influences.
❖ Environmental factors can inactivate genes.

Genes do not directly produce behaviors. Genes produce proteins that increase the probability that a behavior will develop under certain circumstances. Genes can also have an indirect effect. Genes can alter your environment by producing behaviors or traits that alter how people in your environment react to you.

Evolution refers to a change in the frequency of various genes in a population over generations regardless of whether helpful or harmful to the species. Evolution attempts to answer two questions:

How species did evolve involves the tentative construction of "evolutionary trees".

How species do evolve rests upon some assumptions:
❖ Offspring generally resemble their parents for genetic reasons.
❖ Mutations and recombination of genes introduce new heritable variations.
❖ Certain individuals successfully reproduce more than others do.

Artificial selection refers to choosing individuals with desired traits and making them parents of the next generation. Therefore,

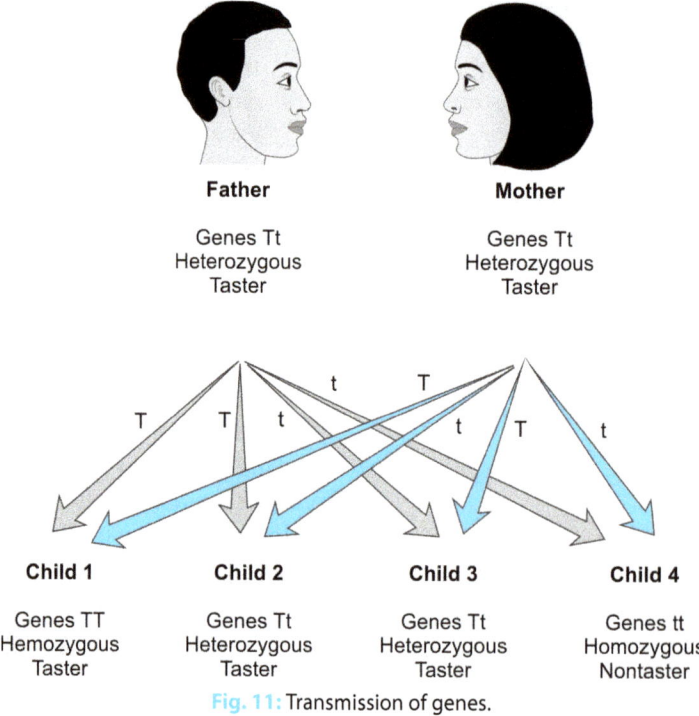

Fig. 11: Transmission of genes.

evolutionary psychology focuses upon functional and evolutionary explanations of how behaviors evolved. It assumes that behaviors characteristic of a species have arisen through natural selection and provide a survival advantage.

Examples: Differences in peripheral/color vision, sleep mechanisms in the brain, eating habits, temperature regulation.

Heredity and Environment

Heredity

It is the transmission of mental and physical traits from parents to offspring. Heredity contains those traits that are present at the time of birth of the child. It is seen that through heredity, particular variations among individuals prevail and cause the species to exist. For example, traits such as intelligence and personality have evolved over time.

Genetic Diversity

It is the amount of variation seen in a particular population. The difference occurs in different communities, race, or ethnic groups that lead to individual differences among the population. Genes have a significant effect on human beings. For example, Japanese and Chinese have a significant appearance than the whites and the Indians.

For example, diabetes mellitus is inherited as a heterogeneous, multigenic trait. It carries a risk of 25–50% in identical twins, whereas siblings have a 6% risk and offspring a 5% risk.

Genetic variability: It is a measure of the tendency of individual genotypes in a population to vary from one another. Genetic variability describes the susceptibility of organisms to diseases and sensitivity to toxins or drugs. There are various sources of variability in population which are as follows:

- ❖ Genetic recombination is one source of variability—during meiosis, recombination of gene occurs causing more variability in a population.
- ❖ Immigration and translocation is movement of an individual into or out of a population which increases genetic variability in next generations.
- ❖ Polyploidy—more than two homologous chromosomes allow even more genetic variability.
- ❖ Diffuse centromeres—chromatids split apart in many ways allowing chromosome fragmentation and polyploidy.
- ❖ Genetic mutations
- ❖ Correlated traits—changes in a single gene have effect on many traits.

Environment

Some of the changes in human behavior have not been explained by the genetic influence and its variability and many researchers believed the effect of environment on behavior and personality of an individual. The environment can be natural, built or artificial, social, or internal/external. It is any external force which influences us or our behavior. It refers to all those things which surround an individual.

The pollutants in the environment have been linked to chronic diseases such as cancer, asthma, and cardiovascular health problems. For example, relationship exists between global warming and malaria, ozone depletion and cancer.

Nature versus Nurture

This concept ignores the separate effects of genes and environment on individual difference. In reality, gene expression is environment-dependent and one could not exist without the other. For example, the phenotypic value (P) of an individual is the combined effect of the genotypic value (G) and the environmental deviation:

$$P = G + E$$

Example: Phenylketonuria is a human genetic condition caused by mutations to a gene coding for a particular liver enzyme which causes delayed brain development and other metabolic changes.

Importance of Genetics in Nursing

- Nurses need to understand the language of genetics and its disorders, are able to take history over three generations, and recognize the possibility of a genetic disorder in an individual or family.
- Nurses often come in contact with children and adults with childhood genetic disorders and will have to deal with how these disorders will influence their future outcomes.
- Nurses plan, implement, administer, and evaluate the screening or testing programs and explain and interpret correctly the purpose, implications, and results of genetic tests.
- The nurse serves as an advocate for a client or family with genetic disorders.
- She monitors and evaluates clients with genetic disorder and works with families having children with genetic disorders.
- The nurse assesses the client and family's cultural and ethnic health beliefs and practices as they relate to the genetic problems.

PSYCHOLOGY OF SENSATION

Sensation is the process by which sensory organs collect information and send it to the brain. At a particular time, a large amount of information is being sensed by any one at one time such as someone talking, distant sound of a vendor, smell of perfume, temperature of room, and brightness of light. With lots of information coming through various sense organs, majority of our world never gets recognized or interpreted. We sense only that thing we are able to and what human beings can sense. Our threshold is different from each other and from other species too.

Sensation is our window to the world. It is the passive process of bringing information from outside world into the body.

Sensation is extension of the physiological aspect of the psychology and physiology of the sensory system provides an understanding of thresholds and psychophysiological concepts. This consists of neural pathways and the ways in which sensory information is processed within the nervous system.

Definition

Sensation is the process of informing the brain about some experience occurring outside the central nervous system. These experiences can be visual, auditory, somatosensory (touch, temperature, pain), olfactory, gustatory, kinesthetic (movement), and vestibular (orientation) senses.

Sensation occurs when special receptors in the sense organs such as the eyes, ears, nose, skin, and taste buds are activated allowing various forms of outside stimuli to become neural signals in the brain.

(This process of converting outside stimuli such as light into neural activity is called transduction.)

Attributes of Sensation

Quality: Sensation of sound differs from sensation of color in quality. Sensation through the same sense organs differs in quality.

Intensity: Strength of sensation depends on the objective strength of stimulus and the mental state of the individual.

Duration: It depends on the continuity of the stimulus or its effect.

Extensity: It means voluminousness or spreadoutness of sensation. As this increases, the sensation appears to be bigger. For example, the touch of a palm is more extensive than the touch of fingers.

Types of Sensation

Sensation is felt through sense organs. We receive sensation through the eyes, nose, tongue, skin, and ear—popularly known as five sense organs. Various types of sensation are as follows:

- **Visual sensation (sense of sight):** Visual sensations which are stimulated by light waves are experienced through the sense of the eye. The sense of sight is regarded as an evolution of the elementary sense of touch or feeling. The eye is comprised of complex sensory system; when light energy reaches photoreceptors (rods and cones), neural signs are sent through the visual system, providing sensations. They are two types of sensation—sensation of brightness and sensation of color.
- **Auditory sensation (sense of hearing):** These are received through the ears. The eardrum or "tympanum," vibrates in response to the air vibrations or sound waves reaching it from the outside. These vibrations are intensified, and the auditory nerve ends take up the impression and pass it to the brain. Sound waves are sensed according to their characteristics of pitch, intensity, quality, and harmony.
- **Taste sensation (sense of taste):** It is the tongue which acquires these sensations. There are many papillae in the tongue. Mostly, there are taste pores in these papillae. There are bag-like structures called taste buds. The taste buds are stimulated chemically by objects brought in contact with them, the impulse being conveyed to the nerves and transmitted to the brain. The sensations of the taste are classified into five classes, i.e., sweet, sour, bitter, salty, and hot. The central portion of the tongue cannot receive sensations of different tastes. The tip of the tongue acquires the sweet taste, the rear the bitter taste, the edges the sour taste, while saline taste is spread uniformly all over the tongue.
- **Olfactory sensation (sense of smell):** Receptor cells for the olfactory sensations are located in the nose at its apex. As only a part of the breath reaches them, it is necessary to draw a deeper breath in order to smell the odor. The odor-carrying air, which is drawn in, activates these cells by touching them. We smell the rose only because minute particles of its substance are carried into our nostrils. We smell gas because some of its particles enter our nostrils.

Tactile sensations (sense of touch): The skin contains the receivers of somesthetic sensations. There are two types of sensations:
1. Cutaneous sensations include the sensations of pressure, warmth, cold, and pain. There are different areas for these sensations interspersed with insensitive areas. They are different from each other and they have different areas of the body assigned to them.
2. Kinesthetic sensations are felt in muscles, bones, and various nervous joints and their covering membrane. Tension, contraction, pulling, etc., are examples of motor sensations. They are caused by the muscles, tendons, and joints. The nerves embedded in these give the sensations of motion when the muscles contract or the joints move. The brain receives information of these sensations through the sensory nerves whose parts are in muscles, tendons, and joints. The motor sensations put pressure upon the skin.

Motor Sensations

Motor sensations are a means of the knowledge of the primary qualities of objects, e.g., their position, distance, direction, weight, etc.; these sensations take part automatically and generally pass by unnoticed. The kind of motor sensations are as follows:

Sensations of position: Such a sensation is generated when the arms are held motionless in a fully extended position.

Sensation of free movement: If the arms are moved in all directions, then the arising sensations are those of free movement.

Sensation of impeded movement: These can be experienced by lifting some heavy weight.

Abnormal Sensation

Abnormalities related to vision:
- ❖ **Hyperopia/farsightedness:** In this, distant objects are visible with clarity but near objects appear blurred because of the distance between lens and retina.
- ❖ **Myopia/near-sightedness:** In this, near objects are visible with clarity but distant objects appear blurred because of the distance between lens and retina.
- ❖ **Astigmatism:** It is the defect in the curvature of cornea or lens which causes light rays to refract unevenly and defects in vision develop.
- ❖ Tunnel vision, squint or strabismus, diplopia, presbyopia, and color blindness (total or partial) are some of the visual defects which can cause abnormal vision.
- ❖ **Cataract:** It develops because of opaqueness in cornea.

Abnormalities related to hearing: Conductive deafness (corrected by conventional hearing aid) and sensorineural deafness, otitis media, tinnitus.

Abnormalities related to olfaction: Anosmia (inability to smell), dysosmia (things smell different from how they should), and hyposmia (decreased ability to smell).

Abnormalities in other sense organs are also experienced like in gustatory sensation problem can occur due to changes in taste sensation due to stomatitis, gingivitis, glossitis, dental caries, leukoplakia, plaque formation on tongue, ageusia (complete loss of taste), etc.

Some people report of strange sensation of crawling on the body, unpleasant sensation, and lack of control over body movements.

QUESTION BANK

MULTIPLE CHOICE QUESTIONS

1. Mind is also referred to as _____ in psychology.
   a. Mental processes
   b. Interest
   c. Idea
   d. Will
2. The _____ receive(s) incoming signals from other neurons.
   a. Soma
   b. Terminal buttons
   c. Myelin sheath
   d. Dendrites
3. The central nervous system is comprised of _____.
   a. Sympathetic and parasympathetic nervous systems
   b. Organs and glands
   c. Brain and spinal cord
   d. Somatic and autonomic nervous systems
4. Sympathetic activation is associated with _____.
   a. Pupil dilation
   b. Storage of glucose in the liver
   c. Increased heart rate
   d. Both a and c
5. The _____ is a sensory relay station where all sensory information, except for smell, goes before being sent to other areas of the brain for further processing.
   a. Amygdala
   b. Hippocampus
   c. Hypothalamus
   d. Thalamus

UNIT II: Biological and Behavior

6. **Which of the following is not a structure of the forebrain?**
   a. Thalamus
   b. Substantia nigra
   c. Hippocampus
   d. Amygdala
7. **The types of sensation are:**
   a. 2
   b. 3
   c. 4
   d. 5
8. **Myopia refers to:**
   a. Nearsightedness
   b. Double vision
   c. Farsightedness
   d. Squint
9. **Individual difference is influenced by:**
   a. Heredity
   b. Environment
   c. Personality
   d. Both a and c
10. **Neurotransmitters are classified as:**
    a. Excitatory only
    b. Inhibitory only
    c. Both excitatory and inhibitory
    d. None of the above

ANSWER KEY
| 1. a | 2. d | 3. c | 4. d | 5. d | 6. b | 7. d | 8. a |
| 9. c | 10. c | | | | | | |

SHORT ANSWER TYPE QUESTIONS

1. Explain the components of body–mind interaction.
2. What are the levels of awareness?
3. Explain functions of lobe of the central nervous system.
4. What are the functions of endocrine glands? Describe their impact on behavior.
5. What is sensation? Classify various senses.
6. What are motor sensations?
7. How genetics is closely related to behavior?
8. Explain the role of nurse in genetic counseling.

LONG ANSWER TYPE QUESTIONS

1. Describe the importance of studying genetics in nursing.
2. Explain the working of various senses in detail.
3. Describe the role of muscles and glands on the individual's behavior.
4. Explain theories of body–mind relationship.
5. What are abnormalities in sensory process?

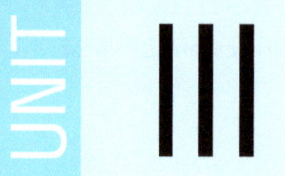

Mental Health and Mental Hygiene

OUTLINE

- ❑ Concept of Mental Health and Mental Hygiene
- ❑ Characteristics of Mentally Healthy Person
- ❑ Warning Signs of Poor Mental Health
- ❑ Mental Hygiene
- ❑ Promotive and Preventive Mental Health Strategies and Services
- ❑ Defense Mechanism and its Implication
- ❑ Dealing with Ego
- ❑ Frustration and Conflict—Types of Conflicts and Measurements to Overcome
- ❑ Role of Nurse in Reducing Frustration and Conflict and Enhancing Coping

■ CONCEPT OF MENTAL HEALTH AND MENTAL HYGIENE

Introduction

Human being in today's perspective is becoming more and more materialistic and due to increase in modernization and urbanization, complexity of life is increasing day by day. Increasing demands and needs make it difficult to achieve the desired goals. Therefore, failure in achievement leads to frustration and stress and therefore causes a rise to various mental disorders.

Mental illness and mental retardation together affect about 1 to 10 persons and constitute the greatest health problem all over the world. According to global burden of disease and WHO report 2020, there are different types of mental illness with different presentations present worldwide. They are generally characterized by a combination of abnormal thoughts, emotions, behavior, and relationship with others. Depression is the most common mental illness which will come at the first place in the world by the year 2030. There are effective strategies for preventing mental disorders and treatments are available to alleviate the mental disorders. Access to health care and social services is the major key for conserving mental health.

During the early times, the mentally ill were chained and tortured because they were feared, and their illness was believed to be caused by demons or evil spirits. It was found treated with medical care, kindness and given more freedom; later patients became less disturbed, and some were even healed. Because of medical and scientific discoveries, professional treatments are more prevalent.

Mental Health

The concept of mental health is as old as human beings. Our ancient scriptures are full of references to mental diseases. But this concept is comparatively new even in the West. Burmham who emphasizes the importance of integration or wholeness of personality said "**a mentally healthy person is one who has a balanced personality, free from schism and inconsistencies, emotional and nervous tension, discords and conflicts. A well-adjusted person can deal with his potentialities as well as he can accept** his limitations." It is a process of optimal functioning that characterizes successive stages of development throughout life.

Through meaningful interpersonal relationships and participation in significant interactive system such as family, the individual is confronted with tasks of socialization and self-development. To the extent of mastering these tasks, a person will adjust to each stage of development and thus be prepared for the tasks of later stages. Mental health plays an important role in all life situations.

Definition

Mental health can be defined as the presence of healthy reactions or the absence of pathological reactions. It is a person's state of well-being where the individual adequately adjusts to situations he/she is subjected to.

Mental health is a state of balance between the individual and the surrounding world, a state of harmony between oneself and others, a coexistence between the realities of the self and that of the other people and that of the environment.

According to Karl Menninger (American psychiatrist and a member of the Menninger family of psychiatrists who founded the Menninger Foundation and the Menninger Clinic in Topeka, Kansas), defined mental health as "adjustment of human being to the world and to each other with a maximum of effectiveness and happiness." It is a state of balance between the individual and the surrounding world, a state of harmony between oneself and others.

According to Mary Townsend in *Psychiatric/Mental Health Nursing*, "Mental health is the successful adaptation to stressors from the internal and external environment, evidenced by thoughts, feelings and behaviors that are age-appropriate and congruent with local and cultural norms."

For example, individuals express their mental state through their relationships with friends, associates, and groups. If an individual's behavior does not conform to the norm or standard behavior of his/her cultural group, the person exhibits certain patterns of behavior which are symptomatic of mental illness or abnormal behavior.

According to American Psychiatric Association, 1950: "Simultaneous success at working, living and creating the capacity for mature and flexible resolution of conflicts between instincts, conscience and reality."

According to WHO: Mental health is defined as a state of well-being in which the individual realizes his/her own abilities, can cope with the normal stresses of life, can work productively and fruitfully, and is able to make a contribution to his/her community.

Dimensions of Mental Health

Marie Jahoda (1958) has identified six dimensions **(Fig. 1)**:
1. **Positive attitude toward self:** It includes an objective view of self, knowledge, and acceptance of strengths and limitation. A positive attitude toward one's, self-acceptance of weakness and pride in strengths, motivation toward inner stability.

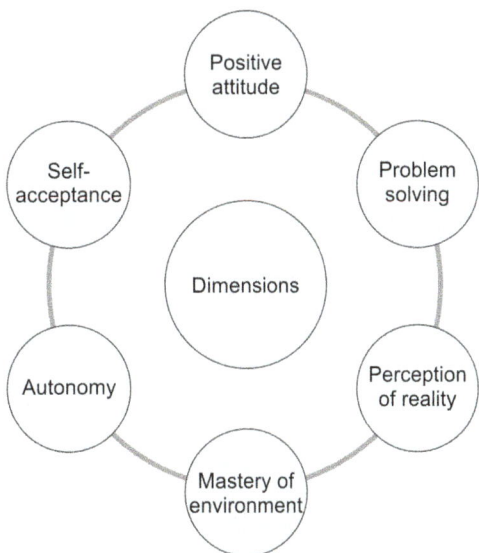

Fig. 1: Dimensions of mental health.

2. **Growth and development and the ability of self-actualization:** It relates to the achievement of the tasks associated with each level of development. It is the growth toward self-realization of one's potential toward achieving the best of one might become.
3. **Integration:** It is the ability to show adjustability to the environment. It involves a balance of psychic forces, unified outlook as life, and some capacity for withstanding anxiety and stress.
4. **Autonomy:** It is an ability to perform independent activities and actions which the individual determines behavior.
5. **Perception of reality:** It includes perception of the reality without distortion which is free from wishes, desires, and concerned with the welfare of others.
6. **Environmental mastery:** It suggests that the individual has achieved a satisfactory role within the group, society, or environment. He is able to love and accept the love of others.

CHARACTERISTICS OF MENTALLY HEALTHY INDIVIDUAL (BOX 1)

1. **Free from internal conflicts:** Individual's thoughts, feelings, and actions will function harmoniously toward the common end. He feels that he is wanted and loved by others. He has positive philosophy of life and he plans his life goals according to that. He maintains daily routine of planned activities and practices healthy lifestyle. He is free from inner conflicts, anxiety, and stress and lives productively and satisfactorily.
2. **Adjusting capacity:** Mentally healthy individual is able to get along with others easily. He shows better adjustment in all areas of life, i.e., physical, social, and emotional. He accepts criticism and is easily upset; appreciates other's efforts; establishes relationships with fellow beings which promote the sense of belongingness; learns to tolerate frustrations and disappointment in daily life; and utilizes effective coping mechanism to meet the life stresses. He also accepts and respects the decision of others.
3. **Self-confidence and identity formation:** He has sense of personal worth, sense of security, and self-respect. He is also satisfied with sexual identity. He deals with threats and complexities of life with confidence. He has a sense of self-worthiness and self-acceptance. He is aware of his strength and weaknesses.
4. **Mature and responsible:** Mentally healthy individual exhibits maturity at all levels, especially emotional maturity. He behaves in responsible manner and takes responsibilities of his behavior. He lives according to the societal norms. He is ready to face challenges of his own and make decisions.
5. **Clarity of life goals:** Mentally healthy individual defines goals of life more realistic. He is in touch with reality and feels pleasure in doing the tasks. He feels satisfaction and self-worth in accomplishing life goals.
6. **Positive philosophy of life:** Mentally healthy individual has a positive view about future and knows himself and has self-actualization needs to fulfill. He is able to evaluate his own behavior objectively. He has the ability to form hobbies to enjoy leisure time and enjoy a sense of humor

Box 1: Characteristics of mentally healthy person.

- Punctual
- Emotionally stable
- Positive attitude
- Self-appreciation
- Accept criticism
- Competent and independent
- Control of thoughts and imagination
- Adequate contact with the reality
- Efficiency in work and play
- Social acceptance
- Positive self-concept

that contributes to the welfare of the society.
7. **Rational attitude**: He promotes healthy living by rational attitude toward it. He ensures productive form of behavior and faces realities rationally and objectively. He is able to understand environmental forces with which he deals.
8. **Sense of autonomy:** He is independent of his choices and is self-directed. He is able to take responsibility of his decisions. He possesses competence to face the problems in real life and reach the highest competency level. He feels adequate and self-reliant.

Factors Affecting Mental Health (Table 1)

There are various theories or models suggesting factors influencing mental health. Some of the models are described below.

- **Sociocultural model** emphasizes the role of social condition, such as poverty discrimination, casteism, violence, etc., as the basic causes of poor mental health.
- **Medical model** emphasizes the role of various organic conditions that affect our brain functioning.
- **Psychoanalytical model** emphasizes the stress situations that involve a threat to the individual's psyche. It gives importance to early childhood experiences as a major factor for mental ill health.
- **Behavioristic model** gives importance to faulty learning such as the failure to learn necessary adaptive behavior.
- **Interpersonal model** emphasizes the unsatisfactory interpersonal relationship among human beings.

Other Factors

- **Hereditary:** Genetic defects, chromosomal defects, faulty genes, constitutional liabilities—physique, physical handicap, etc. Physical deprivation—malnutrition, sleep disturbances, emotional disruption, brain pathology
- **Psychological factors:** Mental deprivation, deprivation in home, defective family pattern structure, etc. Early psychic trauma, chronic stress, strained interpersonal relationship, boredom, and isolation, insecurity feelings, lack of self-esteem and confidence. Economic and employment problems.
- **Physical factors:** Physical factors such as good looks and positive personality aid to positive mental health. Physical illness, chronic disease condition, seasonal variations, neurodevelopment defects, physical disability, etc., cause frustration and in turn lead to abnormal mental health.
- **Sociocultural factors:** Societal and cultural norms, unemployment, urbanization and modernization, social problems, family conflicts, social or environmental crisis, cultural variations, war and violence, group prejudices.

These are the various factors leading to alteration in mental health and further cause serious mental disorders and illness. So we

Table 1: Factors affecting mental health.

Predisposing factors	Precipitating factors	Perpetuating factors
• Heredity	• Biological stressors	• Harmful illness beliefs
• Chronic disease	• Acute physical illness	• Labeling effects
• Early life adversity	• Psychosocial stressors	• Misinformation
• Chronic illness	• Acute psychiatric disorders	• Workplace and compensation factors
• Chronic distress or mental illness	• Epidemic health concerns	• Social support factors
		• Negative health habits, deconditioning
		• Chronic illness
		• Poor integration in treatment system

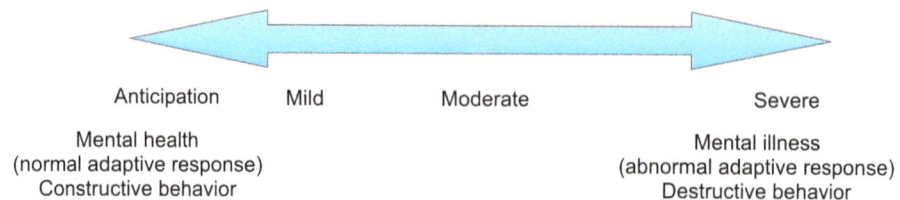

Fig. 2: Mental health illness continuum.

should have perspectives regarding what is mental illness and how these factors cause changes in mental health.

There is no obvious and consistent line between mental illness and mental health. In fact, all human behaviors lie somewhere along continuum of mental health and mental illness.

Mental Illness

A universal concept of mental illness is difficult. As per the continuum model, there is no obvious or consistent line between mental health and mental illness. Mental illness is a maladjusted way of behavior, which produces disharmony in the person's ability to meet human needs comfortably or effectively and function within a culture **(Fig. 2)**.

Definition

Mental illness or mental disorders are clinically significant behavioral or psychological syndrome or pattern that occurs in a person and that is associated with present distress or disability or impairment in one or more important areas of functioning, especially social and occupational functioning associated with significantly increased risk of suffering death, pain, disability, or an important loss of freedom and is not merely an expectable response to a particular event.

—*American Psychiatric Association (APA), 1994*

"Mental illness is maladaptive response to stressors from the internal and external environment, evidenced by thoughts, feelings and behaviors that are incongruent and not age-appropriate and incongruent with local and cultural norms and interfere with the individual's social, occupational and/or physical functioning."

—*Mary C Townsend*

WARNING SIGNS OF POOR MENTAL HEALTH

Mental health often gets imbalanced due to various factors as discussed above. This imbalance is often reflected in the form of behavior and daily activities of the individual who gets disturbed or altered. Behavior may range from mild alteration to severe symptoms leading to mental illness. These variations show different symptomatology as per the different age groups. Some of the changes are as follows:

In children
- Unable to cope with daily life situations
- Maladjustment in social, emotional, and educational areas
- Often crying and sadness
- Phobias, nightmares or night terrors, sleep difficulties
- Temper tantrum, nail biting, enuresis, encopresis, etc.
- Preoccupation, worried, confused
- Anxious and fearful attitude
- Declined school performance
- Lack of interest and isolation
- Loss of eye contact and low self-confidence

In adolescents
- Substance use most common problem
- Inability to cope with daily life situations
- Changes in eating and sleeping pattern
- Feelings of inadequacy and insecurity
- Aggressive and defiant behavior most common among teenage boys

- Juvenile delinquency and truancy
- Emotional liability
- Adequate academic performance
- Lack of interest, inattentive behavior
- Involvement in antisocial activities
- Physical or mental health problems such as somatic complaints, headaches, loss of appetite, sadness, and depression.
- Fantasy or daydreaming due to excessive use of social media

In adults
- Inability to make decisions and cope with daily life situations
- Lack of touch with the reality
- Confused or distorted thinking
- Emotional disturbances
- Disturbance in mental processes such as thinking, perception, and affects.
- Changes in sleeping and eating patterns
- Delayed grief processing
- Social withdrawal and isolation
- Dependent behavior on others
- Decreased self-concept and self-confidence
- Pessimistic behavior
- Adapting maladaptive behaviors such as use of drugs and alcohol to relieve stress, anxieties, and worries
- Suicidal ideations and thoughts, homicidal behavior
- Personality disorganization
- In old age
- Social withdrawal and isolation
- Frustrated or irritable behavior
- Suicidal behavior or ideations
- Feelings of inadequacy due to dependence on others
- Psychosomatic illnesses
- Psychosocial problems such as maladjustment and decreased self-esteem
- Impaired interpersonal relationship
- Cognitive, emotional, intellectual, and personality changes due to elderly process lead to behavioral changes
- Memory impairment, cognitive distortions leading to hallucinations
- Grandiose delusions, irrelevant talk, irrational behavior

MENTAL HYGIENE

Introduction

Mental health just like physical health needs restoration and promotion and has to be taken care of. We often focus on physical health and neglect mental health which is affected by certain factors as discussed before. So it is necessary to preserve mental health to prevent mental illness. Therefore, concept of mental hygiene is taken into consideration as mental hygiene denotes "care of mind." It equips a person to master tasks, to overcome obstacles, and to avoid reactions that lead to frustrations and stress. It is composed of principles and practices for the promotion of mental health and the prevention of mental illness.

Mental hygiene is a science which deals with the process of attaining mental health and preserving mental health in the society. The term "mental health" is closely related to the term "mental hygiene" as the main objective of mental hygiene is to attain mental health. In other words, mental hygiene is a means of mental health. That is why we can say that mental hygiene is the means and mental health is the end.

Definitions

There are many definitions of the term "mental hygiene." Some of the definitions are mentioned below:

According to Klien: "Mental hygiene is an endeavor to aid people to ward off trouble as well as to furnish ways of handling trouble in intelligent fashion when it cannot be warded off." To him, these troubles may be: illness, finances, social position, religion, sex, economic security, old age, inadequate shelter, etc.

According to Rivillin: Mental hygiene means the application of a body of hygiene information and technique. It is taken from the sciences of psychology, child psychology, education, sociology, psychiatry, medicine, and biology. It cares for the purpose of the preservation and improvement of mental health of the individual and community. It is meant for prevention and cure of minor and major mental diseases and defects of mental, educational, and social maladjustment.

According to English and English: Mental hygiene is the science and art of preserving and maximizing the mental health.

According to Bhatia BD and M Craig: Mental hygiene is organized attempt to effect human adjustment through the application of principles and practices of living.

According to Hadfield JA: Mental hygiene is concerned with the principle and practice in promotion, maintenance of mental health, and prevention of mental disorders.

History

The history of mental hygiene is as old as our civilization. In India, Ayurveda successfully developed a full-fledged system for treating the mentally ill people long back. But in the West, the mental hygiene movement started in the first decade of the 20th century. Clifford Beers, a graduate of Yale University, can be regarded as the father of mental hygiene. He being frustrated with his life once attempted to commit suicide in the year 1908. But luckily he was saved and treated for his mental illness. After recovery, he wrote a book entitled "A Mind That Found Itself" where he described about his illness and the type of treatment he had received. This book created a revolution among the general public for the necessity of mental hygiene. Gradually, many institutes of mental hygiene were established in India as well as in many other parts of the world to train personnel in the field of mental hygiene.

Objectives of Mental Hygiene

- **To help to realize one's potentiality:** Every individual possesses certain potentialities. Mental hygiene tries to help each individual to develop his/her potentialities.
- **To develop self-respect and respect for others:** Loss of self-respect is one of the factors for the great majorities of emotional disorders. A person who likes himself can like others and one who dislikes himself cannot like anybody. Hence, the main aim of mental hygiene is to help one to respect oneself.
- **To understand one's limitations and tolerate the limitations of others:** Mental hygiene helps one to understand his own limitations as well as to tolerate others' limitations.
- **To cause harmonious development:** Mental hygiene aims at the harmonious development of the physical, mental, and spiritual capacities of the individual so that he can adjust himself in the environment.
- **To create happiness:** Another objective of mental hygiene is to develop a positive attitude toward life so as to create a sense of happiness in a person who can live happily in this world.
- **To enable one to make effective adjustment:** Mental hygiene also prepares an individual for effective adjustment in all spheres of life and all situations such as in school, home, society work, and also with self.
- **To enable one to know his/her self:** Many of us do not know our own self. We are not at all aware about our potentialities, weaknesses, limitations, etc., for which many individuals suffer from different types of confusion. Mental hygiene helps an individual to know himself.

Functions of Mental Hygiene

Mental hygiene has four important functions. These are:

1. **Prevention or preventive:** The most important function of mental hygiene is to prevent mental health problems by developing some programs. Individual adopts preventive methods and

understands the relationship that occurs between development of personality and life experiences.
2. **Creative:** Another function of mental illness is to develop program such as counseling and psychotherapy to treat an individual or a group or to treat a mental patient.
3. **Preservative:** Not all people are mentally ill; rather some of them possess sound mental health. So the third function is to develop program through education for preserving mental health.
4. **Training:** Another function of mental hygiene is to train a set of personnel who can help the people with psychological problem by trying to understand their problems and then helping them to meet their needs.

Principles of Mental Hygiene

To formulate general principles of mental hygiene is a really difficult task as there is a wide range of differences among the individuals. Some of the reasons for this are that human beings have multiple needs which grow in the course of development. These needs are contradictory in nature. There is no single and absolute standard to judge human behavior or action. However, in spite of these difficulties, we can formulate some general principles. These are:

- **Adjustment at home:** Every child should develop such type of behavior at home so that he can adjust himself in any type of situation. Parents should take utmost care because the behavior patterns that develop in early childhood leave permanent impression on the child. Parents should try to develop the desirable traits in their children and develop competence, security, adequacy, self-esteem, and discipline by catering to their basic needs.
- **Adjustment in school:** After home, school plays an important role in the development of personality. The school through its various activities can go a long way in creating an environment for the children to preserve and develop their mental health.
- **Adjustment in society:** Man is a social animal and he has to adjust himself with the society. Without proper social interaction, harmonious development of personality cannot occur. Hence, parents, teachers, and society must provide socially acceptable channels for the release of pent-up emotional feeling so that the children and adolescents develop healthy personality.
- **Adjustment at work:** According to Freud, one is mentally healthy, if one can work successfully. School through its program, should develop the proper mental state toward work in child.

Limitations of Mental Hygiene

Though mental hygiene is an important aspect in our educational system, yet there are many limitations in implementing the principles of mental hygiene. Some of these are:

- Majority of our parents are not aware of mental hygiene. Hence, they do not give importance how to keep their children's mental health preserved and unimpaired.
- Teachers in our school system are so overloaded with work that they cannot devote time to organize different types of programs which help the students in helping their mental health intact.
- There is also a dearth of trained personnel to deal with the mental health problems of our population.

Mental Hygiene Movement

In 1909, the National Committee for Mental Hygiene was established in New York as a result of efforts made by leading psychiatrists such as Clifford W Beers. Lightner Witmer from Liepzig University started psychological clinic in 1907. The National Mental Health program in India was launched in 1982. The District Mental Health Program was launched in 1996 during 9th Five-year Plan.

PROMOTIVE AND PREVENTIVE MENTAL HEALTH SERVICES

Introduction

The terms "mental health promotion" and "prevention" are different aspects having the same goal. Mental health promotion is an essential topic in today's scenario as more mental problems are prevailing and the World Health Organization in 1946 under Bhore Committee laid the basis for infrastructure of health service. Mental health services form a part of complex health services and should not be separated from other services. Majority of the mentally ill patients do not reach the existing mental health services. Preventive mental health services are the part of a general health delivery system. Therefore, preventive psychiatry is the use of theoretical knowledge and skill to plan and implement programs designed to achieve primary, secondary, and tertiary prevention of onset of psychiatry disorders.

Levels of Prevention

Caplan in 1974 introduced a public health model which incorporates three levels of preventive interventions among clients with emotional disturbances and psychiatric illness.

Primary Prevention

Primary prevention refers to reducing the incidence of disorder that is preventing disorder from occurring in the first place. It is the first stage of case and it involves using measures that prevent mental illness and provide cost-effective interventions.

Aims/Goals of Primary Prevention

- Lowering the occurrence of new cases by identifying high-risk group, stressful situations, stressful life events which predispose for mental illness.
- Educating the community to utilize coping strategies to overcome stress or attacking problem to solve the problematic situation.
- Strengthening the individual's capacity by lowering stress, tensions, and anxiety which precipitate mental illness and its symptoms.

Characteristics

- It builds adaptive strengths, utilizes coping resources, and preserves the mental health of the people.
- It is concerned with whole population, especially focusing high-risk population.
- Main tools are education and social change.
- Utilization of community welfare agencies and other personnel
- Provision of psychosocial support
- Promoting appropriate tasks related to specific age groups
- Developing a sense of control over one's own fate
- Achievement of satisfaction with oneself and his existence
- Health education
- Motivation to utilize the stress reduction activity
- Promotion of positive healthy lifestyle
- Maintaining high standards of living
- Effective interpersonal relationships
- Equipping the individual with personal and environmental resources
- Implementing national health policy—preventive aspect

Preventive Factors in Primary Prevention

Cowen in 1944 described the protective factors in primary prevention.

- Forming wholesome early attachment wellness programs have to be organized, e.g., good antenatal care, efficient obstetrical assistance, parenting, and child-rearing practices.
- Positive scholastic environment
- Enhancing social competence, e.g., teaching problem-solving techniques to prevent and control social problem and to

reduce occurrence of social pathological conditions
- Fostering empowerment:
  - To develop interaction and behavioral pattern
  - To enhance citizen participation
  - To gain control over and to make critical decision in their lives
- Effective coping strategies to handle stressful situations for adaptation and readjustment in life
- Stress avoidance and stress management
- Providing emotional and social support to help the people in stressful situations

Role of Nurse in Primary Prevention

Nurse has to find themselves in different situations in various roles as a counselor, educator, facilitator, role model, and advocate in the implementation of primary prevention activities.

Prenatal or perinatal period
- Educate the women about regular exercises and the side effect or ill effects of self-medication, etc.
- Provision of good antenatal care to pregnant women includes regular antenatal checkup, vaccination, iron and folic acid supplementation, high-caloric diet, screening, hygienic care, rest, and sleep.
- Identify the high-risk pregnant women and provide institutionalized services.
- If the child is unwanted, then tell about the termination of pregnancy which can be done according to law.
- Motivate the community to have institutional delivery.
- Meet the needs of newborn, e.g., cord care, warmth, protection, feeding, bath, clean environment, rooming-in or latching-in, etc.
- During natal period, efficient timely obstetrical assistance has to be provided; it will protect the child from ill effects of anoxia and birth injuries.

During infancy
- Educate the parents regarding the growth and development of the child.
- Advice the parents to take proper precautions to prevent the occurrence of infections and accidents, e.g., immunization, adopting safely universal precautions.
- Involve siblings in care of infant.
- Provision of safe motherhood and child survival activities
- Enriching the child-mother relationship
- Avoid the prolonged separation of child.

During childhood
- Advice the parents to provide healthy nutrition for child.
- Encourage to have open communication within the family related to child's growth and development.
- Help the parents to learn the procedures which will strengthen their child's self-esteem.
- Promote the initiatives among children.
- Consult parents in implementation of appropriate disciplinary measures.
- Identify the problems related to scholastic performance and emotional disturbances among the children and advise them to provide timely interventions and referring the cases to appropriate agencies.
- Training programs have to be organized to school teachers and parents in early identification of behavioral problems.

During adolescence
- Encourage the child to identify themselves among other group members by their abilities and achievement of goal.
- Promote the adolescent to perform their roles effectively.
- Motivate the children to fulfill their internal thoughts and desires.
- Encourage the children to follow the rules, customs, and regulations related to every aspect of behavior.
- Healthy family and peer relationships to assist the adolescent to internalize values and beliefs and attitudes.

- Sex education will help the child to accept the physiological changes and perform effectively social roles.
- Encourage the child to achieve the independence in family and society.
- Promote the child's interest and level of industry.
- Conducive home environment has to be provided.
- Parents have to be role model to their children. They should not use physical punishment.
- Involve the adolescent to participate in family functions and activities.
- Provide congenital and conflict-free environment.
- Meet the health needs of child.

During adulthood and old age
- Avoid isolate and withdrawal feelings.
- Motivate the young adults to adopt control, commitment, and challenges in fulfilling activities.
- Motivate the adults to guide the next generation with creative ideas to generate relative working goals to overcome that they are stagnated in activities.
- Enhance the intimate relationship and interactions to exchange information and feelings among family members and friends.
- Promote the adult to develop alternative strategies in meeting psychosocial needs.
- Guide the adults in their career path and in developing job reputations.

In crisis situations
- Provide emotional support through guidance and counseling services in the transitional periods of life in every aspect and give valuable helping hand to solve their problems utilizing their own resources.
- Counsel the bereaved family to accept the loss.
- Crisis intervention, anticipatory guidance, and reassurance services have to be provided for needy group.

Secondary Prevention

- Secondary prevention refers to the decrease in the prevalence or severity of mental disorders. So it is the second stage in which measures are used to control the disease process.
- They focus on early detection and case finding and priority interventions.

Role of Nurse in Secondary Prevention

1. **Early diagnosis and case finding:** Educate the community about early manifestations of mental illness. Motivate the community leaders, industrialists, voluntary agencies, e.g., Mahilamandal, Youth clubs to involve activity in identification of mental illness. Organize workshops, orientation training programs, and awareness campaigns for various focus groups.
2. **Screening programs:** Organize community screening programs to identify the mental illness. Prepare questionnaires in simple local language to identify the symptoms of mental illness. These can be used in schools, colleges, industries, etc.
3. **Provision of effective therapeutic activities:** After identifying the case, therapeutic activities will be planned early to prevent complications, e.g., group therapy, family therapy, psychotherapy, and guidance and counseling. After the patient is discharged from the hospital, referral will be made to community mental health center; then community mental health (CMH) nurse visits the individual at home.
4. Through this visit, the mental health nurse is able to evaluate the situation. It provides an opportunity for the client and his family to ventilate their feelings and concerns freely. The nurse will discuss her observation with other health team members and initiates therapeutic interventions and continuity care in relation to social situation. She motivates the family members to take the client for follow-up services. If the client is

not adjusting to the family or community circumstances normally, the nurse can refer the client for re-admission to mental health hospital. Nurse can guide the community welfare agencies to provide its services to needy clients.

5. **Early reference and follow-up services:** A nurse has to refer the cases from community to the hospital for seeking therapeutic activities; follow-up services can be planned to prevent occurrence of complications.
6. **Mental health education:** Educating the general public regarding mental health, mental illness, and misconceptions related to mental illnesses is very important. This could be carried out by conducting mass camps and through films, shows, flash cards, and mass communication.
7. **Consultation services:** A nurse has to provide consultation services to peripheral health workers to identify psychiatry-related problems among the illnesses such as anxiety, psychosis, psychosomatic illnesses, etc.

    Training of health professionals: Orientation training programs, conferences, workshops in service training, etc., have to be organized to update the knowledge of health professionals.
8. **Crisis intervention:** The essential factor responsible for occurrence of crisis is imbalance between difficulty in problem-solving and resources available to deal with it. So crisis coping depends on the situational support and utilization of own resources. If crisis is not tackled properly, it may lead to psychiatric emergencies such as suicide. The community mental health nurse needs to identify the available outpatient and inpatient treatment within the community and partial/short-term hospitalization such as day-care center.

    Hot lines service link: It is telephone service link through which help can be extended.

    Walk-in clinics: It is a 24-hour psychiatric emergency room in which diagnostic and therapeutic services are available without an appointment.

Tertiary Prevention (Fig. 3)

Tertiary prevention refers to decreasing the severity of mental disorders and associated disability by means of rehabilitative intervention.

It is the third stage of prevention and measures are used to minimize relapse and chronic disability and to restore client to their optimal level of function. Adaptation, restoration, reintegration, and aftercare are major components of tertiary prevention.

Role of Nurse in Tertiary Prevention

Programs in mental hospital: In mental hospitals, the main aim should be prevention of chronicity by energetic treatment of fundamental illness in all admitted patients.

Treatment and follow-up: Nurse needs to ensure the type of psychotropic drugs the patient is taking. She also needs to ensure maintenance dose, supervision of safe intake of drug, and educate the family members to

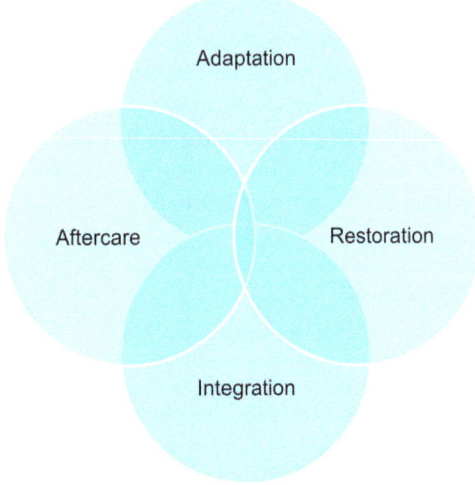

Fig. 3: Components of tertiary prevention.

observe for side effects of the drugs and for regular checkups for the adjustment of the dose of drugs.

Individual and family therapy: The patient has to go back to his family, so it is very essential that the family is helped to meet the stress and make the client physically, mentally, socially, vocationally, and economically useful so a nurse has to educate the family and community for treating the client as an individual.

Interactional skill training: Social skill training can be given to develop effective interaction and communication abilities.

Occupational training: Ensure the harmonious relationship among family members to adopt the healthy behavior. Re-equip the mentally restored with daily living care abilities and to plan usual day-to-day activities. The patient needs to be rehabilitated and helped to become socially productive. His interest area can be exploited and he can be helped to pick a job. So refer the client to appropriate agencies for employment thereby achieving independence (vocational rehabilitation).

Rehabilitation: Rehabilitation is an essential aspect of mental illness. Patients need to readjust themselves outside the hospital. So family and community resources are used for long-term rehabilitation of the patients. Various community facilities for the mentally ill person are as follows: Day hospital center, Group homes, Half way houses, Foster home **(Table 2)**.

DEFENSE MECHANISM

Introduction

Defense mechanisms are psychological strategies brought into play by the unconscious mind to manipulate, deny, or distort reality. Defense mechanism is also known as ego defense mechanism or ego coping mechanism. Healthy persons normally use different defenses throughout life. An ego defense mechanism becomes pathological only when its persistent use leads to maladaptive behavior such that the physical and/or mental health of the individual is adversely affected. Sigmund Freud in 1961 identified the ego component as discussed in personality. Ego governs our rational thinking, and when anxiety occurs ego comes into functioning and utilizes defense mechanism to restore balance. Defense mechanisms were identified by Anna Freud (1953).

If these defense mechanisms are used consciously or unconsciously as protective device by ego to relieve mild-to-moderate anxiety they become adaptive but if are overused and person is not able to perceive reality then they become maladaptive. Defense mechanisms are a type of process or coping that results in automatic psychological responses exhibited as a means of protecting the individual against anxiety.

Definition

These are defined as any group of mental processes that enables the mind to reach compromises and solutions to conflicts that are unable to resolve.

Table 2: Mental health services and agencies at various levels.

National level	International level
• National Mental Health Program (1982) • District Mental Health Program (1996) • National Institute of Mental Health and Neurosciences, Bengaluru • Central Institute of Psychiatry, Ranchi • The Banyan, Chennai • AASRA, NGO, Mumbai • Ranchi Institute of Neuropsychiatry and Allied Sciences, Ranchi	• World Federation for Mental Health, United Nations • SAMHSA, USA

UNIT III: Mental Health and Mental Hygiene

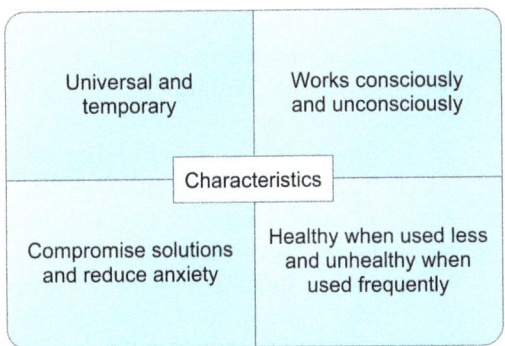

Fig. 4: Characteristics of defense mechanism.

According to Freud, these are unconscious resources used by the ego to reduce conflict between the id and superego, as a reflection of how individual deals with the conflict and stress **(Fig. 4)**.

Functions of Defense Mechanism

1. Defense mechanism provides accurate perception of the reality and environment.
2. It helps to modulate, regulate, and control drives, affects and impulses to keep in touch with reality and adapt to the daily life situations.
3. It regulates the thought processes and helps to relieve anticipatory anxiety.
4. It helps ego to balance superego and id components of personality and helps to integrate the personality of an individual.
5. Defense mechanisms are adaptive if used less frequently to relieve anxiety or tension and they are only temporary solutions.

Classification of Ego Defense Mechanism

Mentally healthy people normally use different defense mechanisms throughout life. They become pathological when use is persistent and become maladaptive behavior such that physical or mental status of an individual is adversely affected. George Eman Vaillant introduced a four-level classification of defense mechanism.

Level 1 (psychotic/pathological): Psychotic defense mechanism eliminates the need to cope with reality of daily life situations. These mostly operate at unconscious level. In this, the individual tries to avoid conflicts encountered in his relationships and the external world. Some of the defense mechanisms which fall under this level are as follows:

- **Psychotic denial:** It is the refusal to accept reality or fact, acting as if a painful event, thought, or feeling did not exist. It is considered one of the most primitive of the defense mechanisms because it is characteristic of early childhood development. Many people use denial in their everyday life to avoid dealing with painful feelings or areas of their life they do not wish to admit. For instance, a person who is a functioning alcoholic will often simply deny that they have a drinking problem, pointing to how well they function in their job and relationships.
- **Delusional projection:** This defense mechanism is specific for mental illnesses such as schizophrenia, delusional disorders etc.; it involves attributing unacceptable thoughts, emotions, and impulses to another source that is not based in reality. These are mostly of persecutory nature. For example, a person projects that his family is planning to kill him and capture his property.
- **Distortion:** It is gross reshaping of external reality to meet the internal needs. Individual often believes something to be true which is not real. For example, a student thinks that he failed examination because questions were tough and not because he did not prepare well.
- **Autistic withdrawal:** An individual lacks sense of relatedness and decreased social interaction and communication to avoid anxiety related to any threat. It is mostly seen in psychotic conditions such as schizophrenia, in which patient withdraws into his own world.

Level 2 (immature): These defense mechanisms are most often used by the adolescents. These mechanisms lessen the anxiety provoked by threatening situation temporarily. People who use these excessively are seen socially undesirable and a person is not able to cope up effectively with daily-life situations. These are also seen in severe depression and personality disorders. Some of the immature defenses are described below:

- **Projection:** It is the misattribution of a person's undesired thoughts, feelings, or impulses onto another person who does not have those thoughts, feelings, or impulses. Projection is used especially when the thoughts are considered unacceptable for the person to express or when he feels completely ill at ease with having them. For example, a spouse may be angry at their significant other for not listening, when in fact it is the angry spouse who does not listen. Projection is often the result of a lack of insight and acknowledgment of one's own motivations and feelings.
- **Fantasy:** It refers to the channeling of unacceptable desires or wishes into imagination and often can lead to daydreaming if not directed. The person images himself in scene or view which is mostly acceptable and gives him satisfaction.
- **Acting out:** It is performing an extreme behavior in order to express thoughts or feelings that a person feels incapable of expressing otherwise. Instead of saying, "I'm angry with you," a person who acts out may instead throw a book at the person or punch a hole through a wall. When a person acts out, it can act as a pressure release, and often helps the individual feel calmer and peaceful once again. For instance, a child's temper tantrum is a form of acting out when he/she does not get his/her way with a parent. Self-injury may also be a form of acting-out, expressing in physical pain what one cannot stand to feel emotionally.
- **Regression:** It is the reversion to an earlier stage of development in the face of unacceptable thoughts or impulses. For example, an adolescent who is overwhelmed with fear, anger, and growing sexual impulses might become clingy and start exhibiting earlier childhood behaviors he has long since overcome, such as bedwetting. An adult may regress when under a great deal of stress, refusing to leave his bed and engage in normal, everyday activities.
- **Passive aggression:** It is aggression toward others expressed indirectly or passively. Most people automatically use to protect themselves and it can be conscious or unconscious. These are associated with feelings of hatred, fear, rejection, low self-esteem, and insecurities which cannot be directly expressed. A person often has hostile attitude.
- **Idealization:** Subconsciously choosing to perceive another individual as having more positive qualities than he/she actually possesses.

Level 3 (neurotic defense mechanism): These are though neurotic and developed during early years of development, these are fairly common in adults. These provide short-term advantages in coping but long-term use can distort the social and occupational functioning and cause problems in decision-making.

- **Displacement:** It occurs when an individual shifts an unacceptable feeling from one object to another more acceptable one. According to Freudian Psychology, displacement is an unconscious defense mechanism in which the mind redirects effects from an object felt to be dangerous or unacceptable to an object felt to be safe or acceptable. For example, parents have a verbally abusive boss at work and does not defend themselves, but when they get home they yell and spank their kids.

- **Reaction formation:** This occurs when we express an unacceptable impulse by transforming into the opposite. It is the behavior that is completely opposite of what one really wants or feels, taking the opposite belief that the true belief causes anxiety. For example, treating someone you strongly dislike in an excessively friendly manner in order to hide your true feelings.
  A staff nurse in her ward faces a fight with another staff member, and she goes to the adjoining ward and shows exactly opposite behavior, i.e., laughing and talking pleasant events.
- **Dissociation:** It is temporary drastic modification of one's personal identity or character to avoid emotional distress, separation, or postponement of a feeling that normally would accompany a situation or thought. Dissociation is a state of acute mental decompensation in which certain thoughts, emotions, sensations, and memories are compartmentalized because they are too overwhelming for the conscious mind to integrate. For example, an adult relates severe sexual abuse experienced as a child but does it without feelings. She says that the experience was as if she were outside her body watching the abuse.
- **Isolation:** It is separation of feelings from ideas and events, avoiding the unpleasant feelings or unpleasant experiences. This mechanism was first proposed by Sigmund Freud and is a defense against harmful thoughts. For example, loss of loved one will be described due to certain medical conditions and associated complications without emotional tone.
- **Repression:** It is another commonly used defense mechanism. It is simply keeping the information out of conscious awareness. Repression is more complex mechanism in which unpleasant or unacceptable experiences, emotions, or motivations are actively forced into the unconscious and kept there and are involuntary. For example, a person suffered from abuse in the childhood has difficulty forming relationships. It is a process of pulling thoughts into the unconscious and preventing painful or dangerous thoughts from entering into consciousness.
- **Intellectualization:** It is separating the self from emotional content of an event and it is avoiding the unavoidable emotions by focusing on intellectual aspects. The defense mechanism allows to avoid anxiety and stressful emotional aspects of the situation and focus only on the intellectual component. For example, a person who has just been diagnosed with terminal illness might focus on learning everything about the disease in order to avoid distress and remain distant from the reality of the situation.

Level 4 (mature defense mechanism): These are commonly found among emotionally healthy adults and are considered more mature. These have been developed through years so as to optimize success in life and relationships. These defenses help the users to integrate conflicting emotions and thoughts while still remaining effective.

- **Altruism:** It is constructive service to others that bring pleasure and personal satisfaction. Altruism is loving others as oneself, behavior that promotes the survival chances of others at a cost to one's own. It is regardless of any interest and pleasure seeking and is done totally for the benefit or sake of others. The act of giving without regard to rewards or the benefits of recognition is called pure altruism. It is self-sacrifice for the benefit of others. Examples are patriots, social workers, etc. Bhagat Singh sacrificed himself for independence.
- **Sublimation:** It is a defense mechanism that allows us to act out unacceptable impulses by converting these behaviors into a more acceptable form, the transformation

or melting down of negative emotions or instincts into positive actions, behavior, or emotions. Freud believes that sublimation is a sign of maturity as it allows people to function normally in socially acceptable ways and according to cultural norms. For example, a person experiencing extreme anger or frustration might vent up it on kick-boxing as a means of venting anger and frustration.

- **Suppression:** It is the conscious or voluntary process of pushing thoughts into the preconscious which are coming into conscious awareness. It is excluding from consciousness those ideas, feelings, and situations that are creating conflict and causing discomfort, e.g., concentrating more on household work and children rather than an argument taken place with husband in the morning.
- **Humor:** Overt expression of ideas and feelings (especially those that are unpleasant to focus on or too terrible to talk about) that gives pleasure to others, e.g., looking at the funny side of a situation can help you forget about the real unpleasant situation.
- **Identification:** It is the unconscious modeling of one's self upon other person's character and behavior. In this, a person adapts the qualities of the person he admires. For example, a person wants to be like a famous celebrity, so he will start wearing clothes like him and behave according to him. To keep failure out of their awareness, people often identify themselves with successful roles they are playing at the time.
- **Introjection:** It is identifying some ideas or objects so deeply that it becomes a part of that person. It is complete acceptance of another's opinion and values as one's own. Incorporating feelings, emotions, values, beliefs, traits and personality of other person. For example, often fathers teach their sons that boys do not cry, so they internalize it.

Implications of Ego Defense Mechanism

1. Anxiety arises when ego is faced with a situation with which it cannot cope. This may be the result of an external situation such as a civilian living in wartime conditions or it may be due to internal threat, related to the demands of id or superego. Thus, various forms of demands can threaten the integrity of the ego, which must protect itself.
2. Defense mechanism exists to protect the ego from anxiety, but people do so at the risk of distorting reality. To the extent the ego is aware of using particular defense, distortion of reality is reduced, but anxiety will increase.
3. Most defense mechanisms (except repression) operate by allowing gratification in some indirect way, typically involving either symbolic gratification or a substitute object. It reduces id's demands to the extent.
4. When we engage in rationalization, we try to justify our actions. It prevents the person from recognizing the true motives of their actions; it represents a form of distortion of reality.
5. The superego helps to live in the society, it represents. We must cope with the demands of the society. Without a superego, a person would face few conflicts since there would be only id and external reality to satisfy. Such individuals, who are lacking normal superego development, show no guilt for their antisocial behavior.
6. A nurse can understand her own way of dealing a situation and also others. She adjusts to the situation, works satisfactorily in a healthy environment, adopts team approach, relieves anxiety, and maintains overall physical and psychological health.
7. As a nurse manager, she identifies the root cause of conflicts and cold war among staff in her ward. She assesses and resolves the conflicts by knowing ego defenses intelligently.

UNIT III: Mental Health and Mental Hygiene

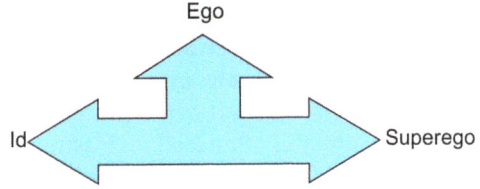

Fig. 5: Ego restores balance between id and superego.

8. A mental health nurse can successfully correlate the mental illnesses such as psychoses and neuroses and analyze various defense mechanisms used by the patient.

DEALING WITH EGO (FIG. 5)

The ego consists of elaborate ways of behaving and thinking which constitute the "executive function" of a person. The ego delays satisfying id and motives and channels behavior into more socially acceptable outlets. It keeps a person working for a living, getting along with people, and adjusting to the realities of life. Freud characterized ego "as working on reality principle."

The ego tries to satisfy the id's urge for pleasure but only in realistic ways that take account of what is possible in the real world. The ongoing tension between the insistent urges of the id and the constraints of reality helps the ego develop more and more sophisticated thinking skills **(Fig. 6)**.

Ego expands through all three topographical dimensions of conscious, preconscious, and unconscious. Defense mechanism resides in the unconscious domain of the ego. It is the executive organ of the psyche and controls motility, perception, and contact with the reality.

FRUSTRATION AND CONFLICT— TYPES OF CONFLICTS AND MEASUREMENTS TO OVERCOME

Individual gets motivated and often tries to fulfill his/her motives and internal urge to act toward a particular goal. Sometimes there are things, objects, or individuals which hinder our pathway toward achieving those particular goals. The course of motivation does not always run smoothly. Things happen that prevent us from reaching the goals toward

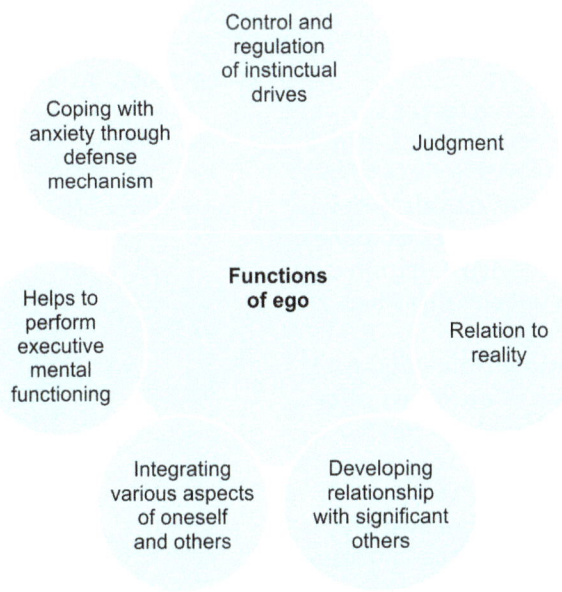

Fig. 6: Functions of ego.

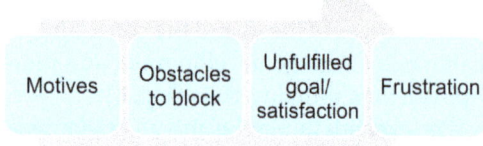

Fig. 7: Process of frustration.

which we are driven or pulled and it causes a common emotional response to opposition called frustration. The word "frustration" has been derived from a Latin word "frusta" meaning to obstruct (**Fig. 7**).

Definition

Frustration may be defined as the emotion produced when we are blocked from reaching our goal.

An event thwarting circumstances that block or interfere with the goal-directed activity is frustration.

Frustration refers to blocking of behavior directed toward the goal. It is an emotional tension resulting from the blocking of a desire or need.

Sources of Frustration

a. **Environmental frustration:** Some frustrations are caused by minor or daily life situations such as busy signal, traffic slowdowns, late arrivals, pending assignment to complete, lack of money, limited resources, restriction imposed by society, or actions or behaviors which are not culturally appropriate.
b. **Personal frustration:** Unfulfilled goals, incapabilities, lack of necessary efforts or specific abilities, physical handicaps, personal inadequacy, relationship difficulties, miscommunication
c. **Causes of frustration in students:** Grades, deadlines, expectations, social pressure, peer pressure, examinations.
d. **Conflict leading to frustration:** When there is choice between alternatives and an individual is not able to arrive at a decision, conflict arises which can be internal or external and this often leads to frustration, e.g., workplace conflict, goal differences.

Symptoms of Frustration (Fig. 8)

Signs or symptoms of frustration are much less desperate than those of anxiety. Facial signs accompany the signals of frustration. These signals are withdrawal, fixation, aggression, regression, apathy, rude behavior, throwing the hands into the air, tapping the fingers or feet, disgust or displeasure on the face. More severe the frustration, more will be the movement.

When someone is frustrated, the most typical reaction is anger. When the obstacle is too influential to direct anger, the anger is frequently redirected to something less influential.

As achievement of a specific goal is repeatedly thwarted, many people gradually scum to a loss of confidence. A person with no confidence in her ability to accomplish a goal often creates a self-fulfilling prophecy by putting less effort into achieving the said goal and she may give up at goal entirely. It causes emotional and behavioral disturbances such as depression, anxiety, fear, guilt, etc.

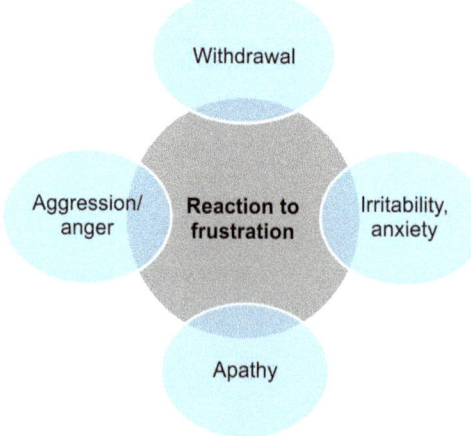

Fig. 8: Reaction to frustration.

Dealing with Frustration

- **Clear communication:** Every individual would do well if he/she develops an attitude of openness to experience and learn from the same. Often conflict becomes severe when we do not communicate that leads to frustration. Therefore, clear, direct, and assertive communication approach is to be used.
- **Realistic goal settings:** If individual knows about his strengths and limitations and set goals accordingly which are achievable. Focus on what you want to happen.
- **Sharing views:** When dealing with a stressful situation, reach out to a person who has faced a similar situation to reduce frustration. That person can offer you valuable insights and advice which will leave you feeling encouraged, supported, and inspired.
- **Problem-solving strategies:** Ask yourself what is working in this situation. Focus on what you want to happen and analyze the problem systematically and rationally. Visualize the outcome to the situation and adopt multiple alternatives and work on the best one.
- **Relaxation techniques:** When you feel irritated or frustrated, take a deep breath and relax. Use various relaxation techniques such as progressive muscle relaxation, yoga, meditation, and exercise and inculcate in your daily life.
- **Journal writing:** If you are dealing with the frustration where you cannot think about the solution, try writing in a diary or journal. This can help to analyze your situation stepwise and calm down your brain.
- **Manage your expectations of others:** Most common reason of frustration in daily life is expectation from others and when they are not fulfilled, we often feel disheartened and angry. Recognize that you cannot fully anticipate anyone else's behavior. Change your own mental framework so that you are not holding them to the standards they will not meet.

Teacher's Role in Decreasing Frustration among Students

- Develop positive teacher–student relationship.
- Provide learning aides.
- Talk politely to the students and do not yell or shout at them.
- Help them communicate what their frustration is about.
- Encourage students to describe calmly what he/she is feeling.
- Guide the students to brainstorm solutions to the problem.
- Help the students to determine whether the situation is important enough to address or something he/she could forget about.
- Give students achievable targets.

Role of Nurse in Dealing with Frustration

- Nurses play an essential role in dealing with frustration which patients often face during hospitalization. The nurse acts as a good facilitator and communicator in resolving day-to-day problems of patients.
- The nurse administers deep breathing and relaxation techniques to patients who have become stressed and anxious due to frustration of being hospitalized.
- Nurse must have a clear communication and express her concerns with the team members.
- She must educate patient regarding his disease condition and treatment regimen and can present patient with the literature about his disease or conducting group therapies.
- She must resolve the conflicts arising with the patient, his family members, and the health workers by acting as a mediator.

- She must create a therapeutic environment around the patient so that causes of frustration can be reduced.
- She must coordinate with all the health team members in providing systematic and organized care to the patient in order to avoid frustration in patients.

Conflict and its Resolution

Conflict

The most common cause of frustration is conflict of motives—a struggle to resist to overcome contest of opposing forces, state or condition of opposition, antagonism, and discord; a painful tension set up by a clash between opposed and contradictory impulses. It is the state of indecisiveness which arises when two equally strong and fairly identical drives compete with each other resulting in anxiety.

Definition

Conflict is a process that begins when one party perceives that another party has negatively affected or is about to negatively affect, something that the first party cares about. It is that point in an ongoing activity when an interaction crosses over to become an interparty conflict. For example, two equally attractive jobs, meeting best friends, long-awaited functions in the college.

Causes of Conflict (Fig. 9)

Given below are the five main causes of conflict.

Recognizing these causes is the first step in dealing with conflict situations.

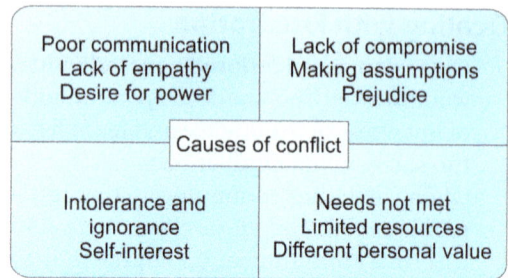

Fig. 9: Sources of conflict.

1. **Differing values can lead to conflicts:** When people have differing values, conflicts can result. If one of your personal values in life is that your family comes first, and if your boss's personal value is that work comes first, conflict can be the result when they ask you to stay late at work or to give up a planned family vacation due to project deadlines.

2. **Making assumptions can lead to conflicts:** If the husband assumes that his wife will have a hot meal waiting for him when he gets home from work (after all he works so hard at bringing home the bacon) and when that hot meal is not ready, conflict between the husband and the wife can result.

   When one person assumes anything about another person, well you know the saying about when you assume anything. If the wife assumes her husband will remember their anniversary every year (*how can he forget the most important date in their relationship, after all?*), a conflict can result when the husband not only does not make special plans to celebrate the day but does not even remember that it is their anniversary.

3. **Differing expectations can lead to conflict:** We expect people to know things without us telling them. What do you mean they cannot read our minds? Well, they should be able to, is not that obvious? Well, no. A lot of things are not obvious to many people.

   Having differing expectations of people, such as expecting a single person in the office to work during the Christmas vacation while the married people with children expect to have the vacation time to spend with their family. Is it not obvious that those with children have the special holidays and March break off each year? Uhm, no, it is not obvious.

Just because that may be your expectation, that does not mean that it is the expectation of other people. No wonder there is so much resentment and conflict at work, if you have that kind of expectation.

4. **Differences in the way you were brought up can result in conflict:** The way that you were brought up, your religion, your gender, your race, and your ethnicity can result in conflict with people who are different from you.

   If you are a woman born in the 1930s and who grew up during the Great Depression, someone who was grown up during in free-loving 1970s may have a conflict with you regarding marriage and its vows.

   Also, how many of us remember the Cold War and grew up believing that a nuclear war was inevitable? How can we relate that fear to today's youth who have no concept of what it was to live during those times?

   We see this all the time between men and women, too. We say that a man can act aggressively at work, but the same actions by a woman are viewed as her being a bitch. Gender can play a major role in conflicts.

5. **Knowledge and ability to deal with conflict can result in conflict:** If you do not know how to resolve conflict or are unwilling to try to resolve conflict, this in itself can conflict with someone else who has more knowledge and is more willing than you are. If two nations are unwilling to resolve their differences, they are bound to keep that conflict alive for future generations. We see this in the news every day. Neither side is willing to give an inch to the other side and so the conflict continues.

Types of Conflict

Conflict comes in several forms. They are:

Internal: The conflict a person has with himself. Moral dilemmas, overcoming trauma, and psychological problems. This conflict is not with other characters, though it can affect other characters in the story.

Personal: The conflict is between a person and his closest people—his family, his lover, his close friends. It is about interpersonal relations between individuals.

Social: The conflict is between the parent and the child, between the doctor and the patient, between the Hero and the society. When you are dealing with larger issues than just interpersonal relationships, this is the conflict of choice.

Elemental: The conflict between man and the environment, between the hero and a force of nature. It could be anything from a giant meteor heading toward earth or a pack of rabid Chihuahuas.

Kurt Lewin has given other four types of conflict based on daily life frustration and on the basis of motives.

1. **Approach–approach conflict:** In this type of conflict, individual will have two desires with positive valence which are equally powerful. For example, a person has two attractive job offers and he has to choose any one of them—tension arises.

   Such conflicts are not so harmful because after selecting one, the other one automatically subsides or loses its importance to him. But in some situations, choice will be very difficult. For example, a girl has to choose either loving parents or a boyfriend for intercaste marriage. Such cases are like "you cannot have the cake and eat it too."

2. **Avoidance–avoidance conflict:** This conflict involves two goals with negative valence. At times, the individual is forced to choose one among two negative goals. In such conflicts, both are unwanted goals; this is also known as a no-win situation. For example, a woman must work at a job which she dislikes very much or else she has to remain unemployed.

Here the individual is caught between two repelling threats, fears or situations. When she cannot choose either of them, she may try to escape from the field itself. But the consequences of the escape may also be harmful. For example, a person who cannot convince the mother or the wife may resort to alcohol consumption which is otherwise dangerous or some people may even commit suicide.

3. **Approach–avoidance conflict:** This is also a very complex conflict and very difficult to resolve because in this type of conflict a person is both attracted and repelled by the same goal object. Here the goal object will have both positive and negative valences.

   The positive valence attracts the person, but as he approaches, the negative valence repels him back. Attraction of the goal and inability to approach it lead to frustration and tension.

   For example, a person is approaching to accept a job offer because the salary is attractive, but at the same time he is repelled back as the job is very risky. A man wants to marry to lead a family life but does not want the responsibilities of family life.

4. **Multiple-approach–avoidance conflict:** Some of the situations in life we come across will involve both positive and negative valences of multiple nature. Suppose a woman is engaged to be married. The marriage to her has positive valences such as providing security to life and marrying a person whom she loves very much.

   Suppose, on the other hand, if the marriage is repellent to her because she has to quit her attractive job and salary, recognition of which makes her dependent, the situation builds up tension in her.

   The resolution of this conflict depends upon the sum total of both valences. If the sum total of attractive valence takes upper hand, she will quit the job and go for marriage; otherwise she may reject marriage and continue the job if the sum total of negative valence is powerful.

Conflict Resolution

The nursing profession is one that is based on collaborative relationships with both colleagues and patients. It requires individuals to work closely with others with varying backgrounds or cultures. Individuals can hold diverse values, potentially affecting these relationships, which may result in conflict. Good communication or conflict resolution skills can decrease the risk of conflict. Conflict resolution is a process of working through opposing views in order to reach a common goal or mutual purpose.

There are five main conflict-resolution scenarios.

1. **Ignore the conflict:** If you have a tendency to avoid or postpone talking about the conflict, you are trying to ignore it and hope it goes away. This rarely works with serious conflicts. If you want to leave a relationship because of the conflict, that is your choice. But, putting your head in the sand and not dealing with the problem means that you will not learn from the experience either. What you fail to learn, you are bound to repeat in other relationships.

2. **Smooth over the conflict:** Do you try to accommodate the other person and suppress your desires? Smoothing over any conflict just to avoid confrontation or dealing with both sides of the argument can also result in a temporary reprieve. The conflict may still be there, but resentment is also underlying as one person has given up his/her values in order to smooth over the conflict.

3. **Use your authority to settle the conflict:** This is the way that it is going to be because I said so! Parents say this all the time to

their children when they want them to go to bed and the child wants to stay up and watch TV.

Is not this the boss's favorite way, too? After all, they are the boss and they have authority over you. Right? Yes? No? How does it make you feel when someone has perceived authority over you and tells you the way it is going to be?

4. **Negotiate a resolution to the conflict:** Ah, I love a good negotiation. You get what you want and I get what I want. Most of the time, this works out really well. But with all negotiation, I have to give up something and so do you. If you want me to work this weekend, then I want more money. You may not want to pay me more money because it is not in the project budget, but that is what I want. If you do not pay my rate, then you do not get what you want. I want to make more money, so you have to give me something in return. Working on that cool upcoming project would be good, too.

5. **Use collaboration to resolve the conflict:** This is your typical win–win scenario. Both parties win when they use collaboration.

But collaboration only works when people trust each other to come to a mutually beneficial agreement. If you do not trust the other person (*and it does not have to be blind trust, either*), you would not believe that he is coming to the table to put an end to the conflict between you.

However, if trust is there, this conflict-resolution scenario can be the best way to resolve conflicts once and for all. When both parties come together, communicate, and trust each other, a definitive resolution to their conflict can occur.

Ways People Deal with Conflict (Fig. 10)

There is no one best way to deal with conflict. It depends on the current situation. Here are

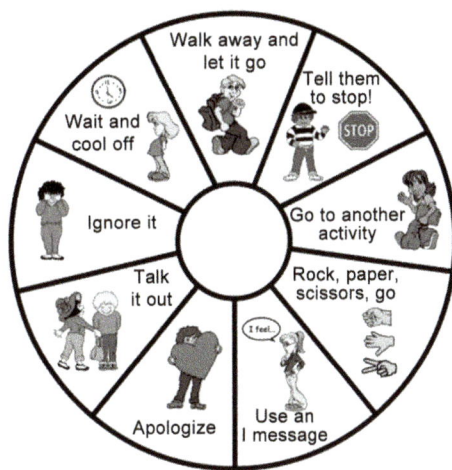

Fig. 10: Ways to deal with conflict.

the major ways that people use to deal with conflict.

1. Avoid it. Pretend it is not there or ignore it.
   a. Use it when it simply is not worth the effort to argue. Usually, this approach tends to worsen the conflict over time.
2. Accommodate it. Give into others, sometimes to the extent that you compromise yourself.
   a. Use this approach very sparingly and infrequently, for example, in situations when you know that you will have another more useful approach in the very near future. Usually, this approach tends to worsen the conflict over time, and causes conflicts within yourself.
3. Competing. Work to get your way, rather than clarifying and addressing the issue. Competitors love accommodators.
   a. Use when you have a very strong conviction about your position.
4. Compromising. Mutual give-and-take.
   a. Use when the goal is to get past the issue and move on.
5. Collaborating. Focus on working together.
   a. Use when the goal is to meet as many current needs as possible by using

mutual resources. This approach sometimes raises new mutual needs.

b. Use when the goal is to cultivate ownership and commitment.

NURSES AS A FACILITATOR OF CONFLICT RESOLUTION

- Nurses need to become proactive and learn how to effectively communicate with their patients, the patients' families and friends, as well as their colleagues.
- Good communication skills allow the nurse to resolve his/her own conflicts or facilitate conflict resolution between other individuals.
- As a facilitator, the nurse must protect each person's self-respect by focusing on the issue(s) and not the personality of the party involved.
- It is also important not to blame the participants for the problem. This hinders open and complete discussion of the issue.
- Encouraging discussion of both positive and negative feelings will increase the chances of both parties expressing all of their concerns.
- Fostering active listening and understanding enhances this. The facilitator must allow for equal time for all parties to participate expressing their opinions.
- The nurse must summarize key themes in the discussion and assist in developing alternative solutions to the issue. At a later date or time, the facilitator must follow up on the progress of the conflict resolution and give positive feedback to both parties related to the use of problem-solving skills.

QUESTION BANK

MULTIPLE CHOICE QUESTIONS

1. Mental health education is discussed in _____ levels of prevention.
    a. Primary
    b. Secondary
    c. Tertiary
    d. All of the above
2. Signs of mental illness are:
    a. Abnormal changes in thinking, perception, and judgment
    b. Abnormal changes in feeling and memory
    c. Both a and b
    d. Abnormal changes in behavior toward others
3. Signs of mental illness are:
    a. Abnormal changes in thinking, perception, and judgment
    b. Abnormal changes in feeling and memory
    c. Both a and b
    d. Abnormal changes in behavior toward others
4. Which one is not involved in mental illness?
    a. Hereditary factors
    b. Childhood experiences
    c. Changes in brain
    d. Rheumatic fever
5. A mentally healthy individual has:
    a. Independent personality
    b. Comfortable placing in social hierarchy
    c. A purposeful life
    d. All of the above

UNIT III: Mental Health and Mental Hygiene

6. **What is an example of regression?**
   a. Feelings of an ex-boyfriend
   b. Denying something ever took place
   c. Returning to an earlier age to cope with situation
   d. Telling the truth
   e. Holding your anger in
7. **Forcing thoughts to remain unconscious to avoid the anxiety that would result if they were conscious—is the definition of which Freudian defense mechanism?**
   a. Denial
   b. Isolation
   c. Regression
   d. Repression
   e. Projection
8. **Which of the Freud's three main structures of personality is described to be "unconscious" and "pleasure seeking"?**
   a. Superego
   b. Id
   c. Projection
   d. Ego
   e. Subliminal perception
9. **Frustration can be defined as a feeling of irritation or annoyance when something or someone is preventing a person from:**
   a. Becoming stressed
   b. Achieving a goal
   c. Fighting
   d. Calming down
10. **Constructive and destructive conflicts are distinguished from each other in which of the following ways?**
    a. Constructive conflict is "we"-oriented; destructive conflict is mental-oriented
    b. Constructive conflict is characterized by de-escalation of the conflict; destructive conflict is characterized by escalation of the conflict
    c. Constructive conflict is characterized by cross-complaining; destructive conflict is characterized by flexibility
    d. Both a and b
11. **Which of the following is not a characteristic of conflict?**
    a. Expressed struggle
    b. Independent parties
    c. Perceived incompatible goals
    d. Perceived interference from outside parties
12. **Which of the following is a tactic of avoiding conflict?**
    a. Competing
    b. Stonewalling
    c. Autonomy
    d. Compromising

ANSWER KEY

| 1. d | 2. c | 3. c | 4. d | 5. d | 6. c | 7. d | 8. b |
| 9. b | 10. d | 11. b | 12. b | | | | |

SHORT ANSWER TYPE QUESTIONS

1. Define mental hygiene and mental health.
2. What are levels of prevention?

UNIT III: Mental Health and Mental Hygiene

3. Enlist warning signs of mental illness.
4. Enlist components of tertiary prevention.
5. Define rationalization, sublimation, and projection.
6. What are the negative effects of defense mechanism?
7. Define conflict and conflict resolution.
8. What are the functions of ego?
9. Enlist causes of conflict.

LONG ANSWER TYPE QUESTIONS

1. Define mental health and discuss characteristics of mentally healthy person.
2. Describe the principles of mental hygiene.
3. Discuss the factors affecting mental health.
4. Classify defense mechanism and explain mature defense mechanism.
5. Discuss the implications of defense mechanism.
6. Discuss the role of nurse in secondary prevention.
7. Discuss the types of conflict.
8. Elaborate the causes of frustration.
9. Enumerate normal and abnormal behavior in details.

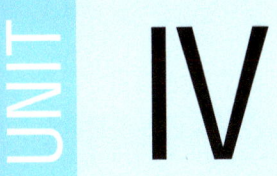

UNIT IV

Developmental Psychology

OUTLINE

- ❑ Physical, Psychosocial and Cognitive Development Across Life Span—Prenatal Through Early Childhood, Middle to Late Childhood Through Adolescence, Early and Mid Adulthood, Late Adulthood, Death and Dying
- ❑ Role of Nurse in Supporting Normal Growth and Development Across the Life Span
- ❑ Psychological Needs of Various Groups in Health and Sickness—Infancy, Childhood, Adolescence, Adulthood and Old Age
- ❑ Introduction to Child Psychology and Role of Nurse in Meeting the Psychological Needs of Children
- ❑ Psychology of Vulnerable Individuals—Challenged, Women, Sick, etc.
- ❑ Role of Nurse with Vulnerable Group

■ INTRODUCTION

Developmental psychology is a scientific approach that aims to explain growth, change, and consistency through the life span. Developmental psychology looks at how thinking, feeling, and behavior change throughout a person's life.

A significant proportion of theories within this discipline focuses upon development during childhood, as this is the period during an individual's lifespan when the most changes occur.

Developmental psychologists study a wide range of theoretical areas, such as biological, social, emotional, and cognitive processes.

■ DEVELOPMENTAL THEORY

- ❖ Freud theory (sexual development) (Discussed in Unit V)
- ❖ Piaget theory (cognitive development)
- ❖ Erikson theory (psychosocial development)

Jean Piaget Theory

Piaget's theory is based on the idea that the developing child builds cognitive structures. He described the mechanism by which the mind processes new information. He said that a person understands whatever information fits into his established view of the world. When information does not fit, the person must re-examine and adjust his thinking to accommodate the new information. Piaget described four stages of cognitive development and relates them to a person's ability to understand and assimilate new information. Piaget's theory identifies four developmental stages and the processes by which children progress through them **(Table 1)**. The four stages are:

1. **Sensorimotor stage (birth to 2 years):** The child builds a set of concepts about reality and how it works through physical interaction with their environment. This is the stage where a child does not know that physical objects remain in existence even when these are out of sight.
2. **Preoperational stage (age 2–7 years):** The child is not yet able to think abstractly and needs concrete physical situations. He/she learns to use language and to represent objects by images and words. Thinking is

Table 1: Jean Piaget theory.

Stages	Features
Preoperational stage (2–7 years)	• Emergence of symbolic thought, egocentrism, lack of the concept of conservation, animism
Concrete operational stage (7–12 years)	• Increasingly logical thought, classification and categorization, less egocentric, conservation, no abstract or hypothetical reason
Formal operational stage (age 12 to adulthood)	• Hypothetico-deductive reasoning, emerges gradually, continues to develop into adulthood

still egocentric and has difficulty taking the viewpoint of others. He or she classifies objects by a single feature, e.g., groups together all the red blocks regardless of shape or all the square blocks regardless of color.

3. **Concrete operations (age 7–11 years):** As physical experience accumulates, the child starts to conceptualize, creating logical structures that explain their physical experiences. Abstract problem-solving is also possible at this stage. For example, arithmetic equations can be solved with numbers, not just with objects.
4. **Formal operations (beginning at ages 11–15 years):** By this point, the child's cognitive structures are like those of an adult and include conceptual reasoning.

Erikson's Theory of Psychosocial Development (Table 2)

Psychosocial Stage 1: Trust versus Mistrust

It occurs between birth and 1 year of age and is the most fundamental stage of life. Because an infant is utterly dependent, the development of trust is based on the dependability and quality of the child's caregivers. If a child successfully develops trust, he or she will feel safe and secure in the world. Caregivers who are inconsistent, emotionally unavailable, or rejecting contribute to feelings of mistrust in the children they care for. Failure to develop trust will result in fear and a belief that the world is inconsistent and unpredictable.

Psychosocial Stage 2: Autonomy versus Shame and Doubt

It takes place during early childhood and is focused on children developing a greater sense of personal control. Like Freud, Erikson believed that toilet training was a vital part of this process. However, Erikson's reasoning was quite different from that of Freud's. Erikson believed that learning to control one's body functions leads to a feeling of control and a sense of independence. Other important events include gaining more control over food choices, toy preferences, and clothing selection. Children who successfully complete this stage feel secure and confident, while those who do not are left with a sense of inadequacy and self-doubt.

Psychosocial Stage 3: Initiative versus Guilt

During the preschool years, children begin to assert their power and control over the world through directing play and other social interactions. Children who are successful at this stage feel capable and able to lead others. Those who fail to acquire these skills are left with a sense of guilt, self-doubt and lack of initiative.

Psychosocial Stage 4: Industry versus Inferiority

This stage covers the early school years from approximately the age of 5–11 years. Through social interactions, children begin to develop

UNIT IV: Developmental Psychology

Table 2: Erikson development stages.

Stage	Age (years)	Psychosexual	Psychosocial crisis	Virtue	Danger
Infancy	Birth to age 2	Oral/sensory	Trust versus mistrust	Hope	Withdrawal
Early	2–3	Muscular/anal	Autonomy versus shame	Will	Compulsion
Play age	3–5	Locomotor	Initiative versus guilt	Purpose	Inhibition
School age	6–12	Latency	Industry versus inferiority	Competence	Inertia
Adolescence	12–18	Puberty	Identity versus identity confusion	Fidelity	Role repudiation
Young	19–35		Intimacy versus isolation	Love	Exclusivity
Adulthood	35–65		Generativity versus stagnation	Care	Rejectivity
Old age	After 65		Integrity vs. despair	Wisdom	Disdain

a sense of pride in their accomplishments and abilities.

Children who are encouraged and commended by parents and teachers develop a feeling of competence and belief in their skills. Those who receive little or no encouragement from parents, teachers, or peers will doubt their ability to be successful.

Psychosocial Stage 5: Identity versus Confusion

During adolescence, children explore their independence and develop a sense of self. Those who receive proper encouragement and reinforcement through personal exploration will emerge from this stage with a strong sense of self and a feeling of independence and control. Those who remain unsure of their beliefs and desires will be insecure and confused about themselves and the future.

Psychosocial Stage 6: Intimacy versus Isolation

This stage covers the period of early adulthood when people are exploring personal relationships. Erikson believed it was vital that people develop close, committed relationships with other people. Those who are successful at this step will develop relationships that are committed and secure. Erikson believed that a strong sense of personal identity was important to developing intimate relationships. Studies have demonstrated that those with a poor sense of self tend to have less committed relationships and are more likely to suffer emotional isolation, loneliness, and depression.

Psychosocial Stage 7: Generativity versus Stagnation

During adulthood, we continue to build our life, focusing on our career and family. Those who are successful during this phase will feel that they are contributing to the world by being active in their home and community. Those who fail to attain this skill will feel unproductive and uninvolved in the world.

Psychosocial Stage 8: Integrity versus Despair

This phase occurs during the old age and is focused on reflecting back on life. Those who are unsuccessful during this phase will feel that their life has been wasted and will experience many regrets. The individual will be left with feelings of bitterness and despair. Those who feel proud of their accomplishments will feel a sense of integrity. Successfully completing this phase means looking back with few regrets and a general feeling of satisfaction. These individuals will attain.

DEVELOPMENT OF INDIVIDUAL ACROSS LIFE SPAN (TABLE 3)

1. **Prenatal period:** The human body, like that of most animals, develops from a single cell produced by the union of a male and a female gamete (or sex cell). This union marks the beginning of the prenatal period, which in humans encompasses three distinct stages. The prenatal period ends with parturition and is followed by a long postnatal period.
2. **Infancy:** Infancy is the period between birth and the acquisition of language 1-2 years later. Within a few months, the infants are able to identify their mothers by sight, and they show a striking sensitivity to the tones, rhythmic flow, and individual sounds that make up human speech. Even young infants are soon able to organize their experience by creating categories for objects and events (e.g., people, furniture, food, animals) in the same way as older people do **(Table 4).**
3. **Toddler:** The toddler period is usually considered from age 1 to 3 years, enormous changes take place in the child and consequently in the family. During the toddler period, the child accomplishes a wide array of development tasks **(Table 5).** Promoting toddler health and maintaining wellness

Table 3: Different stages of development of an individual.

Stages	Features
Pre-embryonic stage	The first 2 weeks of development, which is a period of cell division and initial differentiation (cell maturation)
Embryonic period	This is a period of differentiation (cell maturation), of organogenesis, which lasts from the third to the 8th week of development
Fetal period	This is characterized by the maturation of tissues and organs and rapid growth of the body
Emotional bonding	Fetus is emotionally attached to the mother in the womb and hears the mother's sound; if the mother is having any stress that will affect the fetus and cause prematurity and if the mother consumes any alcohol during pregnancy this will cause damage to the fetal brain and leads to fetal alcohol syndrome.

Table 4: Development stages of an infant.

Stages	Features
Mental development	Infants make rapid advances in recognition and recall memory, developing curiosity, and questioning attitude and are capable of complex perceptual judgments involving distance, shape, direction, and depth
Physical growth	• **Height:** Double their weight at 4–6 months, triple it by 1st year. Infant increases in height during the 1st year by 50% from their average birth length. Head circumference increases rapidly. Teeth erupt at the age of 6 months • **Weight:** They lose 5–10 % of weight by 3–4 days after birth
Sexual development	Infants will often fondle their genitals. Many children enjoy sensual non-sexual experiences, i.e., breastfeeding, thumb sucking, rocking to bed, and cuddling
Motor development	• **Motor development:** The newborn's movements are random, diffuse, and uncoordinated. Reflexes carry out bodily functions and are responses to external stimuli • **Fine motor development:** Holds hand in fist. When crying, the newborn draws arms and legs to the body

Contd...

Contd...

Stages	Features
Sensory development	• **Vision:** A 1-month-old infant regards an object in the midline of vision. Eye movement, coordinated most of the time, follows a light to the midline. Follows a light to the periphery and has binocular coordination • **Hearing:** Hearing is demonstrated by the 1-month-old infant who quiets momentarily at a distinctive sound such as a bell
Emotional development	The newborn infant expresses his emotion just through cry for hunger, pain, or discomfort sensation
Cognitive development	The cognitive development of a newborn infant is difficult to understand or observe
Common health problems	• **Teething:** Most infants have little difficulty with teething. Generally, gums are sore and tender before a new tooth breaks the surface • **Thumb sucking:** Infants begin to suck a thumb or finger at about 3 months of age and continue the habit through the first few years of life • **Headbanging:** Some infants rhythmically bang their heads against the bars and crib for a period of time before falling asleep • **Sleeping problems:** Sleep problem develops in early infancy because of colic
Psychological needs	• **Deep sleep:** The baby sleeps quietly without moving, and breathing is regular • **Light sleep:** The baby might move, may have irregular breathing, and even startle at noises, or may experience eye movements in the dreamy sleep of rapid eye movement (REM) sleep

Table 5: Development stages of a toddler.

Stages	Features
Physical growth	A child gains only about 5–6 lb (2.5 kg) and 5 inches (12 cm) a year during toddler. Physical growth is slow during a toddler's decline in appetite and erratic eating habits. After 2 years chest circumference becomes larger than the head circumference
Physiological development	Brain growth continues slowly, corresponding to advancing intellectual skills and fine motor development. By 2 years toddler had completed improved coordination and equilibrium. Respiration slows slightly but continues to be mainly abdominal. Stomach capacity increases to the point that the child can eat three meals a day. The sense of hearing, smell, taste, touch, and vision develop. Bladder and bowel control are typically achieved during this time period
Sexual development	According to Freud, toddlers are in the anal stage of development. Freud first pointed out the tension revolving around a toddler, bladder training, and viewed toilet training as a possible way of resolving conflict and handling stress. Toddlers recognize gender differences at the age of 2 years
Psychosocial development	Toddlers learn self-control, develop autonomy, and increase independence. Able to socialize
Spiritual development	Children in this stage attend religious programs and follow the rituals carried by older ones
Emotional development	In this period if autonomy is not developed toddlers feel shame
Cognitive development	Language ability develops in this period, toddler interest in trying to discover new results, and different actions can achieve. They learn about different shapes
Common health problems	**Sibling rivalry:** It is defined as an intense feeling of jealousy between siblings **Temper tantrums:** It is an outward explosive reaction to inward stressful or frustrating situations that are a normal part of toddler life
Psychological needs	• Unconditional love from family. Self-confidence and high self-esteem. The opportunity to play with other children • Encouraging teachers and supportive caretakers. Safe and secure surroundings. Appropriate guidance and discipline

involve knowledge of normal growth and development processes, an understanding of common significant milestones, and the ability to anticipate deviations.

4. **Child (preschooler):** The preschool years span from 3 to 6 years. Although physical growth slows, this is a time characterized by reinforcement of the cognitive and social skills that begin during the toddler years **(Table 6).** As children grow into early childhood, their world will begin to open up. They will become more independent and begin to focus.

5. **School children:** Greater ability to concentrate and participate in self-initiating quiet activities that challenge cognitive skills, such as reading, playing computer, and board games **(Table 7).**

6. **Adolescence:** Physically, adolescence begins with the onset of puberty at 12 or 13 and culminates at age 19 or 20 in adulthood. Intellectually, adolescence is the period when the individual becomes able to systematically formulate hypotheses or propositions, test them, and make rational evaluations. The formal thinking of adolescents and adults tends to be self-consciously deductive, rational, and systematic. Emotionally, adolescence is the time when individuals learn to control and direct their sex urges and begin to establish their sexual roles and relationships **(Table 8).** The second decade of life is also a time when individuals lessen their emotional (if not physical) dependence on their parents and develop a mature set of values and responsible self-direction.

7. **Adulthood:** It is a period of optimum mental functioning when the individual's intellectual, emotional, and social capabilities are at their peak to meet the demands of career, marriage, and children. Some psychologists delineate various periods and transitions in early to middle adulthood that involves crises or reassessments of one's life and results in decisions regarding new commitments or goals **(Table 9).** During the middle 30s, people develop a sense of time limitation, and previous behavior patterns or beliefs may be given up in favor of new ones.

8. **Older adult:** Elderly people often have limited regenerative abilities and are more susceptible to disease, syndromes, injuries, and sickness than younger adults. The organic process of aging is called senescence, the medical study of the aging process is called gerontology, and the study of diseases that afflict the elderly is called geriatrics. The elderly also face other social issues around retirement, loneliness, and ageism **(Table 10).**

Table 6: Development stages of a preschooler.

Stages	Features
Physical growth	In this stage children grow relatively slowly; they become taller and thinner without gaining weight. Children at this age gain 1.8 kg per year. Skeletal maturation develops in this stage
Physiological development	By the age of 4 years, heart size is four times of birth size, now similar to that of the adult heart. Fat replaces the red marrow of the long bones. The length of the respiratory tract is increased, muscle fiber increases in strength and size
Sexual development	The sexual behavior of the children at this stage is characterized by the development of an attitude of antagonism and indifference toward the opposite sex. Sexual identity is more recognized. They want to play with their same sex
Psychosocial development	Egocentric, tolerates short separation, less dependent on parents, may have dreams and nightmares, attachment to opposite-sex parent, more cooperative in play

Contd...

Contd...

Stages	Features
Spiritual development	The preschooler has a concrete conception of God, who has physical characteristics and can understand simple religious stories. They have strong faith in God
Emotional development	Fears the dark. Tends to be impatient and selfish. Expresses aggression through physical and verbal behaviors. Shows signs of jealousy of siblings. Preschooler watches adults and imitates their behavior. They learn roles and responsibilities from their parents
Cognitive development	At this stage the child acquires new experiences and tries to adapt themselves to their environment and prepare themselves to solve the problems. They developed reasoning, perception, imagination, thinking observation, etc.
Common health problems	Accidents, dental caries
Psychological needs	Unconditional love from family. Self-confidence and high self-esteem. The opportunity to play with other children. Encouraging teachers and supportive caretakers

Table 7: Development stages of school children.

Stages	Features
Physical growth	Weight and height during the school years show a sex-related difference. Boys tend to gain slightly more weight through 12 years. The yearly height gain is similar in boys who tend to be taller
Physiological development	The heart assumes a more vertical position in the chest because of left ventricular development and downward placement of the diaphragm. The immune system continues to develop. Skeletal growth increases muscle strength and size also increases
Sexual development	This is the period of latency, learned about sex-role behavior and identify by observing caregiver instructions, the media, and friendship with children of the same gender
Spiritual development	During these years, children learn specific things about their religion that will develop into a religious philosophy to be used in their interpretation of the world
Emotional development	Fears injury to body and fear of the dark. Jealous of siblings (especially 6–8 years old child). Curious about everything. Has short bursts of anger by age of 10 years but is able to control anger by 12 years
Cognitive development	Piaget suggested that around 6 years of age, children start to move from the egocentric view of the preschool age to the more open and flexible thought of the school-aged child. By 7–11 years, during concrete operational stage characterized by considerable growth in thinking, imagination, and language, which allows school-age children to expand and understand their world. Children think not only of the present but also the past and future. Since children can recall events that happened in the past, they become aware that exist over a period of time
Common health problems	School phobia, stealing, recreational drug use, obesity
Psychological needs	Motivation, sense of belongingness and love, feeling useful, feeling potency, need for optimism. Respect and appreciation, attention, acceptance

Table 8: Development stages of an adolescent.

Stages	Features
Physical growth	Most of the girls are 1–2 inches taller than boys when coming into adolescence and generally stop growing within 3 years from menarche. Thus, those girls who start menstruating at 10 years of age may reach their adult height by age 13. The skeletal system grows faster than the muscles and muscle mass increases more rapidly than the height
Physiological development	The sebaceous glands of the face, neck, and chest become more active. Brain growth continues during adolescence, the cell that supports and nourishes the nervous system proliferate even though the number of neurons does not increase. The heart is almost double in size. The lungs increase in length and diameter. Gastric acid capacity increases up to 1,500 mL
Sexual development	Adolescence is the physiological period between the beginning of puberty and the cessation of bodily growth. Girls begin dramatic development and maturation of reproductive organs at an approximate age of 10–13 years; for boys 12–14 years
Psychosocial development	He needs to know "who he is" in relation to family and society, i.e., he develops a sense of identity. If the adolescent is unable to formulate a satisfactory identity from the multi-identifications, a sense of self-confusion will be developed. According to **Erikson:** Adolescent shows interest in other sex. He looks for close friendships
Emotional development	This period is accompanied usually by changes in emotional control. Adolescent exhibits alternating and recurrent episodes of disturbed behavior with periods of quiet one. He may become hostile or ready to fight, complain or resist everything
Spiritual development	Adolescents question the existence of God and any religious practices they can think. They are more oriented toward spiritual and ideological matters, and less oriented toward practice, rituals, and strictly observing religious costumes
Cognitive development	In this, they think in abstract terms and use the scientific method to reach a conclusion and solve the problems. Adolescents generally become more sophisticated in their ability to understand words and their related concepts
Common health problems	Anorexia, anger issues, alcohol abuse, homosexuality, suicide, etc.
Psychological needs	These are the needs for orientation and control, pleasure gain/distress avoidance, self-esteem protection, and attachment. Taking these needs into account in various areas of pedagogical and psychosocial work gives good opportunities to help children and adolescents develop in a desired direction

Table 9: Development stages during adulthood.

Stages	Features
Physiological development	The young adult has completed physical growth by the age of 20. Young adult is usually quite active, experiences severe illnesses less commonly than older adults
Sexual development	Adult establish sexual orientation and integrate love and sex in their life. They make commitments and from intimacy. Make fertility and child bearing decisions. Practice safer sex to protect against STDs.

Contd...

Contd...

Stages	Features
Psychosocial development	The young adult is usually caught between wanting to prolong the irresponsibility of adolescence and wanting to assume adult commitments. The years from 35 to 43 are the time of vigorous examination of life goals and relationships; alterations are made in personal, social, and occupational lives. They take major decisions concerning career, marriage, and parenthood
Emotional development	This is the period of intimate relationships, interaction, and emotional regulation. During this time important life decisions are made about career and living arrangements
Cognitive development	Rational thinking habits increase steadily through the young and middle adult years. Formal and informal educational experiences, general life experiences, and occupational opportunities dramatically increase the individual's conceptual, problem-solving and motor skills. Young adults are continually evolving and adjustment to changes in the home, workplace, and personal lives; their decision-making processes should be flexible
Common health problems	Obesity, drug and alcohol, medical illnesses
Psychological needs	Basic psychological needs satisfaction, motivation, and exercise in older adults. A predominant motivation theory used to predict exercise behavior is self-determination theory, which posits that motivation is driven by the satisfaction of three basic psychological needs—autonomy, competence, and relatedness

Table 10: Development changes in an older adult.

Stages	Features
Physical changes	People typically reach the peak of their physical strength and endurance during their twenties and then gradually decline. Changes in gait
Physiological changes	There are changes in vision, hearing, more joint pain. Some degree of atrophy of the brain and decrease in the rate of neural processes. The respiratory and circulatory systems are less efficient, and changes in the gastrointestinal tract may lead to increased constipation. Bone mass diminishes, especially among women, leading to bone density disorders such as osteoporosis. The muscle becomes weaker and skin dries and becomes less flexible
Psychosocial changes	During middle adulthood, personality tends to stabilize and relationships become more intimate. While some adults may face marital struggles, many find family ties, marriage, and parenting to be sources of generativity
Spiritual development	People tend to become more involved in prayer and religious activities as they age. This provides a social network as well as a belief system that can combat the fear of death
Emotional development	Emotion regulation skills appear to increase during adulthood. Older adults report fewer negative emotions as well as more emotional stability and well-being than younger people. Older adults may also be savvier at navigating interpersonal disagreements than younger people
Cognitive changes	The study of cognitive changes in the older population is complex. The type of memory most likely to decline with age is working memory or short-term memory
Common health problems	Immobility, instability (falls), incontinence, intellectual impairment, psychological problems
Psychological needs	The elderly have a basic need to remain connected to family members, friends, and like-minded seniors. This is psychologically beneficial because such connections can minimize issues with depression and loneliness and boost emotional stability

DEATH AND DYING

Psychological death occurs when the person begins to accept his/her death and to withdraw from others psychologically. These five psychological stages include denial, anger, bargaining, depression, and acceptance. We know that there is no right way to grieve or to come to grips with one's own death.

Kübler-Ross originally developed stages to describe the process patients with terminal illness go through as they come to terms with their own death; it was later applied to grieving friends and family as well, who seemed to undergo a similar process. The stages, popularly known by the acronym **DABDA**, include **(Fig. 1)**:

1. **Denial**: The first reaction is denial. In this stage, individuals believe that the diagnosis is somehow mistaken and cling to a false, preferable reality.
2. **Anger**: When the individual recognizes that denial cannot continue, he/she becomes frustrated, especially at proximate individuals. Certain psychological responses of a person undergoing this phase would be: "Why me? It's not fair!"; "How can this happen to me?"; "Who is to blame?"; "Why would this happen?".
3. **Bargaining**: The third stage involves the hope that the individual can avoid a cause of grief. Usually, the negotiation for an extended life is made in exchange for a reformed lifestyle. People facing less serious trauma can bargain or seek compromise. Examples include the terminally ill person who "negotiates with God" to attend a daughter's wedding, an attempt to bargain for more time to live in exchange for a reformed lifestyle, or a phrase such as "If I could trade their life for mine."
4. **Depression**: "I'm so sad, why bother with anything?"; "I'm going to die soon, so what's the point?"; "I miss my loved one; why go on?" During the fourth stage, the individual despairs at the recognition of his/her mortality. In this state, the individual may become silent, refuse visitors, and spend much of the time mournful and sullen.
5. **Acceptance**: "It's going to be okay."; "I can't fight it; I may as well prepare for it." In this last stage, individuals embrace mortality or inevitable future, or that of a

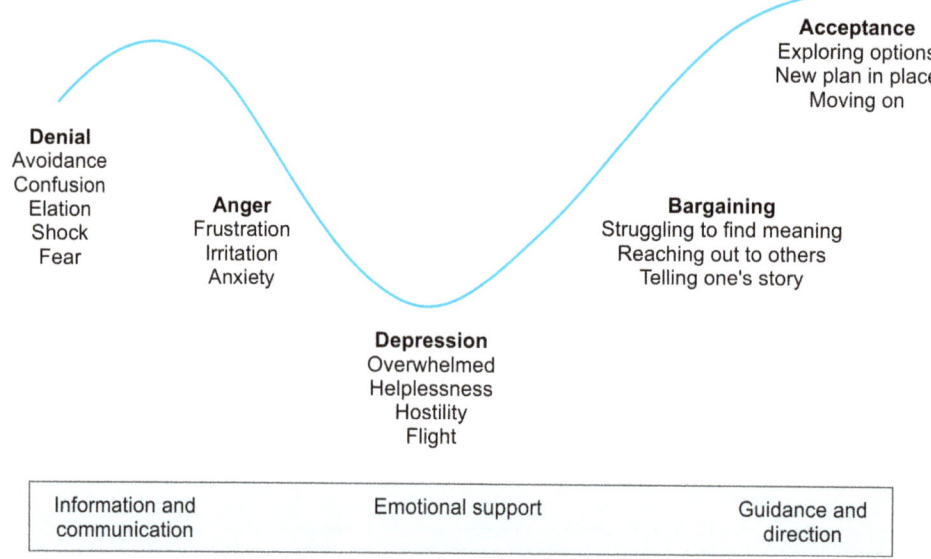

Fig. 1: Kubler–Ross grief cycle.

loved one, or other tragic events. People dying may precede the survivors in this state, which typically comes with a calm, retrospective view for the individual, and a stable condition of emotions.

Role of a nurse in supporting normal growth and development across the life span
1. Recognize the psychological development of all the stages
2. Guidance and support for the implementation of physical health care
3. Guidance for promoting a safe environment
4. Application of theories, principles, and methods of maternal and child programs
5. Development of therapeutic relationships
6. Implementation of developmental education to all the stages
7. Promotion of access to support network
8. Provide education for each group for their better development
9. Use of scientific evidence to guide practice
10. Help the individual to find out the solution of his/her problem which affects his/her developmental stages.

PSYCHOLOGY OF VULNERABLE GROUPS

Vulnerable individuals are often most of the important and at-risk population and often have to face devastating situations. Vulnerable individuals are the persons who can be minors and also are not able to protect themselves and have dysfunction related to all aspects of life.

Vulnerability is the susceptibility of being physically or emotionally wounded. These are the individuals more vulnerable or exposed to the possibility of being attacked, harmed, or wounded either physically or psychologically.

Vulnerable individuals are often considered to have some physical or mental disability or having psychological disorders. Mental or psychological disorders can arise in any age group, in any kind of people. People with these disabilities fall under certain categories of vulnerable group. At-risk population such as children, women, and elderly are also considered as vulnerable groups.

Psychology of Challenged

Physically disabled, previously called physically handicapped, can be due to congenital or acquired due to illness or injury. Their physical aspect affects their psychology in many different ways. The mild reactions often go unrecognized and whatever they are not well-understood, taken for granted, and no effort is made to correct these reactions.

Mentally challenged or disabled has been replaced by the term intellectually disabled and it is impairment of function at the level of the whole person which will affect activities of daily living and disturbed social and occupational functioning.

Developmental disability: It is a substantial handicap in mental or physical functioning with onset before the age of 18 years, e.g., autism, attention deficit hyperkinetic disorders, epilepsy, mental retardation, cerebral palsy. This loss of function is due to prenatal or postnatal events in which predominant disturbance is in the acquisition of cognitive, language, motor, or social skills.

Types of Disabled/Challenged

- **Orthopedically handicapped**—due to injury, poliomyelitis, diabetes mellitus, falls, osteomyelitis, etc.
- **Visually handicapped**—blindness partial or total, squint, nystagmus, visual acuity, etc.
- **Neurologically handicapped**—stroke, brain injury, brain tumor, neurological disease, cerebral palsy, Parkinson's disease, etc.
- **Speech and hearing handicapped**—deaf, mutism, stammering, cleft lip or palate
- **Disfigurement**—due to infections such as leprosy, burns, injury, and postoperative conditions, hare lip, facial asymmetry, dental conditions

- **Mentally challenged**—intellectually disabled, autism, pervasive development disorders, cerebral palsy, vision impairment, attention-deficit/hyperactivity disorder (ADHD)
- **Socially challenged**—social maladjustment, delinquents, antisocial people, criminals, robbers and gamblers, alcoholics, drug addicts

Some of the psychological problems of challenged are as follows:

1. **Ambivalent attitude:** Many physically disabled individuals have ambivalent attitudes. They want both to be treated as normal individuals and at the same time, need to be treated as handicapped persons. Such attitudes fluctuate and may be presumed to be a function of the possibilities of realizing certain goals in different social situations.
2. **Fear related to adjustment:** Because of the lack of sufficient understanding of the meaning of their disabled conditions, many physically disadvantaged individuals impose unnecessary restrictions upon themselves and their activities with considerable loss to themselves and their adjustment to the social environment.
3. **Resent sympathy:** Like a non-handicapped person, a handicapped individual feels that expressions of sympathy place him in a position of social and personal inferiority, force him to entertain ideas of inequality and inadequacy, and disturb his level of self-confidence and hence he/she develops resentment to sympathy shown by others.
4. **Feeling of social isolation:** A handicapped individual is inclined to be lonely, morose, self-conscious, sensitive, and suspicious of the opinions of others. For all his efforts at maintaining himself in the social community and identifying fully with the non-handicapped, the physically disabled person finds it exceptionally difficult, just as the non-disabled person does, to see the world through the eyes of someone else whose physical status is different from that of his own.
5. **Disturbed personality:** Individuals often are prone to develop personality disorders like avoidant. Since they have certain personality traits such as shyness, aloofness, attention-seeking and aggressive behavior patterns, inferiority complex, depressive and anxious, antisocial and dissocial behavior, overactive and agitated, over-dependent, etc.
6. **Frustration and aggressive behavior:** Physically or mentally disabled often feel frustrated and show impulsive, aggressive, and stubborn behavior. Psychiatric disorders related to low self-esteem, such as depression often occur in these individuals.

These individuals are often prone to have a psychiatric illness such as paranoid states, reactive depression, suicidal tendency or attempts, or substance use disorders.

Role of Nurse

- She must identify and assess an individual's disability and plan care accordingly.
- She must make the community aware of various disabilities and how to prevent them.
- She has to speak or communicate to the patients directly and if they do not respond as in mentally challenged, it is still important to address them.
- She must be patient and allow extra time to make sure she assessed the patient's full history and do investigations accordingly.
- She needs to talk to the patient and clear doubts of the patient as he/she feels happy that others understand his/her condition.
- She must speak to the disabled person as she is talking to a normal individual and give him/her respect and maintain his/her dignity.

Psychology of Elderly People

Old age is the time of stress and strain. It is usually referred to as the stages of the life cycle that begins at the age of 65. The number of individuals over age 65 is rapidly increasing. In the year 2020 the number of elderly has outnumbered children younger than 5 years and 16.9% of the total population is elderly. Old age can be considered as developmental phase in the life span of a person and is characterized by deficits in physical and psychosocial functioning.

Psychological Problems in Elderly

Psychosocial problems of the elderly arise due to personality changes of old age, family disorganization, and interpersonal difficulties with family members. These problems are as follows:
- Affective disorders such as depression and mania
- Organic mental disorders such as senile dementia, Alzheimer's disease, and delirium
- Suicidal attempts and tendencies
- Alcohol and drug abuse
- Adjustment disorders related to changes in the aging process
- Psychiatric illness including emotional reactions to physical illness
- Retirement and reduced income which may create a feeling that one's usefulness is essentially over and activities are restricted
- Reduction in physical attractiveness
- Isolation and loneliness
- Elderly abuse in the form of financial, physical, sexual, emotional, neglect, abandonment, etc., is the most prevalent psychosocial problem
- Loss of identity or ego disintegration

Role of Nurse in Dealing with Elderly

Treatment of older people suffering from mental and other health problems requires a comprehensive use of medical and psychological procedures. Administration of group therapy to older patients would mean creating a social environment in which the person can function successfully. Following measures can be adopted to help the elderly:
- Allow extra time for the elderly and communicate well.
- Make them focus on positive aspects of life.
- Validating their behavior is a good way of coping with the elderly.
- Give needed breaks and spent time with loved ones.
- Take out them in social gatherings.
- Listen to them carefully and attentively.
- Take them for regular health checkups.
- Provide assisted aids if necessary.
- Family members must be explained about the elderly changes and related behavior.
- Hospitalized elderly must be taken care of attentively and should be prevented from falls and accidents.

Psychology of Sick Individuals

Physical illness or mental illness causes a varying degree of stress on the patient and family and other person involved in the care of a sick individual. Physical illness can be acute or chronic and often affects adversely the individual growth and psychosocial adaptation (**Fig. 2**). Mental illness is also a wide range of disorders that affect mood, thinking, and behavior.

Types of common illness include:
- Allergies
- Colds and flu
- Systemic diseases—diabetes, ischemic heart disease, asthma, cancer
- Communicable diseases—coronavirus, hepatitis, HIV (AIDS), measles, skin infections, tuberculosis
- Psychological illness—anxiety, phobias, adjustment disorder, depression, substance use disorders, suicidal attempts

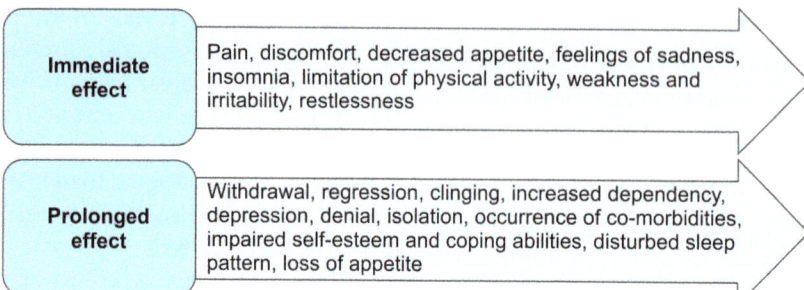

Fig. 2: Effects of illness on sick individuals.

Psychological Problems Related to Hospitalization of Sick Individual

- Hospitalization of sick individuals often involves separation from parents, family, or home environment which causes devastating effects on physical and psychological aspects of the individual **(Fig. 3)**.
- The hospital environment causes anxiety and fear feelings in patients. Often patients feel frustrated and irritable due to the procedures or investigations done on daily basis or as a part of treatment regimen.
- Hospitalization and changes in daily routine of the patient tend to cause physiological disturbances associated with psychological factors such as insomnia, anorexia, frequent urination, lack of communication, inattention and poor concentration, and feelings of detachment from surroundings.
- Hospitalization exacerbates patient's emotions and often causes comorbid mental conditions. For example, patient admitted with substance use disorder can often develop aggressive behavior, depression, or panic attack because of prolonged stay in hospital.

Impact on Family Members

- Hospitalization can represent a time of great vulnerability and imposed stress for both the patient and his/her family members.
- Family members reported to give priority to the welfare of their ill relative and in their heightened emotional state, often adversely put their own health at risk.
- Family members often overcome with feelings of helplessness and worthlessness and they often become irritable and aggressive.
- Anxiety, exhaustion, burnout feelings of guilt and shame, disturbed sleep pattern, and ineffective coping can also develop among family members.

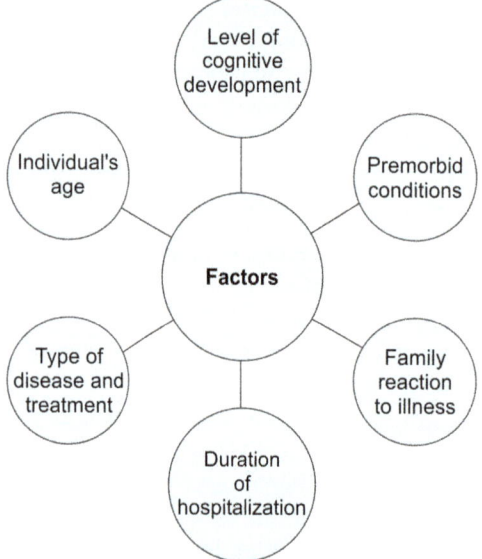

Fig. 3: Factors affecting individual's adaptation to hospitalization.

Role of Nurse

- A nurse must orient and guide the patient and family members to the ward and routine of the hospital to reduce anxiety.
- The nurse should provide proper quality care and develop therapeutic relationship with the patient.
- She must listen attentively to the patient and family members.
- She should educate the patient and family members regarding disease condition and provide appropriate health education.
- The nurse must be empathetic, compassionate and must be understanding and able to resolve problems faced by patients.
- She must act as an advocate for patients and family members and work for the well-being of the patients.
- She must collaborate with the health team members to provide quality care to the patients and reduce hospital stay of the patients and provide cost-effective care.
- She must also teach additional home care treatment to patients and family members and about follow-up and discharge planning.

Psychology of Women

Women are considered at-risk population as they often deal with varying degree of situations throughout their life span and plays multiple roles throughout the life cycle. The issues which are considered during development of women are stereotyped roles, gender discrimination, reproductive rights and related health issues, and empowerment. The psychology of women helps us to explore psychological issues of specific concern to women.

Nowadays so many laws and acts related to women have been come up but still, due to lack of knowledge, discrimination, and ethnic and cultural issues women are deprived of these facilities and become the reason for psychological distress among women. But as compared to previous roles women's roles have been changed and they have become less dependent on men. Men are yet to accept these changes in role relationships.

Common mental health issues in women

- Depression (2:1 ratio) due to multiple role conflicts, menopausal changes, infertility
- Anxiety and specific phobias related to marital or family conflicts, domestic violence, divorce, separation from children
- Post-traumatic stress disorders due to rape, sexual abuse, physical abuse, abortion
- Postpartum depression after giving birth to child
- Postpartum psychosis or blues
- Suicidal attempts
- Eating disorders due to unusual craving and distorted feelings with respect to the body image
- Substance use disorders
- Unusual feelings of inferiority, incapability, inability, and dependability on others

Role of Nurse

- The nurse must educate and make women aware of their rights and responsibilities.
- Community mental health nurses must assess and identify at-risk women who are feeling distressed and depressed due to family conflicts, domestic violence, etc., and must refer them to counseling centers.
- She must lessen the feeling of insecurity and inferiority by straightforward explanations.
- She must identify the psychological and emotional needs of the women and help them to prevent any mental illness.
- She must empower the women by making them aware of different roles of women in different fields.
- She must help women or assist them in assessing basic health needs through various women upliftment programs, e.g., reproductive and child health, janani suraksha yojna.

PSYCHOLOGY OF GROUPS

Groups are the most basic units of any social system. They carry on many organized activities which are necessary for a society. In the course of our lives, all of us are involved with many groups, each of which has the potential for influencing our actions and psychological states. The term "group" may apply to social units varying in size from two persons to a large organization or major political party. The study of group is a fundamental part of much of the research conducted in social psychology.

Group psychology focuses on how groups form, conform and warp decision-making, productivity and creativity, and achieving goals.

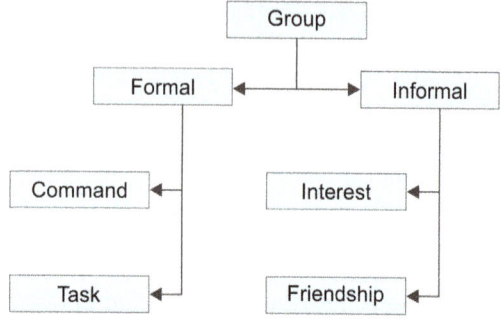

Flowchart 1: Types of a group.

Definition

Two or more individuals who are connected to one another by social relationships.
—*Dohelson*

A group may be defined as a number of individuals who join together to achieve a goal. People join groups to achieve goals that cannot be achieved by them alone.
—*Johnson & Johnson (2006)*

A collection of people who interact with one another, accept rights and obligations as members, and who share a common identity.

A group is an association of two or more people in an interdependent relationship with shared purposes.

Types of Groups (Flowchart 1)

1. **Formal group:** A designated work group defined by the organization's structure
   a. *Command group:* A group composed of individuals who report directly to a given manager
   b. *Task group:* Represents those who work together to complete a job task
2. **Informal group:** A group that is neither formally structured nor organizationally determined; appears in response to the need for social contact. Membership in such groups is voluntary.

   a. *Interest group:* A group of employees who come together to satisfy a common interest; such as improving working conditions, protesting the company's environmental policies, or adjusting vacation schedules
   b. *Friendship group:* A group of people having common beliefs, attraction, or intimacy, e.g., group of friends in a hostel

Other Types

a. **Primary groups**—characterized by small size, face-to-face interaction, and intimacy among members of a group, e.g., family, neighborhood group
b. **Secondary groups**—characterized by large size, individual identification with the values and beliefs prevailing in them rather than cultural interaction, e.g., occupational association and ethnic group
c. **Task groups**—composed of people who work together to perform a task but involve cross-command relationships. For example, for finding out who was responsible for causing wrong medication order would require liaison between the ward in-charge, senior sister, and head nurse.
d. **Social groups**—refers to an integrated system of an interrelated psychological group formed to accomplish defined objectives, e.g., political party with local political clubs, friendship groups

e. **Reference groups**—one in which individual would like to belong
f. **Membership groups**—those where the individual actually belongs
g. **Command groups**—formed by subordinates reporting directly to the particular manager determined by a formal organizational chart
h. **Functional groups**—the individuals working together daily on similar tasks
i. **Problem-solving groups:** It focuses on specific issues in their areas of responsibility, develops a potential solution, and is often empowered to take action.

DEVELOPMENT OF GROUPS

The developmental process of small groups can be viewed in several ways. These are the following stages of group formation **(Fig. 4)**. These were given by Duckman in 1965.

Viewing the group as a whole we observe definite patterns of behavior occurring within a group.

First Stage: Forming
The initial stage in the life of a group is concerned with forming a group. This stage is characterized by members seeking safety and protection, tentativeness of response, seeking superficial contact with others, and demonstrating dependency on existing authority figures. Members at this stage either engage in a busy type of activity or show apathy.

Second Stage: Storming
The second stage in this group is marked by the formation of dyads and triads. Members seek out familiar or similar individuals and begin a deeper sharing of self. Continued attention to the subgroup creates a differentiation in the group and tensions across the dyads/triads may appear. Pairing is a common phenomenon.

Third Stage: Norming
The third developmental stage is marked by a more serious concern about task performance. The dyads/triads begin to open up and seek out other members in the group. Efforts are made to establish various norms for task performance. Members begin to take greater responsibility for their own group and relationship while the authority figure becomes relaxed.

Fourth Stage: Performing
This is a stage of a fully functional group where members see themselves as a group and get involved in the task. Each person makes a contribution and the authority figure is also seen as a part of the group. Group norms are followed and collective pressure is exerted to ensure the effectiveness of the group. The group redefines its goals in the light of information from the outside environment and shows an autonomous will to pursue those goals. The long-term viability of the group is established and nurtured.

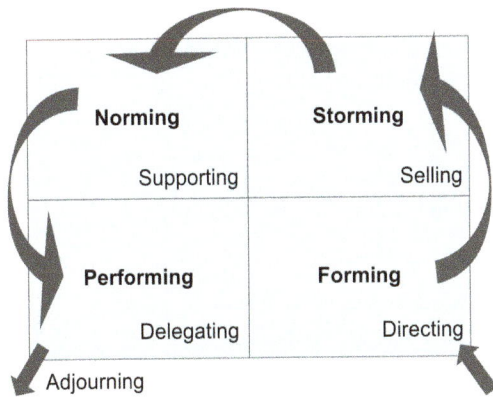

Fig. 4: Five stages of group development.

Psychological Issues in Groups
* Intergroup conflicts and aggression
* Overpowering or dominating a group by any one person causes misunderstanding.
* Role ambiguity causing confusion and distress in a group
* Lack of cohesiveness often leads to group disintegration or group separation.

UNIT IV: Developmental Psychology

- Negative behavior or attitude of some of the group members often causes incoordination in a group.
- Nonconducive work environment often leads to frustration, irritability, and sadness among individuals.
- Rigid rules and regulations of the group cause distress and anxiety feelings in a person.

Implication in Nursing

- Nurses mostly care for one patient at a time, but in the community, they have to deal with an entire population; so it is very necessary that they play effective role in mental health team groups.
- In community and hospital, group integration and group strengthening strategies can be implemented.
- Teamwork is very important while caring for patients in hospitals.
- Nurses should suggest the availability of support groups to patients, e.g., an alcoholic anonymous group for alcoholic patients, Alzheimer's association for elderly, adult children of alcoholic groups, governmental and non-governmental agencies, international agencies such as WHO, UNICEF, etc.
- She must act as leader of the health team and must influence other junior nurses to work cooperatively with coordination.

QUESTION BANK

MULTIPLE CHOICE QUESTIONS

1. **Development refers to:**
    a. Growth
    b. Qualitative changes
    c. Both a and b
    d. Increase in size of body
2. **Growth refers to:**
    a. Development
    b. Qualitative changes
    c. Both a and b
    d. Increase in size of body
3. **Developmental stages are:**
    a. Infancy, toddler, childhood, adolescence, adulthood, older adult
    b. Toddler, childhood, infancy, adolescence, adulthood, older adult
    c. Adolescence, toddler, childhood, infancy, adulthood, older adult
    d. Adulthood, toddler, childhood, infancy, adolescence, older adult
4. **Vulnerable challenges are high in:**
    a. Childhood and old age
    b. Childhood and adolescent age
    c. Adolescence and old age
    d. Adult and old age
5. **What is the name of Erikson's development theory?**
    a. Psychosocial
    b. Cognitive
    c. Moral
    d. Physical
6. **How many stages are there in the psychosocial theory?**
    a. 8
    b. 4
    c. 12
    d. 7
7. **The stage that occurs between birth and 1 year of age is concerned with:**
    a. Initiative versus guilt
    b. Trust versus mistrust
    c. Identity versus role confusion

UNIT IV: Developmental Psychology

8. Intimacy versus isolation occurs at what stage?
    a. Infancy
    b. Young adulthood
    c. Maturity
9. According to Piaget, which one of the following factors plays an important role in influencing development?
    a. Reinforcement
    b. Language
    c. Experience with the physical world
    d. Imitation
10. According to Piaget the second stage of cognitive development is:
    a. Sensorimotor stage
    b. Formal operational stage
    c. Pre-operational stage
    d. Concrete operational stage
11. Not a part of Kubler Ross stages of impending death is:
    a. Shock
    b. Denial
    c. Anger
    d. Aggression
12. The emotional state, an individual experiences to loss of loved objects is:
    a. Grief
    b. Mourning
    c. Bereavement
    d. Agony
13. According to Tuckman (1965) which of the following is NOT a stage of the life cycle of a group?
    a. Performing
    b. Norming
    c. Reforming
    d. Storming

ANSWER KEY

| 1. b | 2. d | 3. a | 4. c | 5. a | 6. a | 7. b | 8. b |
| 9. c | 10. c | 11. a | 12. a | 13. c | | | |

SHORT ANSWER TYPE QUESTIONS

1. Define development psychology.
2. Enlist the stages of development in human being.
3. Enumerate the stages of Erikson theory.
4. Discuss the cognitive development of toddler and childhood.
5. Enlist the psychological needs of adulthood.
6. Explain about vulnerable group.
7. Define women psychology.
8. Define the stages of group.

LONG ANSWER TYPE QUESTIONS

1. Describe different stages of development.
2. What are the development changes in toddler?
3. Describe the various changes in old age.
4. What are different vulnerable challenges at different stages of development?
5. Explain the role of the nurse in health promotion.
6. Explain about the Erikson 8 stages theory.
7. Explain about death and dying.
8. Explain the role of nurse dealing with elderly.

UNIT V

Personality

OUTLINE

- Meaning, Definition of Personality
- Constituents and Traits of Personality
- Determinants of Personality
- Theories and Classification of Personality
- Measurement and Evaluation of Personality—Introduction
- Alteration in Personality
- Role of Nurse in Identification of Individual Personality and Improvement in Altered Personality

■ MEANING AND DEFINITION OF PERSONALITY

People differ from each other in meaningful ways. Personality refers to a person's unique and relatively stable pattern of thoughts, feelings, and actions. Personality is an interaction between biology as genetic studies suggest its heritability and environment which is shown in its learned components.

Personality is derived from the Greek word *"persona,"* meaning the mask used by actors in Greek drama. Personality previously was regarded as the outer appearance of a person. Personality is the total quality of an individual as shown in his habits of thinking, in his attitude, interest in his manners of acting, and his personal philosophy of life. Personality is what characterizes an individual. It includes unique qualities of an individual that influence a variety of characteristic behavior patterns (both overt and covert) across different situations.

What is Personality?

Personality is defined as an enduring pattern of perceiving, relating to, and thinking about environment and oneself.
— *DSM – IV (APA, 1994)*

Personality is the dynamic organization within the individual of those psychosocial systems that determine his unique adjustment to his environment. —*Gordon Allport (1937)*

Personality is defined as persistent, pervasive and deeply ingrained traits or patterns of behavior with which one relates to, perceives and thinks about oneself and environment.
—*DSM – IV – TR (APA)*

Personality is the total quality of individual's behavior. —*RS Woodworth*

Personality is more or less stable and enduring organization of the person's character, temperament, intellect and physique which determine his unique adjustment to the environment. —*Eysenck*

■ TRAITS OR CONSTITUENTS OF PERSONALITY

1. **Personal appearance:** Characteristics such as height, weight, physique, eye color or eye shape, and complexion also determine one's personality. A balanced combination of these characters enhances a positive self-concept.
2. **Intelligence:** The intellectual ability of the individual is a greater part of his

personality. Individuals with higher IQ tend to organize themselves better and in turn have a good personality.

3. **Emotionality:** Human beings often show their reaction based on the emotional component and can be judged based upon that as introvert or extrovert personality only by expressing their emotions.
4. **Sociability:** A human is a social being and his behavior is judged only through social interactions, and without a social component individual personality cannot be completed.
5. **Ascendance (dominate)—submission:** Those having dominant personality traits are self-confident, have leadership qualities, and can take control over others' life easily. Those who have submissive traits are introvert, emotional, and lack control over their life.
6. **Moral character:** It is the evaluation of the moral values of an individual. It involves empathy, fortitude, honesty, loyalty, and good behavior or habits which is inculcated into one's personality.

Various other constituents of personality have been explained through various models and theories, e.g., five-factor model, the big five personality traits, etc.

Nature/characteristics of personality are as follows:

Personality has a very complex nature and there are various characteristics which define its nature and which are as follows:

1. **Unique and specific:** There are no individuals in the world who are alike or have same personality since every individual has a different influence of heredity and environment on his personality.
2. **Self-consciousness:** It is a finely tuned judgment of self-worth and awareness. When the individual is aware of himself, he is able to determine his personality.
3. **Judged by society:** An individual's thoughts and behavior are often influenced by society. Individuals who are social personality type often tend to be leaders, supporters, and motivators.
4. **Include all behavior patterns:** Personality is how individuals tend to think, feel, and have based on their cognitive, connative, and affective domains respectively.
5. **Sum of all traits of an individual:** It is the sum of physical, mental, and social qualities of an individual and is the sum of ideas, attitudes, and values of a person which form an integral part of his character.
6. **Dynamic organization:** As the environment or situation around the individual changes, certain changes in behavior pattern are also determined which in turn influence the personality of an individual.
7. **Unique adjustment to environment:** A well-adjusted person is having a stable personality, high self-esteem, and is contended. If the interaction of all the constituents of personality is accompanied by strain and conflict, then it results in maladjusted personality and if the interaction is harmonious and peaceful then it results in a well-adjusted individual.
8. **Product of heredity and environment:** This means the way genes act depends on the genes which they work. In the same way, the effect of the environment depends on the genes with which they work. For a balanced personality of an individual, there should be harmonious interaction between heredity and environment.
9. **It strives for goal:** Individuals who are goal-oriented must have self-regulation and a stable personality which will help them to manage their thoughts and actions while working toward a particular goal.
10. **It consists of conscious, semiconscious, and unconscious:** Structure of personality is divided into three parts, first is conscious in which individual

is fully aware of the reality, second is semiconscious which records all activities and acts as a filter for thoughts, and the third is unconscious which involves unwanted thoughts, conflicts, and unfulfilled urges and wishes.
11. **Personality functions as a whole:** Personality is a characteristic set of behavior, cognition, and emotions. Personology studies personality as a system and it is a multidimensional, complex, and comprehensive approach to personality.

FACTORS/DETERMINANTS AFFECTING PERSONALITY (FLOWCHART 1)

1. **Biological factors:**
    a. **Heredity:** Heredity is another factor determining human personality. Some of the similarities in an individual's personality are said to be due to his common heredity. Every human group inherits the same general set of biological needs and capacities which explain our similarities in personality. For example, many children behave exactly how their parents do. Twin theories also suggest these similarities. Intelligence is inherited from ancestors.
    b. **Brain:** It is generally believed that the father and the child adopt almost the same type of brain stimulation and later differences are the result of the environment in which the child has grown up.
    c. **Physical factors:** Physical features may involve the height of a person, color, health status, beauty, etc. These factors are involved when interacting with any other person and this contributes to personality development in many ways.
2. **Social factors:** Social factors also play a vital role as the things that surround us daily influence our daily activities and hence get inculcated into our personality. Relationships, coordination, cooperation, communication, and social interactions between and within organizations, families, workplaces, communities, and societies—all contribute in one way or another as personality determinants.
3. **Cultural factors:** It involves traditional practices, customs, beliefs, precedents, and values which in turn determine the moral character of an individual. The creed, religion, status, and beliefs are also important factors affecting personality.
4. **Situational factors:** Situational factors indirectly affect a person's behavior from

Flowchart 1: Determinants of personality.

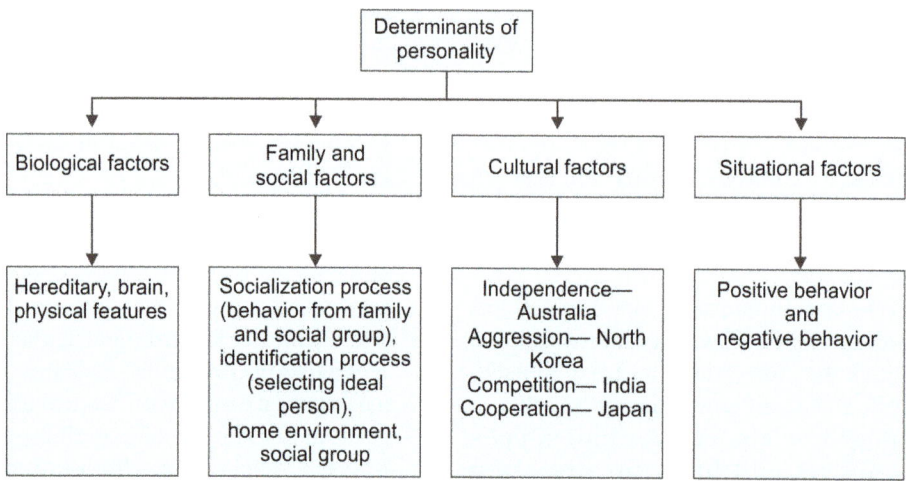

time to time but they often bring out the person's traits that are not commonly seen. For example, in an office, an individual's behavior will be totally different as compared to in parties with friends.

Various other factors which can determine personality are:
- Social characteristics of an individual, societal demands and social economical status being rich or poor, and living conditions whether in good areas versus slums and geographic region
- Educational qualification, career chosen, observation perceived, and experimentation made
- Provision of healthy food and privileges made available such as good parental care and support
- Warmth, love, and acceptance by associated family members, relatives, and friends
- Varying environments such as workplace, home, and society.

THEORIES AND CLASSIFICATION OF PERSONALITY

Type: It is a clump of traits thought to describe a certain kind of individual, e.g., introvert type.

Trait: It is a descriptive characteristic of an individual, assumed to be stable across situations, e.g., shy, brave, reliable, friendly, confident, etc.

Type of Theories

1. Temperament Theory

Temperament theory is also known as "Four humors" theory. According to the Greek physician Hippocrates (460–370 BC), "FATHER OF MEDICINE," certain human moods, emotions, and behaviors are caused by body fluids (called "humors"):
- **Blood** "sanguine": Optimism, cheerful, energetic, bodily strong, emotionally stable, vigorous, confident
- **Yellow bile** "choleric": Active but irritable, emotionally weak, bodily strong, hot-tempered
- **Black bile** "melancholic": Depression, lacks energy, unhappy, pessimistic, emotionally, and bodily weak
- **Phlegmatic:** Sluggishness, unexcitable, happy but lazy, bodily weak, slow-moving

2. Kretschmer Types of Physique

Ernst Kretschmer is a German psychologist who initiated scientific investigations and attempted to correlate physique and characteristics. He also studied mental disorders based on different body types.

Four main body types:
A. **Asthenic:** (thin, small, weak) associated with introversion and timidity, resembling a milder form of the negative symptoms of schizophrenics
B. **Athletic:** (muscular, large-boned) epileptic
C. **Pyknic:** (stocky, fat) friendly, interpersonally dependent, and gregarious, are predisposed toward manic-depressive illness
D. **Dysplastic:** Unproportionate body parts and do not belong to any of the three types mentioned above. Since the body is unproportionate due to hormonal changes, metabolic disturbances, etc., their behavior and personality are also imbalanced.

3. Sheldon Theory

In the 1950s, **William Sheldon** (1899) became interested in the variety of human bodies. He built upon earlier work done by **Ernst Kretschmer** in the 1930s. Kretschmer believed that there was a relationship between three different physical types and certain psychological disorders. His research, although involving thousands of institutionalized patients, was a suspect because he failed to control for age and the schizophrenics were considerably younger than the bipolar patients, and so more likely to be thinner.

Classification according to Sheldon Theory
Few of the classifications given by Sheldon Theory are as shown in **Table 1**.

4. Jung's Classification

Carl Gustav Jung, a prominent Swiss psychologist, was originally a follower of Sigmund Freud but later developed his own concept of analytic psychology. He was also the first to describe the **Introverted** (inner-

Table 1: Classification according to Sheldon theory.

Endomorph	Chubby people, tending to be "pear-shaped." **Viscerotonic**: Sociable types, lovers of food and physical comforts, affectionate, weak somatic structure	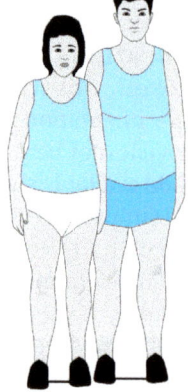
Mesomorph	Self-assertive, with broad shoulders and good musculature, love risk and adventure, balanced body structure **Somatotonic**: Active types, physically fit and energetic	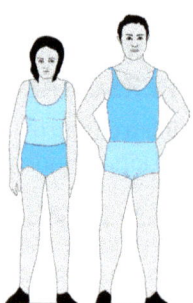
Ectomorph	Slender, unsociable, pessimistic, often tall, people with long arms and legs and fine features **Cerebrotonic**: Nervous types, relatively shy, often intellectual	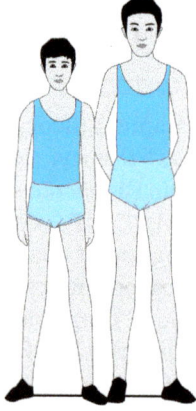

directed) and **Extroverted** (outer-directed) personality types.

Jung's introversion and extroversion attitudes

A. Introvert:
- Most aware of his/her inner world and is aloof and withdrawn
- More concerned with subjective appraisal
- Gives more consideration to fantasies and dreams
- Interested in themselves and their own feelings and emotions
- Are unable to adjust to social situations
- Inclined to worry and get easily embarrassed and are shy and reserved.
- Philosophers, scientists, writers, etc., fall in this category.

B. Extrovert:
- Characterized by the outward movement of psychic energy
- Places more importance on objectivity
- Gains more influence from the surrounding environment than by inner cognitive processes
- Successful in adjusting to the realities of their environment, are socially active, and more interested in leaving a good impression on others
- Sociable, friendly, and not easily upset by difficulties
- Politicians, social workers, lawyers, salesman, etc., come under this category

Trait Theories

A **trait** is a relatively stable characteristic that causes individuals to behave in certain ways. The combination and interaction of various traits form a personality that is unique to each individual (**Fig. 1**).

1. Gordon Allport's Trait Theory

Gordon Allport was the pioneer in personality theories and came up with different synonyms of personality traits and then submerged various traits into three main categories.

Cardinal Traits:
- Dominate an individual's whole life
- The person becomes known specifically for these traits.

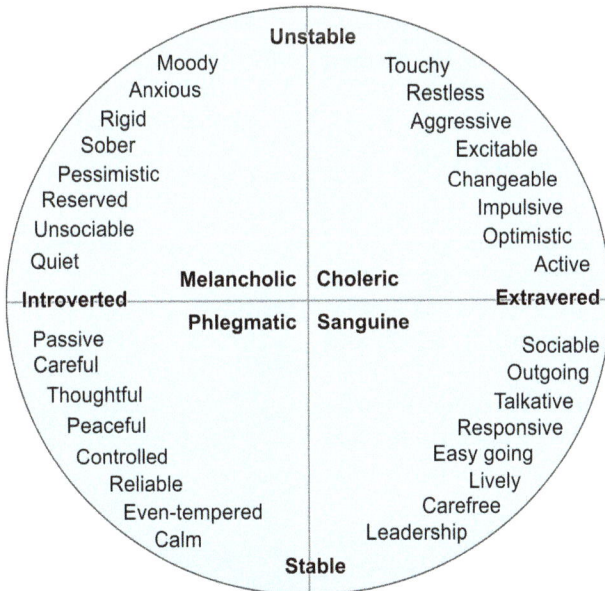

Fig. 1: Traits of personality based on Galen's theory of four temperaments.

- People with such personalities often become well known for these traits.
- Example: Hatred may have been a cardinal trait of Hitler.

Central Traits:
- The general characteristics that form the basic foundations of personality
- While not as dominating as cardinal traits are the major characteristics you might use to describe another person
- Examples: Intelligent, honest, shy, and anxious—are considered central traits.

Secondary Traits:
- Traits that often appear only in certain situations or under specific circumstances
- Example: Getting anxious when speaking to a group or getting impatient while waiting in line

2. Raymond Cattell's Sixteen Personality Factor Questionnaire

Raymond Cattell reduced the number of personality traits from Allport's initial list of over 4,000 to 171. Then, using "factor analysis" he eventually reduced his list to just 16 key personality traits. According to Cattell, these 16 traits are the sources of all human personalities. These factors are listed in **The Sixteen Personality Factor Questionnaire** (16PF).

3. Eysenck's Three Dimensions of Personality

- **Introversion/extroversion:**
  - Introversion focuses attention on inner experiences, while extroversion focuses attention outward on other people and the environment.
  - A person high in introversion might be quiet and reserved, while an individual high in extroversion might be sociable and outgoing.
- **Neuroticism/emotional stability:** Individuals who are high on this trait tend to be irritable, sensitive, ambivalent, or anxious.
- **Psychoticism:** Individuals who are high on this trait tend to have difficulty dealing with reality and may be antisocial, hostile, non-empathetic, and manipulative.

Type A and B
a. Are obsessed with numbers, measuring their success in terms of how many or how much of everything they acquire.
b. Play for fun and relaxation, instead of exhibit their superiority at any cost.
c. Can relax without guilt.

4. The Five-Factor Theory of Personality

Both Cattell's and Eysenck's theories have been the subject of considerable research. As a result, a new trait theory often referred to as the "Big Five" theory emerged. This five-factor model of personality represents five core traits that interact to form human personality. These include **Extroversion, Agreeableness, Conscientiousness, Neuroticism,** and **Openness.**

5. The Psychoanalytical Theory

Sigmund Schlomo Freud (May 6, 1856 to September 23, 1939) was an Austrian neurologist who became known as the founding father of psychoanalysis and psychiatry.

Freud argued that personality is divided into three structures **(Fig. 2)**:
1. The **id** is "the primitive, instinctive component of personality that operates according

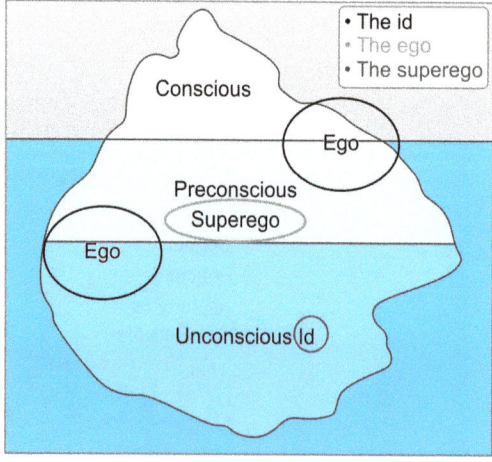

Fig. 2: Freudian components of personality.

to the pleasure principle." The two major drives under Id are—Eros and Thanatos.

2. The *ego* is "the decision-making component of personality that operates according to the reality principle."

3. The *superego* is "the moral component of personality that incorporates social standards about what represents right and wrong."

The id, ego, and superego are arranged into different layers of awareness including the following **(Fig. 3)**:

1. The *conscious* layer: This includes thoughts or feelings we are fully aware of.
2. The *preconscious* layer: This includes information just beneath the surface of our awareness.
3. The *unconscious* layer: This includes thoughts, memories, feelings, and desires that we are not aware of, but that greatly influence our behavior.

Freud believed that behavior is the result of ongoing internal conflict among the id, ego, and superego. Conflicts stemming from sexual and aggressive urges are especially significant. Such conflicts arouse anxiety and we use **defense mechanisms**—"largely unconscious reactions that protect a person from painful emotions such as anxiety and guilt." The ego is always caught in the middle of battles between the superego's desires for moral behavior and the id's desires for immediate gratification. Freud believed that the basic elements of adult personality are in place by the age of 5 and result from the outcome of five psychosexual **stages**. In each stage, children must cope with distinct immature sexual urges that influence adult personality. *Fixation* results if the child fails to move forward from one stage to another, and is usually caused by excessive *gratification*, or *frustration* of needs at a particular stage.

Neurotic anxiety: Caused by id impulses that the ego can barely control.

Moral anxiety: Comes from threats of punishment from the superego.

Defense mechanism: A process used by the ego to distort reality and protect a person from anxiety.

Psychic energy: It is the force or impetus required for mental functioning. The psychic energy originates in id and instinctually fulfills basic physiological needs called libido or libidinal energy. As the child matures it is

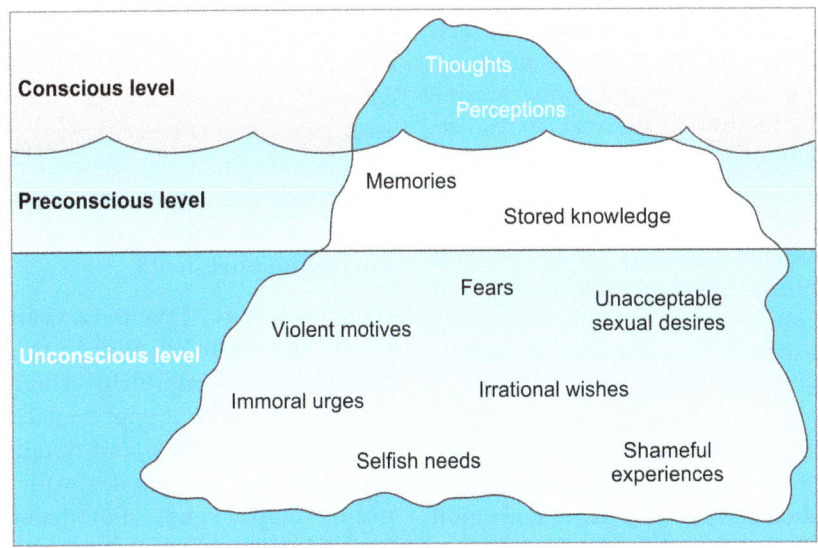

Fig. 3: Freud's view of the human mind: The mental iceberg.

diverted from id to form ego and then from ego to form superego.

Cathexis: It is the process by which id invests energy into an object in an attempt to achieve gratification.

Stages of psychosexual development
1. **Oral stage (age 0-1 year):** Most of an infant's pleasure comes from stimulation of the mouth. If a child is overfed or frustrated, oral traits will develop. Early oral fixations can cause oral dependent personality: Gullible, passive, and need lots of attention. Later oral fixations can cause oral-aggressive adults who like to argue and exploit others
2. **Anal stage (age 1-3 years):** Attention turns to the process of elimination. A child can gain approval or express aggression by letting go or holding on. Ego develops. Harsh or lenient toilet training can make a child anal retentive—stubborn, stingy, orderly, and compulsively clean or anal expulsive—disorderly, messy, destructive, or cruel.
3. **Phallic stage (age 3-6 years):** The child now notices and is physically attracted to the opposite sex parent. The child is vain, sensitive, narcissistic. It can lead to Oedipus conflict: For boys only. Boy feels rivalry with his father for his mother's affection. The boy may feel threatened by father (castration anxiety). To resolve, the boy must *identify* with his father (i.e., become more like him and adopt his heterosexual beliefs). Electra conflict: Girl loves her father and competes with her mother. The girl identifies with her mother more slowly because she already feels castrated. Both concepts are widely rejected today by most psychologists.
4. **Latency (age 6 years to puberty):** Psychosexual development is dormant. Same-sex friendships and play occur here.
5. **Genital stage (puberty-on):** Realization of full adult sexuality occurs here; sexual urges re-awaken.

6. Psychosocial Stages of Personality Development

According to Erik Erickson, there are eight stages of personality development.

Stage 1—oral sensory [birth to 1 year (infancy)]: The basic conflict is trust versus mistrust. The important event is feeding and the important relationship is with the mother and nurse. The infant must develop a loving and trusting relationship with the mother/caregiver through feeding, teething, and comforting. Failure to resolve this conflict can lead to fear and a belief that the world is inconsistent and unpredictable.

Stage 2—muscular-anal [age 1-3 years (toddler)]: The basic conflict is autonomy versus shame/doubt. The important event is toilet training and the important relationship is with the parents. The child's energy is directed toward mastering physical skills such as walking, grasping, and muscular control. The child learns self-control but may develop shame, doubt, impulsivity (rash), or compulsion if not handled well.

Stage 3—locomotor [age 3-6 years (preschool)]: The basic conflict is initiative versus guilt. The important event is independence and the important relationship is family. The child continues to become more assertive in exploration, discovery, adventure, and play. The child may show too much force in this stage causing feelings of guilt. Failure to resolve this conflict can lead to a lack of initiative and self-doubt.

Stage 4—latency [age 6-12 years (school age)]: The basic conflict in this stage is industry versus inferiority. The important event is school and the important relationships are teachers, friends, and neighborhood. The child must learn to deal with new skills and develop a sense of achievement and accomplishment. Failure to do so can create a sense of inferiority, failure, and incompetence.

Stage 5—adolescence [age 12-20 years (adolescence)]: The basic conflict is identity versus role confusion. The important event is the development of peer relationships and the important relationships are peers, groups, and social influences. The teenager must achieve a sense of identity in occupation, sex roles, politics, and religion. In addition, they must resolve their identity and direction.

Stage 6—young adulthood (age 20-40 years): The basic conflict in young adulthood is intimacy versus isolation. The important event is parenting and the important relationships are lovers, friends, and work connections. In this stage, the individual must develop intimate relationships through work and social life. Failure to make such connections can lead to loneliness, isolation, and depression.

Stage 7—middle adulthood (age 40-65 years): The basic conflict is generativity versus stagnation. The important event is parenting and the important relationships are with children and the community. This stage is based on the idea that each adult must finds a way to satisfy, support, and contribute to the next generation; it is often thought of as giving back. Failure to resolve this stage can lead to an unproductive and uninvolved world.

Stage 8—maturity (age 65 years to death): The basic conflict is ego integrity versus despair. The important event is reflection on and acceptance of the individual's life. The individual is creating meaning and purpose of one's life and reflecting on life achievements. Failure to resolve this conflict can create feelings of dislike, regret, bitterness, and despair.

Jean Piaget Theory

Piaget's theory is based on the idea that the developing child builds cognitive structures. He described the mechanism by which the mind processes new information. He said that a person understands whatever information fits into his established view of the world. When information does not fit, the person must re-examine and adjust his thinking to accommodate the new information. Piaget described four stages of cognitive development and relates them to a person's ability to understand and assimilate new information.

Piaget's stages
Piaget's theory identifies four developmental stages and the processes by which children progress through them.

The four stages are:
1. **Sensorimotor stage (birth to 2 years):** The child builds a set of concepts about reality and how it works through physical interaction with their environment. This is the stage where a child does not know that physical objects remain in existence even when out of sight.
2. **Pre-operational stage (age 2-7 years):**
   - The child is not yet able to think abstractly and needs concrete physical situations.
   - The child learns to use language and to represent objects by images and words. Thinking is still egocentric and he/she has difficulty taking the viewpoint of others.
   - The child classifies objects by a single feature, e.g., groups together all the red blocks regardless of shape or all the square blocks regardless of color.
3. **Concrete operations (age 7-11 years):**
   - As physical experience accumulates, the child starts to……
   - Conceptualize, creating logical structures that explain their physical experiences.
   - Abstract problem-solving is also possible at this stage. For example, arithmetic equations can be solved with numbers, not just with objects.
4. **Formal operations (beginning at age 11-15 years):** By this point, the child's cognitive structures are like those of an adult and include conceptual reasoning.

Techniques of Personality Assessment

The techniques of personality assessment can be divided into five categories:
1. Where one can see how the individual behaves in actual life situations
   a. Observational technique
   b. Situational technique
2. Where one can find out what an individual says about himself
   a. Autobiography
   b. Questionnaire
   c. Interview
3. Techniques by which one can find out what others say about the individual whose personality is under assessment
   a. Case history taking
   b. Bibliography
   c. Rating scales
4. Techniques by which one can find how an individual reacts to an imaginative situation involving fantasy
5. Techniques by which one can directly determine some personality variables in terms of a physiological response by measuring instruments

MEASUREMENT AND EVALUATION OF PERSONALITY

1. **Observational method:** Skills play an important part in most assessment procedures. An interview is the most important method of observation. Appearance, bearing, and speech can be noticed. Sometimes the things that we observe confirm the person's self-report, and at other times the person's overt behavior appears to be at odds with what he or she says.
   - Observational procedures may be either informal or formal.
   - Informal observations are primarily qualitative.
   - The body language of the client can be observed during an interview. The body language may be posture, movement of the hands, facial expressions, or voice.
   - The clinician observes the environment in a person's behavior which occurs without attempting to record the frequency or intensity of specific responses.

2. **Personality inventories:** This is the most common method of measuring personality. A personality inventory is a questionnaire in which the person reports his/her feelings in certain situations. Most often, the answers are scored by machines which eliminate the prejudice of the tester **(Table 2)**.

3. **Projected techniques:** This test focuses upon what is inside a person rather than what can be seen in a person's behavior. These tests try to find out more about a person's feelings, unconscious desires, and inner thoughts.
   a. **Thematic apperception test (TAT) (Figs. 4A to F):** TAT was developed by Henry Murray, a psychologist at Harvard (1938). It consists of three sets of pictures, one set is used with both men and women and a second set only for men, and the third set for women. The pictures are shown in a definite sequence and the subject is asked to make up a story based on what he sees in these pictures. It is believed that he would project his own experience, bibliographical data, interest, and problems into his description of pictures.
   TAT throws light in the following areas of life:

Table 2: Examples of questions used in questionnaire.

Sr. No.	Questions	Answers
a.	Would you rate yourself as a quiet person?	Yes No
b.	Do you prefer to work alone rather than with others?	Yes No
c.	Do you frequently feel sad?	Yes No

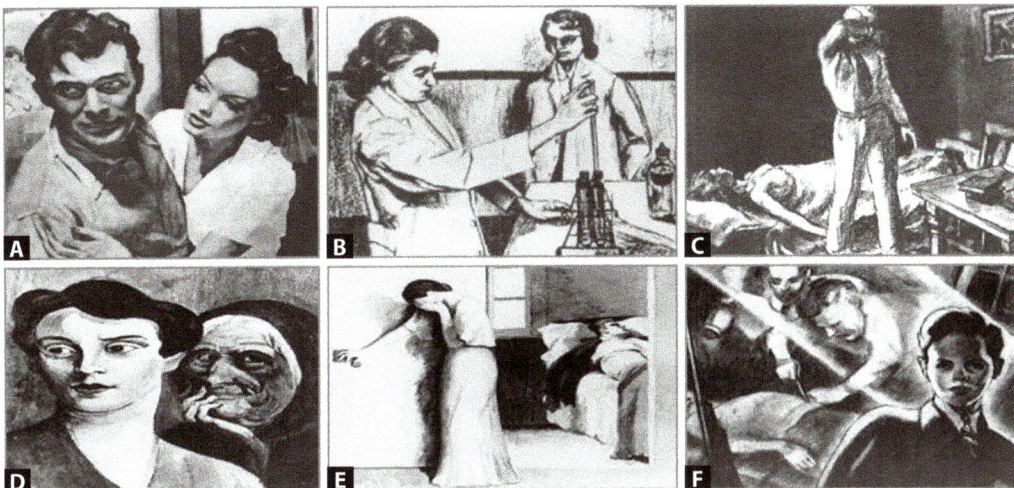

Figs. 4A to F: Thematic apperception test.

- Family relationships
- Motivation of the subjects
- Inner fantasies
- Social relationships
- Emotional conflicts
- Attitude to works
- Outlook toward future
- Frustrations, if any
- Its adherents claim that it taps a subject's unconscious to reveal repressed aspects of personality, motives, and needs for achievement, power and intimacy, and problem-solving abilities.

Children apperception test (CAT) (Figs. 5A to C)

It is the version of TAT being used for children and it consists of only 10 cards. The cards have pictures of animals instead of humans as in TAT. Interpretations and scoring are similar to TAT.

b. **Rorschach's test (Fig. 6)**
- The test takes its name from that of its creator, Swiss psychologist Hermann Rorschach (in 1922).
- **Rorschach's test** (also known as **Inkblot test**) is a psychological test in which subjects' perceptions of inkblots are recorded and then analyzed using psychological interpretation, complex scientifically derived algorithms, or both.
- It has been employed to detect an underlying thought disorder, especially in cases where patients are reluctant to describe their thinking processes openly.
- The response differs from person to person based on the individual's personal experiences. For example, teenaged college students saw inkblot No. 1 as:
  - A bat
  - Two ladies standing back to back
  - Face of an owl
  - A patch of cloud

Rorschach responses can reveal the following information:
- Degree of intellectual control of the subject on his actions
- Emotional aspects
- Mental approach to given problems
- Creative and imaginative capacities
- Security and anxiety
- Personality growth and development
- Phobias, sex disturbances, and severe psychological disorders can be detected which serve as a guide for a treatment program.

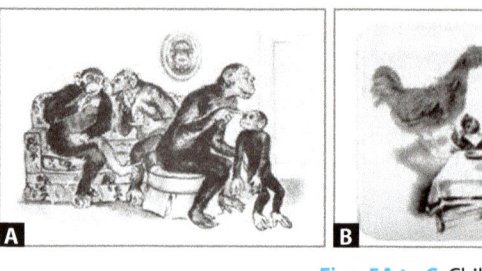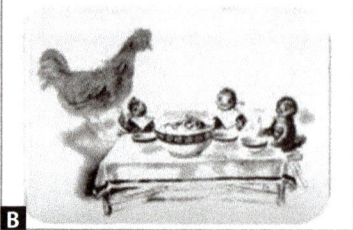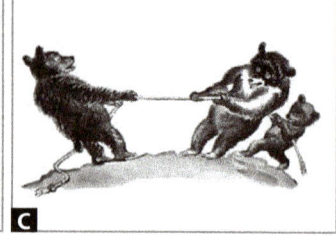

Figs. 5A to C: Children apperception test.

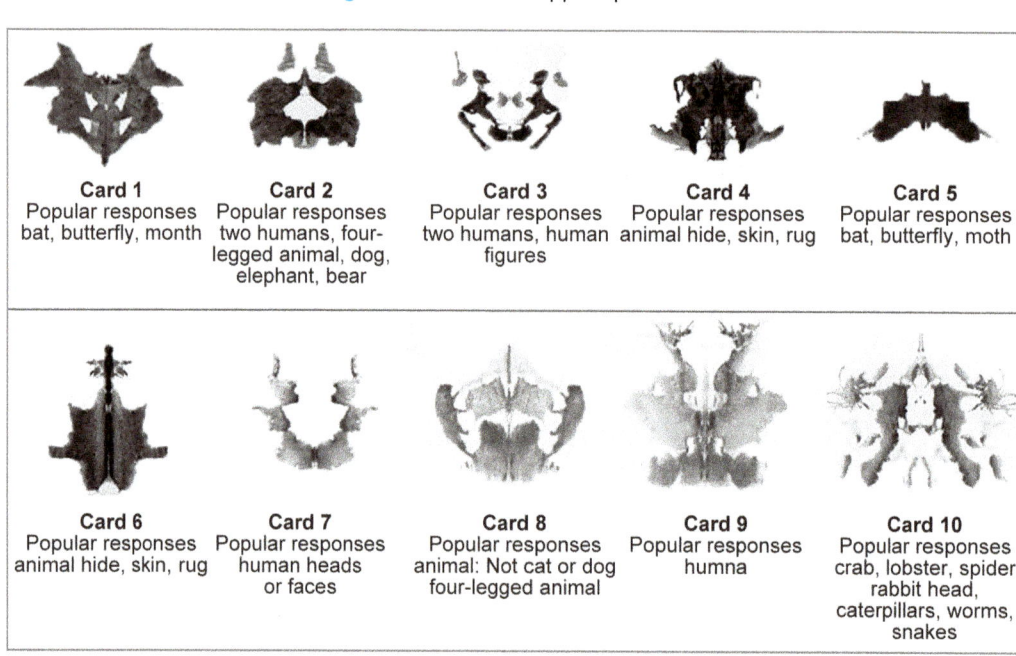

Fig. 6: Rorschach inkblot test.

Goals of Rorschach test
- The general goal of the test is to provide data about cognition and personality variables such as motivations, response tendencies, cognitive operations, affectivity, and personal/interpersonal perceptions.
- There are 10 official inkblots, each printed on a separate white card, approximately 18 × 24 cm in size. Each of the blots has near-perfect bilateral symmetry.
❖ Five inkblots are of black ink, two are of black and red ink, and three are multicolored, on a white background.

Example of Rorschach interpretation:
❖ **Response:** Associated with whole inkblot (location)
❖ **Interpretation:** The subject has the ability to solve his/her problems in a comprehensive manner; he/she possesses high mental ability.
❖ **Word association test (WAT):** When the subject gives a quick response word, he is taken unaware of and his unconscious process directs his association. Here the subject has to answer as quickly as possible with the first word which comes to his mind when he is given a stimulus word.

Projective tests are often used in clinical practice. They are helpful in showing a person's inner areas of conflicts, anxieties, or any problem in relationships because the person is free to describe anything.

Uses
- Individual assessments for employment in fields requiring a high degree such as law enforcement and military leadership positions
- For diagnosis in order to match psychotherapy best suited to patients' personalities
- Forensic purposes in evaluating the motivations and general attitudes of persons accused of violent crimes
- Research into specific aspects of human personality, most often needs for achievement, fears of failure, hostility

ALTERATIONS IN PERSONALITY

The personality of individual changes as the individual grows and it is varied. It is also influenced by the mood changes of a person. Personality traits that are stable over time can suddenly change as life progresses. For example, a person with high temperament and anger will become calm and quiet as he reaches the elderly stage. Alfred Binet has reported these changes in his book titled "Alterations in personality," originally appeared in "Bibliotheque Scientifique Internationale" and was reviewed in the journal Nature in 1892. Since then, a lot of work has been done on finding out the phenomenon behind alteration in personality. In our daily life also, we consistently change our social behavior, mood, and emotions.

Factors causing **SUDDEN** alteration in personality:
- Anxiety, depression, stress
- Various types of mental illness
- Substance use
- Medical conditions
- Malnutrition
- Brain injuries or trauma

Factors causing **GRADUAL** alteration in personality:
- Environmental changes
- Change in living conditions
- Marriage and other life events
- Occupation or profession
- Maturational changes

These factors can change personality in both negative and positive ways and either deteriorate or disorganize individual personality or may lead to a flourishing personality.

Example: When you get admitted to a university course and you have to change your living conditions and adjust to a hostel environment, a lot of changes take place in your mood, habits, and talents and you end up with an independent personality.

Symptoms of Alterations in Personality Due to Illness

- The common behavioral changes due to illness are:
  - Withdrawn, irritable, and ill-tempered behavior can result in schizoid personality disorders.
  - Changes in self-concept, body image, and lifestyle
  - Self-centeredness, resentment, and aggression directed toward himself leading to narcissistic personality disorder
  - Demanding and dependent behavior
  - Non-cooperativeness
  - Hostility
  - Shame and guilty feelings

If these symptoms persist for a longer period of time, it can result in personality disorders or other forms of chronic mental illnesses **(Table 3)**.

Table 3: Categories of personality disorders.

Personality disorder	Symptoms and signs
Cluster A (Odd Cluster)	
Paranoid	Suspicious of other
Schizoid	Inability to form and lack of interest in social relations
Schizotypal	Strange thought patterns, magical thinking, odd perceptions
Cluster B (Impulsive Cluster)	
Histrionic	Tendency to be overly emotional and dramatic
Narcissistic	Overly self-involved, views self as special and deserves special attention
Antisocial	Deceitful, manipulates people, history of conduct problems in childhood
Borderline	Moody, fears abandonment, feels empty, self-mutilates or attempts suicide
Cluster C (Anxious Cluster)	
Avoident	Very sensitive to interpersonal rejection
Dependent	Has difficulty being along, doses not like to end relations
Obsessive	Excessive concerns with details, orderliness and rules, difficulty relaxing and having fun

ROLE OF NURSE IN IDENTIFICATION OF INDIVIDUAL PERSONALITY

1. Nurses need to help patients express their thoughts and feelings and provide care that helps the patient effectively cope with change.
2. Convey an enthusiastic readiness to care for the patient.
3. Nurses have to build up healthy personal relationships such as confidence and cooperation with the patient.
4. Therapeutic relationship establishment leads to lower the feelings of anxiety and stress in patient. Assessment can be done only after building a trustful relationship with the patient.
5. A detailed history can be collected about traits of an individual with an altered personality and changes in the daily routine should be noted.
6. Knowledge about the structure of personality can assist nurses in mental health settings in better understanding of disease condition of the patient.
7. Nurses can plan care to assist the individuals in fulfilling daily tasks which have been disturbed due to changes in behavior.
8. She can assist, teach, advise parents, children, family members and patients regarding different developmental tasks and how to achieve them satisfactorily.
9. Nurses interact with patients, doctors, co-workers, and other important members of society, who need certain behavior patterns, so the nurse should develop and practice well adjustable and balanced personality.
10. Nurses interact with different types of patients every day, so assessment of personality is essential in planning the care of a hospitalized patient.

Qualities of Nurse with Good Personality

- She must be sympathetic, understanding, friendly, kind, and adjustable.
- Effective communication skills
- Emotional stability and should have a high emotional quotient.
- Should be flexible and has good physical endurance.

UNIT V: Personality

- Should have problem-solving skills and should use evidence-based practices.
- Should be well versed with the latest techniques and procedures.

Improvement in Altered Personality

Personality alteration due to medical condition or acute illness subsides when the condition gets treated once. But if the condition is chronic and situations are stressful alteration does not go away.

Mental health conditions may be treated with the help of psychiatric medications and personality disorganization can be dealt.

Mental health professionals and community mental health nurses can identify various personality and behavioral changes in patients and people and can prevent personality disruption.

Psychotherapy or talk therapy can be recommended at the earliest.

Warning signs can be identified at the earliest like disorganized behavior, confusion, agitation, withdrawal, isolation, etc.

Proper diagnosis to be made regarding alteration in personality and related investigations and psychological testing to be carried out by experts.

QUESTION BANK

MULTIPLE CHOICE QUESTIONS

1. A relatively consistent pattern of behavior in the individual is termed:
   a. Traits
   b. Id
   c. Personality
   d. Ego
2. The unique pattern of behavior is termed:
   a. Extrovert
   b. Traits
   c. Personality
   d. Consciousness
3. Which of the following psychologists is associated with psychoanalysis?
   a. Carl Jung
   b. BF Skinner
   c. Sigmund Freud
   d. Ivan Pavlov
4. Who among the following classified personality based on body fluids?
   a. Kretschmer
   b. Hippocrates
   c. Carl Jung
   d. Sheldon
5. Which of the following trait is very much associated with Sanguine personality?
   a. Reserved
   b. Energetic
   c. Sociable
   d. Pessimistic
6. Tall and thin body structure belongs to which of the following personalities?
   a. Ectomorph
   b. Sanguine
   c. Melancholic
   d. Mesomorph
7. Which of the following personality structures are related to pleasure seeking?
   a. Ego
   b. Superego
   c. Id
   d. Unconscious
8. TAT belongs to which of the following methods of assessment?
   a. Interview method
   b. Projective method
   c. Personality inventory
   d. Personality questionnaire
9. The ability to tolerate frustration is an example of one of the functions of the:
   a. Id
   b. Ego
   c. Superego
   d. Unconscious

UNIT V: Personality

10. Personality has been described in terms of traits by:
    a. Cattell
    b. GW Allport
    c. Maslow
    d. Karn Horney
11. Personality is unique for every individual because it is the result of a person's:
    a. Intellectual capacity, race, and socioeconomic status
    b. Genetic background, placement in family, and autoimmunity
    c. Biological constitution, psychological development, and cultural settings
    d. Childhood experiences, intellectual capacity, and socioeconomic status
12. Another term of superego is:
    a. Self
    b. Ideal self
    c. Narcissism
    d. Conscience
13. Which of the following represents the proper order of personality development according to Freud?
    a. Oral, phallic, latency, anal, genital
    b. Anal, oral, phallic, latency, genital
    c. Oral, anal, phallic, latency, genital
    d. Anal, oral, phallic, genital, latency
14. The basic emotional task for toddler is:
    a. Trust
    b. Industry
    c. Identification
    d. Independence
15. Classification into endomorphic, mesomorphic, and ectomorphic was proposed by:
    a. Hippocrates
    b. Ernst Kretschmer
    c. Sheldon
    d. Jung

ANSWER KEY

1. a	2. c	3. c	4. b	5. c	6. a	7. c	8. b
9. b	10. b	11. c	12. d	13. C	14. d	15. d	

SHORT ANSWER TYPE QUESTIONS

1. Define personality.
2. Define type and trait.
3. What is nature or characteristics of personality?
4. What is sentence completion test for assessment of personality?
5. What is psychic energy and cathexis?
6. Enlist various methods to assess personality of an individual.
7. Describe the variables of personality.
8. Discuss various types of personality.
9. Describe the learning theories of personality.

LONG ANSWER TYPE QUESTIONS

1. Discuss stages of psychosocial personality development.
2. Discuss psychoanalytical aspect of Sigmund Freud.
3. What is the importance of studying personality in nursing?
4. Discuss Rorschach inkblot test for personality assessment.

UNIT VI: Coginitive Psychology

OUTLINE

- Cognitive Process: Attention—Definition, Types, Determinants, Duration, Degree and Alteration in Attention
- Perception—Meaning of Perception, Principles, Factor Affecting Perception
- Intelligence: Meaning of Intelligence—Effect of Heredity and Environment in Intelligence,
- Classification, Introduction to Measurement of Intelligence Tests—Mental Deficiencies
- Learning—Definition of Learning, Types of Learning, Factors Influencing Learning—Learning Process
- Habit Formation
- Memory—Meaning and Nature of Memory, Factors Influencing Memory, Methods to Improve Memory, Forgetting
- Thinking—Types, Level, Reasoning and Problem Solving
- Aptitude—Concept, Types, Individual Differences and Variability
- Psychometric Assessment of Cognitive Processes—Introduction
- Alteration in Cognitive Processes

■ ATTENTION

Meaning

Attention is an active part of consciousness. The activity of concentrating mind on a particular matter is called attention. Attention is not possible in the absence of consciousness, but attention and consciousness are not one. The field of consciousness is vast and attention is one of its parts. For example, I am reading at this time. Book, note, table, chair, etc., all this can be under my consciousness, but my attention is on the words being read on the paper.

Definition

Attention is the concentration of consciousness upon one object rather than others.
—*Dumvile*

Attention is the process of getting an object of thought clearly before the mind.
—*Ross*

Attention is the cognitive process of selectively concentrating on one aspect of the environment while ignoring other things.
—*John R Anderson*

Attention is merely conation or striving considered from the point of view of its effects on cognitive process. —*McDougall*

Attention is being keenly alive to some specific factor in our environment. It is a preparatory adjustment for response.
—*Morgan and Gilliland*

Attention can be thought of as the bridge over which some parts of the external world the aspects selectively focused on are brought into the subjective world of our consciousness so that we may regulate our own behavior.
—*Carver and Schuler*

Nature of Attention

- Attention is focusing of consciousness on a particular object.

Flowchart 1: Types of attention.

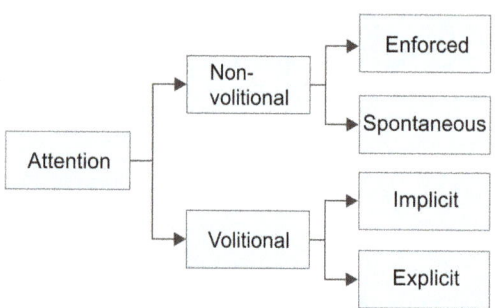

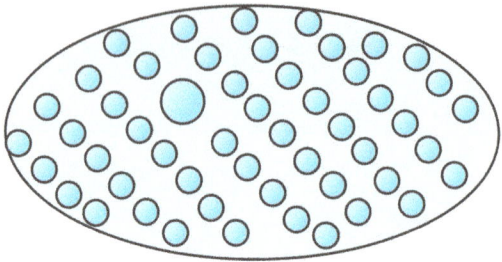

Fig. 1: Effect of size on attention.

- Attention is constantly shifting/changeable.
- Attention is selective.
- Attention is a mental process.
- Attention is a state of preparedness or alertness.
- Attention has narrow range/span.

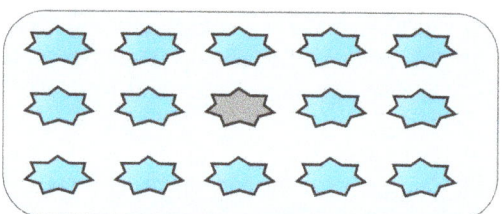

Fig. 2: Effect of intensity on attention.

Types of Attention (Flowchart 1)

1. **Non-volitional:** This is attention aroused without will.
   a. Enforced (sustained by instincts): For example, attraction to the opposite sex
   b. Spontaneous (sustained by sentiment): The mother immediately attended to her child crying.
2. **Volitional:** This is voluntary with will and there is always a goal behind it.
   a. Implicit (obtained by a single act of will and attention without awareness): For example, attending to a mathematical problem when teachers threaten punishment.
   b. Explicit (obtained by a repeated act of will and attention with awareness): It requires strong willpower and strong motives, e.g., attention paid during examinations.

Determinants of Attention

Attention depends upon several factors. These factors may be of two types:
1. **External factors:** External factors are concerned with the environment. These are also called objective factors.

a. **Size:** Size has an effect on attention. It is natural that an unusual size attracts the attention of the people. Very big size or very small size too draws our attention when compared with normal size. For example, a Lilliputian (dwarf man) walking on the road too draws our attention **(Fig. 1)**.
b. **Intensity:** Loud sounds, strong smells, and deep colors are attractive in nature. If a sound is intense, then it would attract our attention. The thunder is louder than a car sound. So, our attention is drawn to thunder **(Fig. 2)**.
c. **Movement:** Moving things draw our attention more than stationary ones. A moving car attracts faster than a stationary car.
d. **Contrast:** Anything that is different from its surrounding is a contrast. Black dust in the milk draws attention quickly. A swan among the crows attracts suddenly **(Fig. 3)**.
e. **Repetition:** If a thing or person or event is repeated several times, then our attention is drawn to it. When an

UNIT VI: Cognitive Psychology

Fig. 3: Effect of contrast on attention.

advertisement is repeated on the walls, it draws our attention.

f. **Duration:** Attention is drawn to a thing that lasts longer. A salesperson draws attention by lengthening his voice.
g. **Change:** Change draws our attention easily. In the midst of continuous noise, a slight moment of silence draws our attention.
h. **Novelty:** Newness attracts quickly than the traditional one. A new teacher attracts the children very much in the school.

2. **Internal factors:** The internal factors are concerned with the individual. So, these are also called subjective factors.
   a. **Interest:** We are interested in some things and disinterested in other things. Interesting things draw our attention soon. An engineer and a botanist going down the same path will attend entirely different things on the way. The engineer's attention will be on the buildings and the botanist's attention will be on the trees.
   b. **Desire:** A person's desire becomes a cause of paying attention to a thing. For example, a person has to desire of buying a hammer. There are many things available in a market, but when he goes to a shop where hammers are available.
   c. **Motives:** Basic motives are important in drawing attention. Human motives, e.g., hunger, thirst, sex, safety, etc., play a vital role in drawing attention. A thirsty person's attention is always on where water is available.
   d. **Aim/goal:** Every man has some immediate aim and ultimate goal in their life. The immediate aim of a student is to pass the examination while his ultimate goal may be to become a doctor. The student, whose goal is not to pass the examination, will not be concerned with textbooks or notes, etc., but who has the aim to pass in the examination, will at once attend to them.
   e. **Habit:** Habit is also a vital determinant of attention. The kind of habit we find in our life, our attention is drawn to such things. If a person has a habit to play cricket, his attention is always drawn to it, and he will listen to cricket commentaries with attention.
   f. **Past experience**: If we know by our past experience that a particular person is sincere to us, we shall pay attention to whatever he advises us. If our experience is contrary, we shall not attend even to his most serious advice.

   Apart from these above factors, *aptitude, attitude, mental set, disposition, temperament,* etc., are also internal factors.

Inattention

As a matter of fact, there are two fields of consciousness—the fields of attention and inattention. The field of *attention is in the center of consciousness* and that of *inattention to the edge consciousness.* The things on the edge of consciousness influence the mind to some extent, but our attention is not diverted to them.

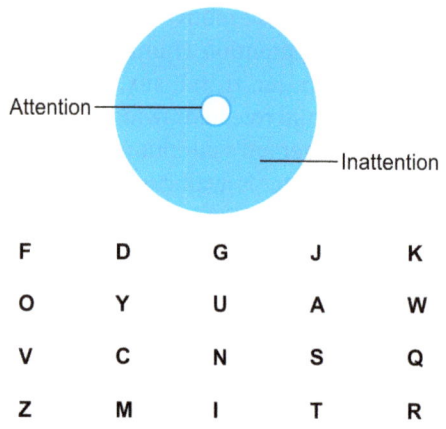

Fig. 4: Example of attention and inattention.

Twenty letters of alphabet are given in **Figure 4**. If we pay attention to the alphabet "N," then other letters are overlooked and if we pay attention to the alphabet "A," then attention is diverted from other alphabets, etc. Now we have attention on alphabet "A" and inattention on other alphabets. Inattention is required for attention. If we want to pay attention to a thing, we will have to overlook other things. If a student wants to pay attention to his lesson, then it is necessary that he diverts his attention from other things.

Theories of Attention

1. **Broadbent's filter theory**: This theory proposes that information from senses passes "in parallel" to short-term store, a temporary "buffer system" which holds information until that can be processed further and effectively extends the duration of the stimulus. Then, the information passes through a selective filter, which operates on the basis of the information's physical characteristics, "selecting one source" for further analysis and rejecting all others. The information allowed through the filter is analyzed in that it is recognized, possibly rehearsed to the motor effectors (muscles), producing an appropriate response (**Fig. 5**).

2. **Treisman's attenuation model:** According to Treisman competing information is analyzed for things other than its physical properties, including sounds, syllable patterns, grammatical structure, and the information's meaning. He suggested that the non-shadowed message is not filtered out early on, but that the selective filter attenuates it. So, a message that is not selected on the basis of its physical properties and would not be rejected completely, its "volume" would be "turned down." Both the non-attenuated and attenuated information undergo further analyses and response is processed (**Fig. 6**).

3. **Deutsch-Norman theory of focused attention:** This theory completely rejected Broadbent's claim that the information is filtered out early on. According to the Deutsch–Norman model, filtering or selecting only occurs after all inputs have been recognized by the memory system and analyzed for meaning. The filter is placed nearer the response end of the processing system. Hence, it is a late selection filter. Some information have been established as more pertinent and have activated particular memory

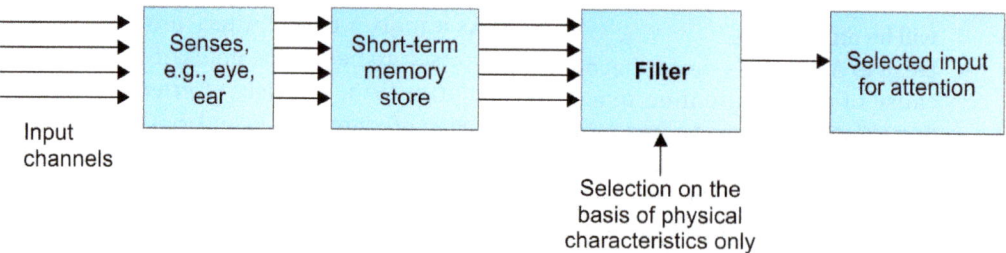

Fig. 5: Broadbent's filter theory.

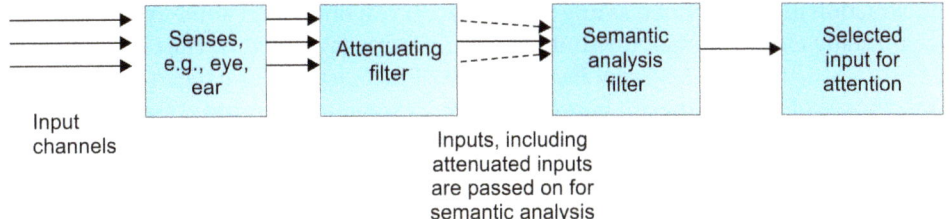

Fig. 6: Treisman's attenuation model.

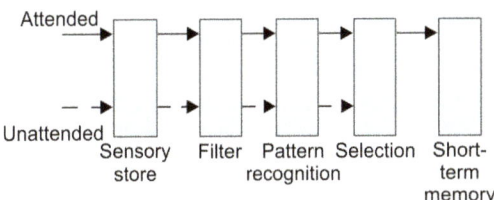

Fig. 7: Deutsch–Norman model of selective attention.

representations. When one memory is selected for further processing, attention becomes selective (**Fig. 7**).

Factors Affecting Attention

a. **Personal factors:** Physical illness, mental illness, fatigue, boredom, restlessness, abnormalities in sense organs, and other health-related issues have great effect on attention.
b. **Environmental factors:** Stressful and challenging situations such as the death of loved ones, parental divorce, and parental separation cause difficulty in focusing.
c. **Personality factors:** Certain kinds of personalities such as avoidant and antisocial types have problems concentrating and focusing.

These factors often lead to inattentiveness and an individual is not able to concentrate and this phenomenon can also be called distraction.

Span of Attention

Span of attention refers to the number of objects, letters, and digits one can attend to in a fraction of a second so as to exclude eye movement or counting. —*Prem Praksh*

The extent or limit of the ability of a person to attend to concentrate on something, the length of time which a reader can concentrate on what he is reading without thinking of anything else is called span of attention.

It varies with age, physical, mental and emotional condition, and nature of material read. Attention brings an object into consciousness. The number of objects that can be brought into consciousness at a time is called the span of attention. On an average, span of attention of a child is limited to 4–5 whereas for adults it is within 6–7 letters or digits.

Tachistoscope is the apparatus used for determining the span of attention. It is a device that displays an image for a specific amount of time. It can be used to increase recognition speed, to show something too fast to be consciously recognized, or to test which elements of an image are memorable.

■ DISTRACTION

Distraction means the driving of attention or some *interference in attention*. For example, when one is studying, the sound of a song or noise breaks in upon attention. The object which causes the distraction is called *distractor*.

Definition

Distraction may be defined as any stimulus whose presence interferes with the process of attention or draws away attention from the object to which we wish to attend.

—*HR Bhatia*

A distraction may be defined as any factor which normally tends to break up attention.
—*Prem Prakash*

The sources of distraction can be roughly divided into external and internal sources.

External factors: These are also called ***environmental factors***. These are more common and prominent. Noise, music, improper lighting, uncomfortable seats, inadequate ventilation, defective method of teaching, improper use of teaching aids, defective voice of the teacher, etc., are the common external distractors in the classrooms.

Internal factors: Emotional disturbances, ill-health, anger, fear, feeling of insecurity, boredom, lack of motivation, feeling of fatigue, lack of interest, unrelated subject matter, etc., are examples of internal distractors.

Forms of Distraction

Continuous distraction: As the name suggests, it is the continuous distraction of attention, e.g., the sound of radio or gramophone played continuously, the noise of marketplace, etc. Experiments say that adjustment to continuous distraction takes place quickly.

Discontinuous distraction: This type of distraction is irregular, being interspersed with intervals, e.g., the hearing of somebody's voice every now and then. It interferes with work because of the impossibility of adjustment.

Methods of Eliminating Distraction

- Much emphasis and importance must be given to the task.
- Create favorable and comfortable situations.
- Make lessons or work interesting and train individuals in concentration.
- Remove the distracting objects from the environment.
- If you encounter some type of distraction every day you must start ignoring it.
- Practice relaxation techniques.
- Use visual reminders and plan things beforehand.
- Stop multitasking.

Nursing Implications

- The nurse must be attentive while taking care of a patient and must receive necessary instructions from the attending doctors, change of shift, etc.
- Overcome the obstacles of attention by removing internal or external distractions.
- Attention is a very essential quality in providing nursing care to the patients, planning the care, and especially for those requiring highly complex care.
- It is very important to pay attention to the subtle changes taking place in patients' health status and report it immediately to the concerned doctor to avoid adverse health events and avoid unnecessary hospitalization.
- It helps the nurse to concentrate by focusing consciousness on one object at a time rather than two.
- It helps the nurse for better organization of the perceptual field for maximum clarity and understanding of the patient's condition.

■ PERCEPTION

Perceptions vary from person to person. Different people perceive different things about the same situation. But more than that, we assign different meanings to what we perceive. And, the meanings might change for a certain person.

Definition

The process by which we recognize, interpret, or give meaning to the information provided by the sense organ is called perception.

Perception is the process by which sensory information is actively organized

UNIT VI: Cognitive Psychology

Flowchart 2: Perception gives meaning to sensation.

and interpreted by the brain, the process of selecting, organizing, and interpreting raw sensory data into useful mental representations of the world **(Flowchart 2)**.

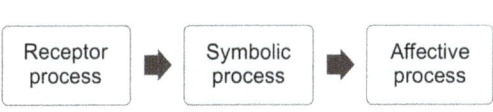

Fig. 8: Process of perception.

Process of Perception

The process of perception involves **(Fig. 8)**
- **Receptor process:** Perception not only depends upon the mental set but also upon the forms of stimulation, the receptor functions (all five senses), and neural functions.
- **Symbolic process:** The sensory stimulations create images, sensations, or ideas (known as symbols) derived from past experiences, e.g., recalling the present situation by learning through past experiences.
- **Affective process:** When we perceive an object, the pleasantness or unpleasantness for the percept (the object which we perceive) may arise due to the past experience or due to the very nature of the percept.

Factors/Determinants Influencing Perceptions

1. **Motivation:** The need and desire of a perceiver strongly influence her/his perception. People want to fulfill their needs and desires through various means. For example, when hungry persons were shown ambiguous pictures, they were found to perceive them as food objects more than satisfied (non-hungry) persons.
2. **Expectation:** The expectations about what we might perceive in a given situation also influence our perception. This phenomenon of perceptual familiarization or perceptual generalization reflects a strong tendency to see what we expect to see even when the results do not accurately reflect external reality. For example, if our milkman arrives daily at 6:00 in the morning to deliver the milk then any knocking at the door at this time is likely to be perceived as the presence of a milkman.
3. **Cognitive sets:** It refers to a consistent way of dealing with our environment. It significantly affects the way we perceive the environment. There are several cognitive styles that people use in perceiving the environment, one most extensively used in the studies is the field-dependent and field-independent cognitive styles. Field-dependent people perceive the external world in its totality, i.e., in a holistic manner. Field-independent people perceive the external world by breaking it into small units, i.e., in a differentiated.
4. **Cultural background and experiences:** Different experiences and learning opportunities available to people in different cultural settings also influence their perception. A person depends on his/her personal, social, and cultural

conditions. Due to these factors, our perceptions are not only finely turned but also modified.

Principles of Perception

1. **The principle of proximity:** The objects that are close together in space or time are perceived as belonging together or as a group. Even if the individual items do not have any connection with each other they will be grouped under a single pattern or perceived as a meaningful picture.
2. **The principle of similarity:** The objects that are similar to one another and have similar characteristics are perceived as a group. Stimuli that have the same size, shape, and color tend to be perceived as parts of the pattern.
3. **The principle of continuity:** This principle states that we tend to perceive objects as belonging together if they appear to form a continuous pattern. Anything which extends itself into a space in the same shape, size, and color without a break is perceived as a whole figure.
4. **The principle of smallness:** According to this principle, smaller area tends to be seen as figures against a larger background.
5. **The principle of symmetry:** This principle states that symmetrical areas tend to be seen as figures against an asymmetrical background.
6. **The principle of surroundedness:** According to this principle, the areas surrounded by others tend to be perceived as figures.
7. **The principle of closure:** We tend to fill the gaps in stimulation and perceive the objects as a whole rather than their separate parts.

Gestalt Principles/Laws of Perception (Fig. 9)

1. **Formation of a figure:** There are some factors that would bring some order to perception.
2. **Nearness:** Stimuli that are near to each other tend to be grouped together.
3. **Similarity:** Stimuli that are similar in size, shape, color, or form tend to be grouped together.
4. **Continuation or continuity:** Perception tends toward simplicity and continuity.
5. **Closure:** It refers to the tendency to complete a figure, so that it has a consistent overall form.

Types of Perception

We perceive objects in different manners as compared to their position in the environment. Objects may be moving or static when we have to perceive motion. We may have to locate sounds and voices in the space around us.

1. **Form perception:** Gestaltists proposed laws of organization that specify how people perceive form. Figure and ground are basic organizational themes for perception **(Fig. 10)**.
   Figure is perceived as distinct from the background. Figure is closer to the viewer than the background. Reversible figures: Figure and ground can be switched.
2. **Size perception:** Three types of constancy are explained briefly here:
   a. **Size constancy:** Size constancy is the tendency to perceive objects in a consistent manner despite the changing sensations that are received by our senses. Visual constancy plays an important role in helping us adapt to our environment successfully. Learning plays an important role in the development of constancy. Once we know that certain objects in our environment have certain characteristics, we tend to perceive them in the same way, regardless of the conditions under which they are perceived. When we know that an object is of a certain size, we tend to perceive it as being that same size, regardless of how far it is from our eyes. In size constancy, the perceiver has the

UNIT VI: Coginitive Psychology

1. Proximity
Elements which are close together seem to be a group

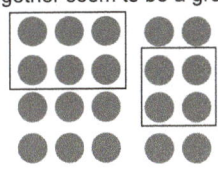

2. Closure
The human brain ingores gaps and tries to understand the bigger context

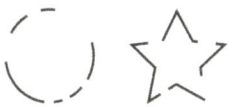

3. Similarity
Elements which look similar seem to be a group

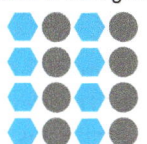

4. Common region
Elements which are close together seem to be a group

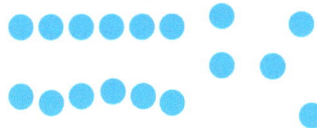

5. Continuity
Elements which are ordered in a line or curve seem to be a group

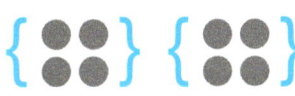

6. Figure and ground
The human brain instinctively recognizes if something is in the fore- or background

7. Symmetry
Symmetric elements give the human brain the feeling that everything is ordered

8. Common fate
Elements which move in the same direction seem to be a group

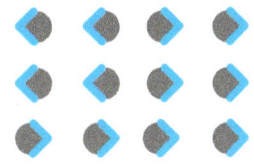

Fig. 9: Gestalt principles.

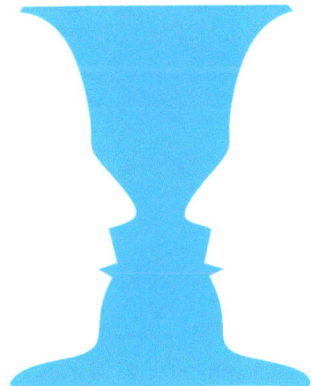

Fig. 10: Figure ground perception.

ability to judge true or measured size, regardless of the distance involved.

b. **Shape constancy:** When we know that the object is a certain shape, we tend to perceive it as the same shape, regardless of the viewing angle.

We have learned to make corrections in our perception depending on the angle from which we observe.

c. **Color constancy:** Colors of objects tend to remain constant in perception when we know their true color. Visual objects also appear constant in their degree of whiteness, greyness, and blackness.

3. **Depth perception**: The ability to view the world in three dimensions and to perceive distance is known as depth perception. "This ability helps to perceive three-dimensional space and to accurately judge distance."

4. **Perception of movement**: When you ride in a moving vehicle and look out the side window, the objects you see outside appear to be moving in the opposite direction. Objects very far away, such as the moon and the sun, appear to move in the same direction as the viewer.

Movement or motion is perceived by following the progressive change of an object's position in space with time. It has two types.
   a. Real movement: The perception of the actual movement of objects in the world is termed as "real motion/movement perception."
   b. Apparent movement: It is the movement perceived in the absence of physical movement of an image across the retina. This can be produced by a rapid succession of motionless stimuli that minimize the changes that occur in real movement.
5. **Time perception:** We perceive time in seconds, minutes, and hours which pass into days, weeks, months, and years and even in centuries. Time is perceived in terms of past, present, and future. Perception of time is less in children than elders.

Factors Influencing Perception

1. **Past experience:** Perception of present stimulus is influenced not only by the immediate stimulus alone but by effects of previous stimuli or past experiences.
2. **Needs, values, and motives:** These organize our perception.
3. **Mental set and attitude:** It is a readiness or alertness to observe a particular stimulus or make a specific response to a stimulus.
4. **Mood and emotions:** Our perception of the world is also influenced by our mood and emotions. For example, in a pleasant mood, the food appears to be delicious.
5. **Cultural influences:** Due to man's psychological level of adjustment, cultural factors cannot be ignored.
6. **Perceptual constancy:** The individual perceives size, color, shape, and brightness of the percept.

Errors/Abnormalities in Perception

Illusion

Our perceptions are not always as they exist. Sometimes we fail to interpret the sensory info correctly. This results in a mismatch between the physical stimuli and its perception. These misperceptions resulting from misinterpretation of information received by our sensory organs are generally known as illusion.

Universal Illusion

Some perceptual illusions are universal and found in all individuals (rail track); these illusions are called universal illusion/permanent illusion as they do not change with experience or practice.

Personal Illusion

Some other illusions are seen to vary from individual to individual; hence they are called personal illusion (**Table 1**).

Table 1: Difference between hallucination and illusion.

Hallucination	Illusion
1. False perception	1. Merely misperceptions
2. Reacts on internal stimuli	2. Responds to real external stimuli
3. Experienced personally and uniquely	3. Often experienced universally
4. Generally abnormal	4. Generally normal
5. Difficult to be researched	5. Can be measured, observed, and researchable
6. Originates internally	6. Originates externally
7. Associated with mental disorders	7. Not associated with mental disorders
8. Has more types	8. Has lesser types
9. Not linked with arts or entertainment	9. Highly associated with the arts and entertainments
10. Has a negative connotation due to its link with pathology	10. Learns toward a +ve connotation with its relevance to design magic, tricks, and the likes

Alterations in Perception

Since so much information in the classroom and at home is presented visually and/or verbally the child with an auditory or visual perceptual disorder can be at a great disadvantage in certain situations.

- Visual processing/perceptual disorder refers to hindered ability to make sense of information taken in through the eyes. This is different from problems involving sight or sharpness of vision. Difficulties with visual processing affect how visual information is interpreted or processed by the brain. The common areas of difficulty are:
  - *Spatial relation:* It refers to the position of objects in space with reference to other objects. For instance, reading and math are the two subjects that rely heavily on the use of symbols (letters, numbers, punctuation, math signs). The child is unable to perceive words and numbers as separate units, directionality problems in reading and math, confusion of similarly shaped letters such b/d/q/p.
  - *Visual discrimination:* This is the ability to differentiate objects based on their individual characteristics. It becomes a disorder when the child is unable to recognize common objects and symbols, with attributes including color, form, pattern, size, and position.
  - *Object recognition (visual agnosia):* Many children are unable to visually recognize objects which are familiar to them, or even objects which are familiar to them, or even objects which they can recognize through their other senses, such as touch or smell.
- **Auditory processing disorder:** It interferes with an individual's ability to analyze or make sense of information taken in through the ears. This is different from problems involving hearing such as deafness or being hard of hearing. This does not affect what is heard by ears but does affect how this information is interpreted or processed by the brain. It can interfere directly with speech and language but can affect all areas of learning, especially reading and spelling.

Implications in Nursing

- The nurse should know the perception, sensation, and its principles.
- She must relate normal with abnormal perception.
- This knowledge will help to identify any perceptual problem in hospital, community, and school health.
- She suspects a problem might be present or developing, in which the concerning behavior is taking place.
- In the school, she speaks to the child's teacher and other professionals who interact with the child to see if they are similar behaviors shown by the child or the child has similar concerns.
- She helps to identify strengths and weaknesses to recommend accommodations and strategies to best facilitate the child's learning. As a nurse educator, she understands the perceptual learning of each student nurse. If needed, she finds the factors influencing perception and provides counseling services.
- She arranges a meeting with the school professionals involved in the child's education to make plans for meeting the specific needs of the child.
- She educates the parents and family members regarding perceptual problems and the ways to improve the perception.
- She identifies and differentiates illusion and hallucination among mentally ill patients and hence provides significant nursing care to them.

■ LEARNING

Learning starts from the moment of birth and continues till death. For successful adjustment with life, an individual has to acquire knowledge about many things and change his behavior according to the needs of the situation. The child starts to understand the world around him through learning.

The language development, development of basic values, and knowledge regarding various aspects of life—all come through learning or training. The process of learning has, therefore, tremendous importance for human beings and for some animals to live and exist. Without learning, life becomes completely meaningless; the capacity to adjust becomes nil.

Definitions of Learning

It is acquiring of knowledge learning is the acquisition of new behavior or the strengthening or weakening of old behavior as the result of experience.—Henry-P-Smith

Learning is the acquisition of habits, knowledge and attitude.

—Crow and Crow

Learning is relatively permanent change in behavior brought about by experience.

—Rod Plotnik

Learning is defined as any relatively permanent change in behavior which occurs as a result of practice and experience.

—Morgan and King

Nature and Characteristics

- Learning is a process.
- It involves all the experiences from birth to death; produces change in behavior.
- Learning makes change in behavior either positive or negative.
- Learning prepares an individual for adjustment and adaptation.
- All learning is purposeful and goal-oriented.
- The slope of learning is too wide.
- Learning is universal and it is continuous.
- Learning does not include those changes that occur as part of maturity, drugs, etc.

Types of Learning

1. **Verbal learning:** It helps to acquire verbal behavior resulting in speaking language and the use of communication devices. Signs, pictures, symbols, words, figures, sounds, voices, etc.
2. **Conceptual learning:** It is a form of mental image which denotes a generalized idea about things, persons, or events.
3. **Motor learning:** Driving a car, flying a plane, drawing using equipment, etc.
4. **Problem-solving:** It is a higher type of learning. It requires the use of reasoning, thinking, imagination, generalization, etc.
5. **Serial learning:** It is learning alphabets, multiplication table, the name of states in the country, list of the prime ministers and presidents, etc.
6. **Paired-associate learning:** Learning of something in association with something else. Ganga = River Ganga, Kishanpur = Lord Krishna.

Factors Influencing Learning

Learning depends upon three main factors.
1. **Nature of the learner**
    a. **Age:** Age can influence the capability of learning. A child cannot learn the things that elders can and an aged person will have difficulty learning modern ways of knowledge.
    b. **Intelligence:** Intelligence effects very much on learning; if the subject has a maximum level of intelligence he can learn more and easily at maximum level.
    c. **Attention:** If a person does not pay attention to how to learn specific knowledge, skill, or experience, he cannot learn easily. But if the individual pays attention, the results are vice versa.
    d. **Interest and motivation:** The subject has intelligence and can also pay attention toward learning but he does not have an interest in how to learn a specific knowledge, skill, or experience. Therefore, the level or process of learning would be very slow.

e. **Mental and physical health:** If an individual does not have mental health or a physical one, the subject can fulfill the demands of the process of learning due to his weak mental and physical capabilities.
   f. **Fatigue and rest:** If an individual is tired, he cannot pay full attention to learning something. So, he/she needs to take rest in between his/her studies.
2. **Nature of learning material:** If the knowledge is interesting in nature, meaningful, clearly printed, and written in easily understandable language and pattern, etc., any individual can learn it efficiently.
3. **Nature of learning method:**
   a. **Definite goal:** It enhances motivation if clear goals are written or are in mind.
   b. **Recitation:** It is a more effective tool of learning, if an individual recites something louder he can learn more effectively.
   c. **Exercise and repetition:** Single act is learned in a single trial but complex acts require repeated trials. If a material is difficult to learn, it can be learned through exercises or repeated trials.
   d. **By parts learning:** If the material is very long, it can be divided into small parts, so an individual can learn specific knowledge, skill, etc., more effectively.
   e. **Reward and punishment:** The presence of reward or punishment can affect learning. Generally, reward is more effective in promoting learning than punishment. Punishment does have some effects on learning. It tends to repress the desired response rather than extinguish it.
   f. **Knowledge of results or psychological feedback:** Frequent and regular review of the amount of progress being made toward the goal acts as a strong motive to promote continuing effort on the part of the learner.

Types of Learning Styles

It is divided based on the type of the learner.

- **Visual learners (learn through seeing):** These learners need to see the teacher's body language, hand gestures, eye contact, and facial expression to fully understand the content of a lesson. They tend to prefer sitting at the front of the classroom to avoid visual obstruction. For example, if a visual learner is only presented with verbal information he/she will absorb and retain less information than if the verbal instructions were combined with visual materials. Tools used are books, videos, computers, posters, etc.
- **Auditory learners (learn through listening):** Individuals learn best through verbal lectures, discussions, talking things through, and listening to what others have to say. They interpret the underlying meanings of speech through listening to the tone of the voice, pitch, speed, and other nuances. Tools used are talks, discussions, and debates.
- **Tactile/kinesthetic learners (learn through moving, doing, and touching):** These learners learn best through a hands-on approach, actively exploring the physical world around them. They may find it hard to sit still for long period and may become distracted by their need for activity and exploration. The tools used are skits, drama, and art.

The Learning Process

Learning is essentially changed behavior due to experience and certain elements must be presented for learning to take place. The elements of the learning process are:

- Goal or goals related to the motivation
- **Stimulus:** The response is produced by the type of stimuli.
- **Perception:** The person learns things by visual, auditory, or kinesthetic learning.
- **Response:** Whether it is a negative, positive, or neutral response.

- **Consequence:** Practice/skill should be able to produce change in behavior.
- **Integration:** Association of new behaviors with previously learned behaviors is related to the transfer of learning.

Theories of Learning

The major classifications are:

1. Trial and Error Theory of Learning

This was the first scientific study of learning by American Psychologist Edward L Thorndike (1874-1949), considered as the father of educational psychology, who conducted a series of experiments on animal learning and came out with conclusion that animals have no rational faculty in learning. They do not learn by reasoning but by trial and error. Animals go on hitting the target by impulse or learn out of "hit and miss," known as trial and error learning.

It is the result of his experiments performed on chickens, rats, and cats. He put a hungry cat in a puzzle box. There was only one door. A fish was kept outside. The door was latched. The repeated movements made the door open. He repeated the experiment many times. The cat learned how to remove the latch and open the door **(Fig. 11)**.

Summary of the experiment
a. **Drive**—intensified hunger due to the sight of the food
b. **Goal**—to get the food from outside the box
c. **Block**—closed-door/latch
d. **Random movements**—trying to get out of the box
e. **Chance success**—first opening of the door
f. **Selection**—recognizing the right movements to open the door/latch
g. **Fixation**—learn to open the door

Laws of learning based on the experiment conducted

a. **The law of readiness:** Learning takes place when the person has the readiness to learn. Motivation is important in learning. The physical and mental readiness is more important in learning.
b. **The law of exercise/use and disuse or practice:** Learning takes place through repetition and practice. Nursing skills

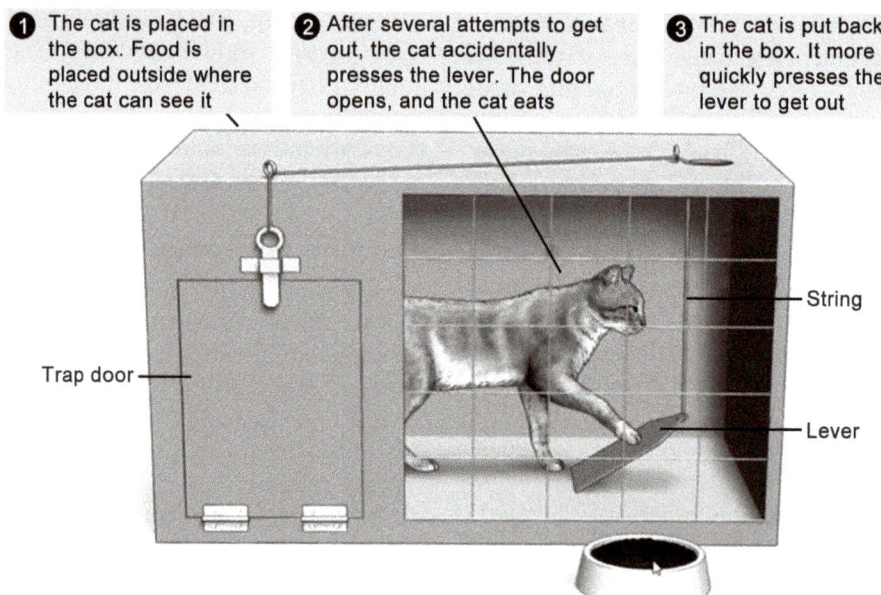

Fig. 11: Edward L Thorndike's law of effect.

learning. Classroom teaching is only an introduction.

c. **The law of effect/satisfaction and dissatisfaction:** Feeling is important, effect is important; satisfaction makes us confident, feeling of self-worth.

2. Theory of Insight Learning

It is typical human learning and includes cognitive processes. It is a type of learning or problem-solving that happens all of a sudden, by understanding the relationships between various parts of the problem rather than through trial and error. Learners have to plan and execute actions before they get endangered. It includes a holistic view of the situation and the generalization of conclusions. The main propagator of this theory is Kohler.

He did an experiment on chimpanzee called Sultan using boxes to reach banana (different sized boxes) and using boxes and stick to reach banana (longer and shorter sticks). This experiment follows some principles such as:
a. Identifying the problem
b. Organizing the pain of action
c. Using insight **(Fig. 12)**

3. Learning by Observation

We learn behavior through observation in addition to trial and error or insightful learning. A child may understand the effect of a wrong behavior by seeing his friend getting punished for the same. Children learn and imitate behavior they observe in other people or family members. Not all observed behavior is learned. Learning by observation mainly includes the aspects such as attention, retention, reproduction, and motivation.

4. Learning by Conditioning

Most of the learning takes place through conditioning such as sucking at the sight of milk bottle, making grimaces in response to a dislike, and smiling in response to other's smile. The mechanism of conditioning is mainly classified into:

a. **Classical conditioning:** It is a learning process that occurs when two stimuli are repeatedly paired. A response that is at first elicited by the second stimulus is eventually elicited by the first stimulus alone.

b. **Operant conditioning:** It is a type of learning where behavior is controlled by the consequences. Key concepts in operant conditioning are positive reinforcement, negative reinforcement, positive punishment, and negative punishment.

A. Classical Conditioning

Classical conditioning was discovered by Ivan Pavlov in the 1900s. Classical conditioning is a form of learning in which people (or any organism) learn to associate two stimuli that occur in sequence. Classical conditioning occurs when a person forms a mental association between two stimuli so that encountering one stimulus means the person thinks of the other (**Fig. 13 and Table 2**).

Similar Experiment by Watson
Watson took one infant called Albert. The baby was given a rabbit to play with. The baby was happy and pleasant. He created a loud noise to frighten the boy as soon as the baby touched the rabbit. The baby was frightened. He repeated it a number of times. Slowly the baby feared the rabbit and never came near it. This supports the theory of classical conditioning.

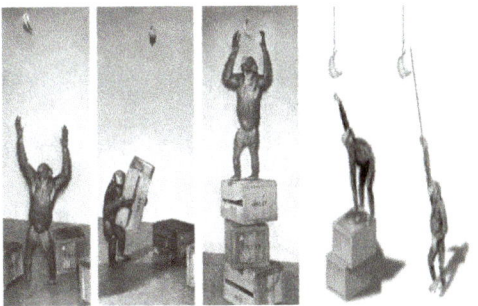

Fig. 12: Theory of insight learning.

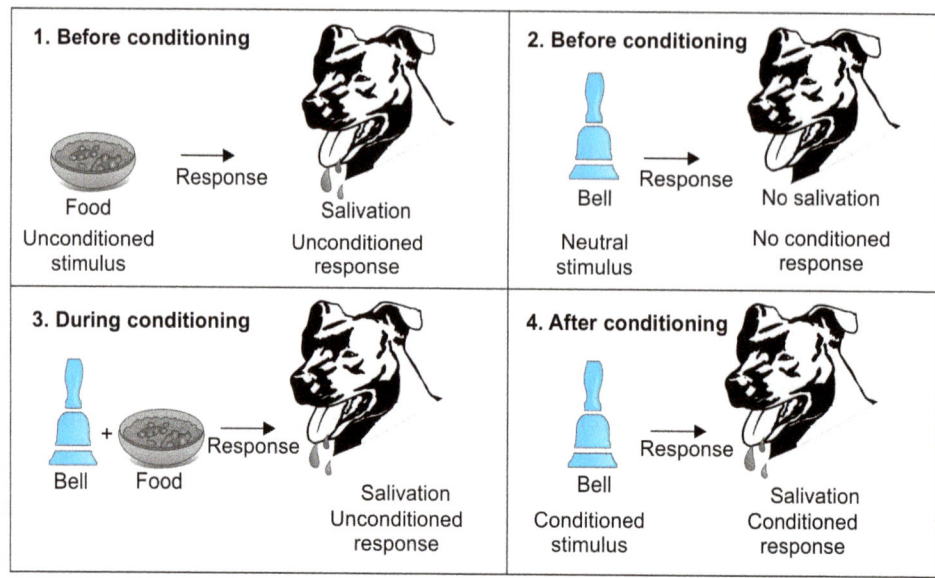

Classical conditioning

Fig. 13: Pavlov's experiments.

Table 2: Terminologies used.	
Condition	To make people or animals act or react in a particular way by gradually getting them used to a specific pattern of events
Neutral stimulus	A stimulus that, before conditioning, has no effect on the desired response
Unconditioned stimulus (UCS)	A stimulus that brings about a response without having been learned
Unconditioned response (UCR)	A response that is natural and needs no training
Conditioned stimulus (CS)	Once neutral stimulus that has been paired with an unconditioned stimulus to bring about a response formerly caused only by the unconditioned stimulus
Conditioned response (CR)	A response that, after conditioning, follows a previously neutral stimulus

Principle of Classical Conditioning Process

- **Acquisition:** The acquisition phase is the initial learning of the conditioned response, e.g., the dog learning to salivate at the sound of the bell.
- **Extinction:** Extinction is used to describe the elimination of the conditioned response by repeatedly presenting the conditioned stimulus without the unconditioned stimulus. If a dog has learned to salivate at the sound of a bell, an experimenter can gradually extinguish the dog's response by repeatedly ringing the bell without presenting food afterward.
- **Spontaneous recovery:** Extinction does not mean, however, that the dog has simply unlearned or forgotten the association between the bell and the food. After extinction, if the experimenter lets a few hours pass and then rings the

bell again, the dog will usually salivate at the sound of the bell once again. The reappearance of an extinguished response after some time has passed is called spontaneous recovery.

- **Generalization:** After an animal has learned a conditioned response to one stimulus, it may also respond to similar stimuli without further training. If a child is bitten by a large black dog, the child may fear not only that dog but also the other large dogs. This phenomenon is called generalization. Less similar stimuli will usually produce less generalization. For example, the child may show little fear of smaller dogs.
- **Discrimination:** The opposite of generalization is discrimination, in which an individual learns to produce a conditioned response to one stimulus but not to another stimulus that is similar. For example, a child may show a fear response to freely roaming dogs but may show no fear when a dog is on a leash or confined to a pen.

Application of Classical Conditioning
- Classical conditioning explains some cases of phobias, which are irrational or excessive fears of specific objects or situations.
- Classical conditioning explains many emotional responses such as happiness, excitement, anger, and anxiety that people have to specific stimuli.
- Classical conditioning procedures are used to treat phobias and other unwanted behaviors such as alcoholism and addictions.
- To treat phobias of specific objects, the therapist gradually and repeatedly presents the feared object to the patient while the patient relaxes.
- Through extinction, the patient loses his or her fear of the object.
- In one treatment for alcoholism, patients drink an alcoholic beverage and then ingest a drug that produces nausea.
- Eventually, they feel nauseous at the sight or smell of alcohol and stop drinking it.

B. Operant Conditioning
Operant or instrumental conditioning is a type of learning in which voluntary behavior is strengthened if it is reinforced and weakened if it is punished. The term "operant conditioning" refers to the fact that the learner must operate or perform a certain behavior before receiving a reward or punishment. American psychologist BF Skinner became one of the most famous psychologists in history for his pioneering research on operant conditioning.

BF Skinner experiments: He designed a special puzzle box. It had a lever that when pressed provided a cup of water/food. Each time the lever was pressed a sound also was created. He put a hungry/thirsty rat in the cage. At regular intervals, he used to press the lever and feed the rat. Few a time later the rat started doing it by itself whenever it felt hungry/thirsty. The sound associated with it and food/water acted as positive reinforcement (**Fig. 14**).

Principles of Operant Conditioning
Reinforcement: It refers to any process that strengthens a particular behavior that will occur again.
- **Positive reinforcement:** Positive reinforcement is a method of strengthening behavior by following it with a pleasant stimulus.
- **Negative reinforcement:** Negative reinforcement is a method of strengthening a behavior by following it with the removal or omission of an unpleasant stimulus.

Punishment: Punishment weakens a behavior, reducing the chances that the behavior will occur again (**Fig. 15**).
- **Positive:** Involves reducing a behavior by delivering an unpleasant stimulus if the behavior occurs.

UNIT VI: Cognitive Psychology

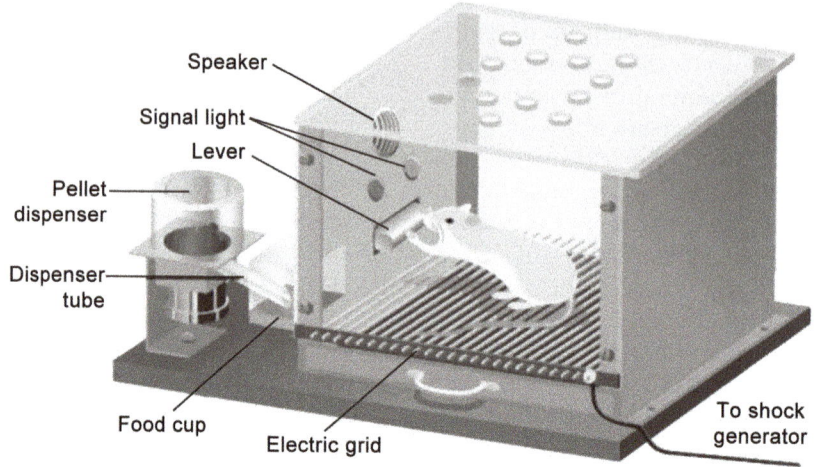

Fig. 14: BF Skinner experiments.

	Positive	Negative
Reinforcement	Positive reinforcement (adding something to the equation to make a behavior more likely to occur in the future)	Negative reinforcement (removing something from the equation to make a behavior more likely to occur in the future)
Punishment	Positive punishment (adding something to the equation to make a behavior less likely to occur in the future)	Negative punishment (removing something from the equation to make a behavior less likely to occur in the future)

Fig. 15: Positive and negative reinforcement.

❖ **Negative:** Involves reducing a behavior by removing a pleasant stimulus if the behavior occurs.

Shaping: It is a reinforcement technique that is used to teach animals or people behaviors that they have never performed before.

In this method, the teacher begins by reinforcing a response the learner can perform easily, and then gradually requires a more and more difficult response.

For example, to teach a rat to press a lever that is over its head, the trainer can first reward any upward head movements, then an upward movement of at least 1 inch, then 2 inches, and so on, until the rat reaches the lever.

Extinction: It is the elimination of a learned behavior by discontinuing the reinforcement of that behavior.
❖ A behavior learned is not always permanent.
❖ If a rat has learned to press a lever because it receives food for doing so, its lever-pressing will decrease and eventually disappear if food is no longer delivered.

Generalization: It occurs in operant conditioning in much the same way that they do in classical conditioning.
❖ In generalization, people perform a behavior learned in one situation in other similar situations.
❖ For example, a man who is rewarded with laughter when he tells certain jokes at a bar may tell the same jokes at restaurants, parties, or wedding receptions.

Discrimination is learning where behavior will be reinforced in one situation but not in another. The man may learn that telling his jokes in church or at a serious business meeting will not make people laugh.

UNIT VI: Coginitive Psychology

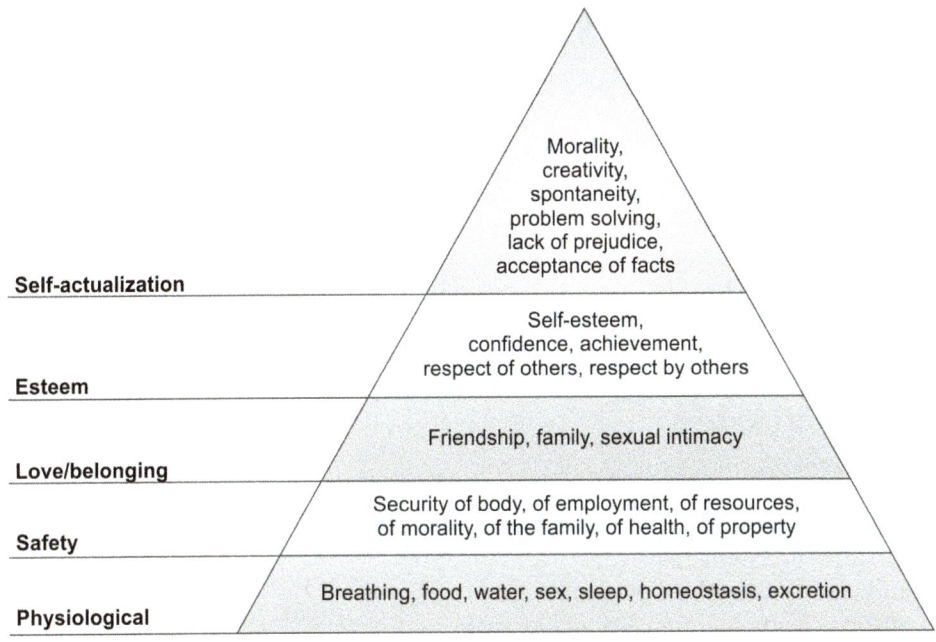

Fig. 16: Humanistic theories of learning.

Application of Operant Conditioning
- Behavior therapists use shaping techniques to teach basic job skills to adults with mental retardation.
- Therapists use reinforcement techniques to teach self-care skills to people with severe mental illnesses such as schizophrenia and use punishment and extinction to reduce aggressive and antisocial behaviors by these individuals.
- To treat stuttering, marital problems, drug addictions, impulsive spending, eating disorders, and many other behavioral problems.

Humanistic Theories of Learning

This theory is propagated by Abraham Maslow. The behavior is the struggle to satisfy the different levels of need as given in **Figure 16**.

Roger's Theory of Learning

It is also basically the subtype of humanistic theory. Roger distinguished two types of learning as cognitive and experimental learning. Cognitive learning is meaningless unless it is applied, e.g., mathematics, history, geography. Experimental learning includes personal involvement. It is self-initiated, self-evaluated. He believed in the strength and potentials of human beings such as natural learning inclination and interest. The role of teachers, parents, and well-wishers in learning is to help the learner in changing desire for personal change and motivation. The learning should care and facilitate growth and development according to their requirement.

Roger classifies the role of a teacher as:
1. Making favorable and positive environment
2. Making clear objectives of the learning
3. Organizing learning resources
4. Balancing intellectual and emotional components of learning
5. Sharing the feeling and thoughts of the learner

The symbols of good learning are:
1. Minimum threat to the learner
2. Good participation of the learner

3. Good performance in practical, social, personal, and research areas
4. Learner develops willingness to learn and utilize self-evaluation.

Laws of Learning

Edward L Thorndike gives the laws of learning. He emphasizes on the laws of learning as essential criteria while learning and retaining and classifies them into primary and secondary laws.

Primary Laws of Learning

a. *Law of readiness:*
   - The degree of preparedness and eagerness to learn
   - Law of action tendency
   - Individuals learn best when they are ready to learn, and they will not learn much if they see no reason for learning.

   Educational implications
   - The teacher should arouse curiosity for learning so that the pupils feel ready to imbibe the new experiences.
   - The teacher should, before taking up the new lesson, arouse the interest and desire of the students to learn.

b. *Law of exercise:*
   - Things that are most often repeated are best remembered.
   - Laws of use and disease
     ◆ Laws of use: Learning is strengthened with repeated trial or practice.
     ◆ Laws of disease: Learning is weakened when trial or practice is discontinued.

   Educational implications
   - The teacher should provide different opportunities for learners to practice or repeat the task, recall, manual drill, reviews, etc.
   - The teacher should have constant practice in what has once been learned.

   Delayed use or long disuse may cause forgetfulness.

c. *Laws of effect:*
   - Learning is strengthened when it is accompanied by a pleasant or satisfying feeling.
   - Learning is weakened when it is associated with an unpleasant feeling.
   - The emotional state of the learner after the learning

   Educational implications
   - As a failure is accompanied by a discouraging emotional state, it should be avoided.
   - Reward and recognition play a great role in encouraging the pupil.
   - Punishments should be avoided as far as possible, punishment produces a negative effect, and it causes discouragement.

Secondary Laws of Learning

a. *Laws of primacy:*
   - Learning that takes place in the beginning is the best and most lasting.
   - Learning should be done correctly for the first time since it is difficult to "unlearn" or change an incorrectly learned material.

   Educational implications
   - The learning on the first day is most vivid and strong. The teacher also should be most serious on the first day of teaching.
   - For the instructor, this means that what they teach the first time must be correct. It is more difficult to un-teach a subject than to teach it correctly the first time.

b. *Law of recency*
   - Things most recently learned are best remembered, while the things learned some time ago are remembered with more difficulty. Frequent review and

summarization help fix in the mind the material covered.

Educational implications
- Instructions recognize the law of recency when they plan a lesson summary or a conclusion of the lecture. Repeat, restate, or re-emphasize important matters at the end of a lesson to make sure that the learner remembers them instead of inconsequential details.

c. *Law of intensity*
- The law of intensity states that if the stimulus (experience) is real, the more likely there is to be a change in behavior (learning).
- A vivid, dramatic, or exciting learning experience teaches more than a routine or boring experience.

Educational implications
- A learner will learn more from the real thing than from a substitute. Demonstrations, skits, and models do much to intensify the learning experiences of the learners.

Subordinate laws of learning

a. **Law of multiple responses**
- Confront with a new situation the learner responds in a variety of ways arriving at the correct response.
- Trial and error
- If the individual wants to solve a puzzle, he is to try in different ways rather than mechanically persisting in the same ways.

b. **Law of set attitude**
- Learning is guided by a total sector attitude of the learner, which determines not only what the learner will do but what will satisfy him/her.
- The learner performs the task well if he has his attitude set in the task.

c. **Law of analogy and assimilation**
- According to this law, the individual makes use of old experiences or acquisitions while learning a new situation. There is a tendency to utilize common elements in the new situation as existed in a similar past situation.

d. **Law of associative shifting**
- According to this law, we may get a response of while a learner is capable, associated with any other situation to which he is sensitive.
- Sometimes, a reaction to a certain stimulus might shift to a different one.

e. **Pre-potency of elements**
- According to this law, the learner reacts selectively to the important things in the situation and neglects the other features or elements which may be irrelevant.

Transfer of Learning

Transfer refers to the transfer of knowledge, training, and habits acquired in one situation to another situation. For example, the ability to play behavior can be transferred to play Tennis.

Types of Transfer

1. **Positive transfer:** Previous learning benefits performance or learning of new things. For example, learning basic sciences helps in learning higher education.
2. **Negative transfer:** Previous learning hinders performance or learning of new things. For example, a child learns to pronounce BUT correctly but finds difficulty pronouncing PUT in the same manner.
3. **Zero transfer:** The previous learning has no influence on other learning, e.g., learning science and arts.

HABIT FORMATION

Habits are learned behaviors and habits such as walking, dressing, eating, sitting, and daily chore activities are the results of learning. Habits are voluntary actions. A habit is extremely automatic, volitional, repetitive, and mechanical behavior of an individual which is generated with conscious effort.

Habit is derived from the Latin word "Habitus" which means to acquire something. It means acquiring any object or action or reaction.

Types of Habits

Good habits: Habits that are socially acceptable and include our routine and enhance our social and occupational functioning such as walking, sleeping pattern, studying, working, etc.

Bad habits: Habits that are not socially acceptable and disrupt one's personality such as stealing, smoking, drinking, etc.

Formation of Habits

Williams James has described certain laws of habit formation.

1. **Begin a new habit with strong and determined initiative:** Any behavior which we desire to turn into some good habit should be started with a commitment and strong efforts. Once the start is good, it will soon become a habit. For example, morning walk with full commitment to oneself and regularity will become a habit.
2. **Never allow an exception to occur till the new habit is formed:** In the formation of habit, continuity and regularity are very essential. Any break in that regularity will turn down the formation of habit. For example, if the morning walk is discontinued for 5-6 days then it is possible that later on, there will be a permanent break.
3. **Seize the opportunity to act:** It means that once the decision is taken to develop a habit it should not be delayed to bring in practical. Delaying with unnecessary excuses will turn into inhibition to perform that activity. For example, a person decided to go for a morning walk daily but keeping on postponing results in never starting of activity.
4. **Keep the faculty of effort alive in you by a little exercise every day:** It simply refers to the practice of the activity desired to develop as a habit. Thorndike's law of exercise also says that if some activity is repeated again and again, it is learned and habit is the final stage of learning.
5. **Start as early in life as possible:** It is well-known fact that activities learned in childhood never fade away. So, it is important to start developing good habits in early childhood. Such habits will be more permanent and stable. For example, good study habits in childhood help in the future.
6. **Use of rewards and punishment:** Any response which results in some kind of reward or benefit is repeated again to become the habit. So, good desirable behaviors should be rewarded to develop good habits. For example, helping others should be rewarded to make a habit. Fear of punishment can also be something that helps in the formation of habits. For example, fear of punishment from the teacher can develop the habit of doing homework daily.
7. **Emotional arousal:** Emotional arousal for certain activities can help in the formation of habits. For example, emotionally arousing a student to work hard for examinations can help to form good habits.
8. **Conditioning:** Conditioning is a method of associating a certain stimulus with a particular response. In the chapter on learning, a detailed explanation has been given. Simply, it can be said that by conditioning an association between a stimulus and response can be established. For example, lying down on the ground when firing, etc., can be associated with the feeling of fear.

Study Habits

One's habitual way of doing one's study in a particular way and style may be termed as his study habit. Scholars and psychologists have found that the following principles are to be followed as good study habits.

a. **Establishing a proper time schedule for study:** Time management is great art. It is useless to make such a comment as you are not getting enough time. We should be quite regular, devoted, and punctual to allot time for study.

b. **Observing desirable healthy habits for carrying out study in the planned time schedule:** This can be understood with the following aspects:
   1. Concentrate attention to study and preparation of study material.
   2. Adopt a desirable mode and time of note/material making.
   3. There should be no stress or dependence on the mechanical memorization of the studied material; use insight.
   4. Practice makes a man perfect. Make a habit of revising and practicing the studied material.
   5. Better to study three or four subjects in a span of time of 3 or 3 hours. The change and variety will help in creating interest.
   6. Love and respect your teachers.
   7. Maintain healthy desirable body posture and position for study. It includes the place selected for the self-study.
   8. Try to observe the principle of work and rest.
   9. Respect the individual difference (studying early morning or late night, studying in silence or in music listening, studying alone or with classmates, reading silently or reciting louder); do not feel jealous of others' ability and do not be inferior.
   10. Study, when you feel motivated, energized, and do not try to study when you feel sleepy or stressed.
   11. The best way to learn is to discuss with colleagues, teach others, and practice what you have learned.

Role of Learning in Sickness and Health

1. When a person is suffering from sickness, it may be mild or severe. So the person has to pay certain adjustments in relation to the sickness and it depends upon the severity of the health problem.
2. The patient learns new habits and new techniques to adjust to the sickness. For example, a patient with hypertension (HTN) or cardiac problem has to learn to avoid the condition of excitement. For example, a patient suffering from diabetes mellitus has to modify his eating habits and lifestyle.
3. Different types of health problems demand different types of learning. In various cases, the patient modifies his already learned pattern and in some cases learns a new behavior pattern.
4. Learning certain adjustment responses is very helpful in the recovery of the patient and in adjustment with the sickness.
5. In normal life, learning bad habits of eating and drinking can expose the body to various health problems. For example, smoking can cause cancer, drinking can develop alcoholic addiction.
6. Some people eat fixed types of food only which lead to a certain deficiency of vital alignment in the body.
7. Being sick sometimes is associated with various rewards such as avoidance of responsibility, getting sympathetic attention of others, and monitory rewards. In such a situation, the patient not only learns the sick role to keep such reward but also tends to delay the recovery (maladaptive behavior).
8. Various personality disorders such as psychopath delinquency, compulsive gambling, and criminal behavior develop with the learning of maladaptive behavior. Drug addiction is also based on learning.
9. Not only the patient learns new behavior but sometimes the people or the closed ones also have to learn to adjust to the

problem of the patient. Parents and closed ones learn to avoid any conversation with the patient which will make him incurious and angry.
10. For the disability to walking one person should always be there to help in the performance of various activities. It is also essential to learn the medication of the patient through it. Put the others also in a condition to learn many things required for the care of the patient. Sometimes the patient develops a negative type of learning in the form of deliberately adapting the sick role.

MEMORY AND FORGETTING

Learning is very important in our daily life. Without it, we cannot move forward to perform the task. Whatever we have learned, must remain in our mind, stored up somehow, and be used when the need arises.

Memory

In psychology, an organism's ability to store, retain, and subsequently retrieve information is known as "Memory." In recent decades, it has become one of the principal pillars of a branch of science called cognitive neuroscience, an interdisciplinary link between cognitive psychology and neuroscience.

Definitions

"Memory is the process of maintaining information over time." —*Matlin, 2005*

"Memory is the means by which we draw on our past experiences in order to use this information in the present."
—*Sternberg, 1999*

Memory is a key cognitive ability to exercise judgment, make decisions, or even be oriented to time and place; a person must remember past experiences.

Nature of Memory

- It is a special ability of our mind to conserve or store what has been previously experienced or acquired through learning.
- It is a complex process that involves factors such as learning, retention, recall, and recognition.
- The process of memory begins with the learning or experiencing something and ends with its revival and reproduction. Therefore, memory is said to involve four stages—learning or experiencing something, its retention, and finally its recognition and recall.

Memory Process (Fig. 17)

- **Sensory input:** Memory starts with the sensory input or stimulus from the environment. The input is received through sensory channels such as vision, hearing, or touch and is held briefly in a sensory register.
- **Short-term memory (STM):** The information is passed through the sensory register to the short-term memory store

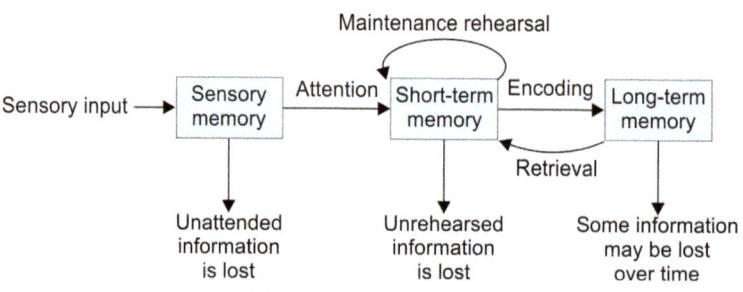

Fig. 17: Memory process.

where it is held for 20–30 seconds. Some part of the information from STM is further processed as rehearsal buffer, i.e., information is repeated and in some way linked with other information already stored in memory.

❖ **Long-term memory (LTM):** From the rehearsal buffer, the processed information is passed on to the long-term memory store where it is organized in categories and stored for years. The information not so processed is forgotten. This process can be compared with your day-to-day experiences. To learn new technical words or names, you have to rehearse several times.

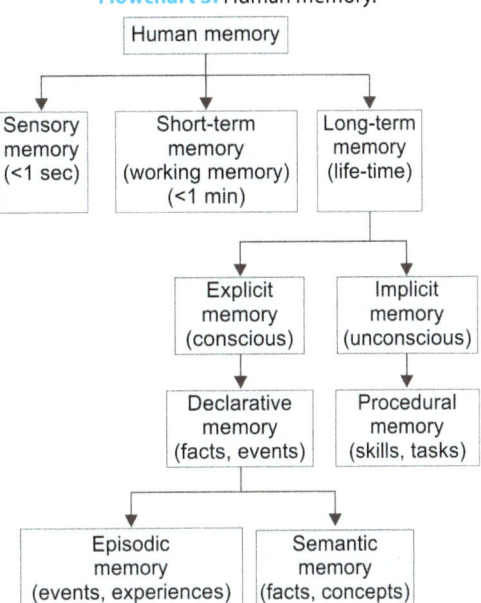

Flowchart 3: Human memory.

Types of Memory

Types of memory are classified based on various aspects such as duration (**Fig. 18**), storage of information, or as per area of storage. Types can be classified as (**Flowchart 3**):

1. **Sensory or immediate memory (200–500 ms):** It retains the sensory image for only a small part of a second, just long enough to develop perception.
   a. **Iconic memory:** It is sensory memory that holds visual information for almost a quarter of a second or more. It makes the visual world appear smooth and continuous despite blinks and eye movements.
   b. **Echoic memory:** It is a momentary sensory memory of auditory stimulus; if attention is elsewhere, sounds and words can still be recalled within 3–4 seconds.

2. **Short-term memory (STM) or working memory:** Some of the information in sensory memory is then transferred to short-term memory. Its capacity is also very limited. It allows one to recall something from several seconds to as long as a minute without rehearsal.

3. **Long-term memory:** The storage in sensory memory and short-term memory has limited capacity and duration; therefore, long-term memory can store a large quantity of information for a longer duration or whole life span, e.g., birth dates, telephone numbers, etc.
   a. **Explicit memory:** It requires conscious recall, in which some conscious process must call back the information. It is subdivided into the following:

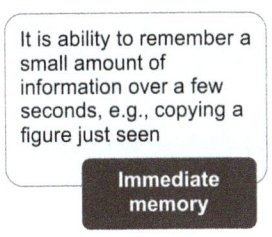

Immediate memory	Recent memory	Remote memory
It is ability to remember a small amount of information over a few seconds, e.g., copying a figure just seen	It is ability to remember information for minutes, hours, or days ago what you heard in yesterday's lectures	It is the ability to remember things that happened years ago, e.g., remembering old school days

Fig. 18: Classification based on duration.

- **Semantic memory:** Semantic memory is used for remembering everyday types of facts and information called knowledge.
- **Episodic:** It concerns information specific to a particular context, such as time and place. It is less organized and hence will be forgotten faster.
- **Visual memory:** It is part of memory preserving some characteristics of our senses pertaining to visual experience. We are able to place memory information that resembles objects, places, animals, or people in sort of a mental image.

b. **Implicit memory:** It is not based on the conscious recall of information. It is used in learning motor skills and is mostly processed in the basal ganglia and cerebellum.

Factors Influencing Memory

1. **Personal characteristics**
   - **Age:** The cognitive development occurs from birth as he grows. But the old age influences memory.
   - **Gender differences:** Studies show that sex and prenatal hormones affect cognitive performance, e.g., estrogen combines with stress to impair memory. Memory problems at menopause. There are gender differences in brain, frontal lobe neuron density.
   - **Development:** Prenatal factors (exposure to cocaine, air pollutants, solvents, lead, etc., and alcohol exposures) influence the memory of an individual.
2. **Food and supplements**
   - Healthy diet and news reports improve cognitive performance.
   - Vegetables, omega-3, antioxidant-rich diets boost memory.
   - Dietary supplements such as vitamin D, long-term β-carotene, vitamin B_{12}, folate, folic acid, and zinc supplements may help to prevent cognitive decline.
   - Natural supplements such as ginkgo biloba may act as a memory enhancer in patients with multiple sclerosis.
3. **Drugs and chemicals:** Hormone therapy, alcohol, nicotine, ecstasy, other illegal drugs (e.g., cannabis, amphetamine, marijuana, cocaine), and metals (lead, solvents, mercury, chemicals in clear plastics) may cause cognitive problems in adults.
4. **Exercise:** Physical activity, aerobic exercise, lifestyle changes, and fitness are associated with mental processes.
5. **Emotion:** Emotion-provoking situations immediately before or immediately after learning have got obliterating effect on memory, e.g., stress.
6. **Environment:** Nuisance distractions can impair learning ability. Aircraft noise may affect children's reading and memory. It can be a place, person, or time that influences one's memory.
7. **Clinical conditions:** Epilepsy, chronic pain, migraine, repeated common infections, high BP, AIDS, cancer, multiple sclerosis, head injury, diabetes, PTSD, and autism are linked to poor memory.

Methods to Improve Memory

Mnemonics: Organization of materials is extremely important to improve memory. The term "Mnemonics" is derived from the Greek word which means "to remember." The mnemonics are short, verbal devices that encode a long series of facts by associating them with familiar and previously encoded information in the recent past. If materials lack natural organization, artificial organizations are necessary to be used by the learner for better memory, e.g., colors of the rainbow are associated with ROY G BIV.

The following mnemonic devices are used to improve memory:
a. **Method of Loci:** "Loci" is the pleural of the Latin word "locus" which means "place." The method of loci says that you visualize

a scene and fit the items to be remembered in that scene. The scene can be a street, a building with rooms, the layout of a college campus, a kitchen, or just about anything that can be visualized clearly and contains a number of discrete items in specific locations to serve as memory pegs. Suppose you want to remember for examination "classical conditioning." Then start by imagining a dog, experimental room, food, bell, and any person as an experimenter. Rehearse this image over and over until it is well-established in your mind. After you have formed your image, associate the events like stimulus substitution, extinction with this. The trick is to make associations with as many concepts as needed.

b. **Rhyming:** Like the method of loci, number- and letter-peg systems are to establish the main idea in your long-term memory, a well-organized set of images to which the to-be-remembered items can be linked. In number systems, you form an image with each number. For instance, a rhyming system can be used for the numbers 1 through 10. For the letter system, you can establish mnemonic pegs by forming strong distinctive images of words that start with the sounds of the letter of the alphabet, e.g., number and letter pegs.
1 is a fan—6 is a disk
2 is a shoe—7 is a pen
3 is a tree—8 is a light
4 is a door—9 is a light
5 is a knife—10 is men and so on

c. **Narrative stories:** You can make a story and in that, you can fit the facts, like you read in elaborate rehearsal. The important thing for a good memory is your motivation and ability to organize the material. One strategy in remembering things well is to organize or arrange the input so that it fits into the existing long-term memory categories, is grouped in some logical manner, or is arranged in some other way that makes sense. The organizational encoding may be inherent in the input itself or it may be supplied by individuals as they learn and remember new things.

d. **Chunking:** This mnemonic technique illustrates systematic ways of encoding information. If you want to remember a long list of digits, e.g., 20061506080, you can break the number into chunks. The first four digits could be remembered as the year of your engagement or associated with any significant thing that happened in that year, the next four digits could be taken as someone's birthday, and the last three digits as someone's weight. Like this, chunks can be associated with some important thing for a lasting memory.

Other ways to improve memory are:
- Keep an active brain.
- Make associations: Creating a mental link between the things you already know and new information
- Visualize and observe: Create a mental picture of what you are interested in.
- Repeat things: Practice makes it perfect.
- Meditation and exercise: These improve blood circulation throughout your body; be more alert and relaxed.
- Eating and sleeping: These keep the brain healthier.
- Organize your life.
- Reduce stress.

Testing Memory

Wechsler Memory Scale

The Wechsler Memory Scale-Revised (WMS-R) is the most widely used memory test battery for adults. It is a composite of verbally paired associate and paragraph retention, visual memory for designs, orientation, digit span, rote recall of the alphabet, and counting backward. The scale yields a Memory Quotient (MQ), which is corrected for age and generally approximates the Wechsler Adult Intelligence Scale Intelligence Quotient (WAIS IQ)—amnestic conditions, such as Korsakoff's syndrome, are characterized by a disproportionately low MQ but a relatively preserved IQ.

Benton Visual Retention Test
It is sensitive to short-term memory loss.

The most frequently used testing condition involves the presentation of each geometric figure for 10 seconds, after which the patient attempts to draw the figure from memory.

Forgetting

Forgetting has positive and negative values in life. It is a great blessing to the mankind. Life would have been very tragic and miserable if memory for all painful events would have been preserved in our mind. The process of forgetting washes away sad and shocking experiences from the mind.

From the negative aspect, forgetting is a very important practical problem in our everyday life, e.g., you have given a book to your friend and searching it at home, a patient forgets to carry his medicine and has a problem on the way. Such other problems pose great botheration for us.

Forgetting is defined as the permanent or temporary loss of the ability to recall or recognize something learned earlier.
—*Munn 1967*

Forgetting is failure to retrieve information from what is already learned.

Causes of Forgetting

The factors responsible for forgetting may be divided into two clear-cut parts.
1. **Factors operating at the time of learning:**
   a. *Strength of original learning:* It has been found experimentally that when the original learning is weaker, the neural traces formed in the brain are fainter and hence are properly retained. But the amount of retention cannot increase indefinitely as a function of the degree of over-learned. A point of diminishing return is to be reached. However, over-learning is always preferable to undertaking.
   b. *Nature of material:* It is found that the meaningful and rhythmic material decreases the rate of forgetting. Ebbinghaus found that any material with an associative value decreases forgetting. The meaningless materials or nonsense syllables need to relate with some meaning or association to these for quick remembering.
   c. *Method of learning:* Various methods are used for learning and memorizing as given under the mnemonics technique.
   d. *Learning under abnormal conditions:* It is one of the major causes of forgetting at the time of learning. Some unpleasant experiences are more quickly forgotten than pleasant ones.
   e. *Speed of learning:* Speed of learning also determines the degree of forgetting. According to Underwood, "When learning is rapid, forgetting will be slow and vice-versa."
2. **Factors operating after learning:** These are the factors that operate between the learning and retention test, and at the time of recall. This is explained on the basis of the theories of forgetting.
   a. *Decay/trace decay/disuse theory:* It tries to explain why forgetting increases with time. The neural traces which are formed in the brain at the time of learning are decayed due to the lack of use. Thus, they grow fainter and fainter with the passage of time. Such fading or decay could be the result of normal metabolic processes of the brain. If we do not use a particular memory trace, it becomes out of use and fades away. It is argued by the disuse theorists that many skills, mathematical formulas, and poems that have been learned in the past and not used for a long time are

forgotten. By relearning these memory traces are strengthened and hence do not fade away.
b. *Displacement theory:* It is given by Waugh and Norman (1965). It explains that in a limited-capacity STM system, forgetting may occur through displacement. When the system is "full," the oldest material in it would be displaced (pushed out) by incoming new material.
c. *Retrieval:* Failure theory and cue-dependent forgetting: According to retrieval failure theory, memories cannot be recalled because the correct retrieval cues are not being used. The role of retrieval cue is demonstrated by the tip-of-the-tongue phenomenon, in which we know something but cannot retrieve it at that particular moment in time (Brown & McNeil, 1966).
d. *Interference theory:* According to this, forgetting is influenced more by what we do before or after learning than by the mere passage of time. It determines the course of forgetting, what we do in the interval between learning and recall. Experimental studies have shown that learning new things interferes with the memory of what is learned earlier and prior learning interferes with the memory of things learned later.
   - Retroactive inhibition: This is a technical name for new learning that may interfere with the material previously learned. This has been demonstrated in experiments as follows. As an example, you may learn one chapter of physiology in activity I, then learn one chapter of anatomy in activity II, then try to recall what you had learned in physiology. The amount of information you forget would be due to interference caused by learning anatomy. Compared to this, if you learn a chapter from physiology, rest for some time, and then recall physiology, you would find that your recall is better than that of the previous chapter.
   - Proactive inhibition: When prior learning interferes with the learning and recall of new material, it is called proactive inhibition. To demonstrate this type of interference experiment is designed as follows. Supposing you learn English, then French, and recall French, you would find that the study of English interferes with your recall of French. Here, what you learned earlier, interferes with the subsequent memory.
e. *Motivated forgetting/repression theory:* Emotional factors also play an important role in forgetting. If we encode information while in one emotional state and try to recall it while in another, our recall suffers. Many lapses of memory in daily life illustrate motivated forgetting. We may forget the names of people we do not like. Repression theory holds that we forget because the retrieval of memories would be painful or unacceptable in some way to the person. Freud, in his book, "The Psychopathology of Everyday Life" had illustrated many examples of repression in forgetting. Repression includes retrieval failure for the associations of threatening, anxiety, and provoking information.

Forgetting During Sickness (Amnesia)

Amnesia refers to loss of memory due to disease. It is of two types.
1. **Biological amnesia:** Forgetting could be due to any of the following reasons—diseases of the brain such as senile dementia, Korsakoff's syndrome,

concussion from blows on the head, brain damage, brain infections, tumor, stroke, temporary disturbances in the blood supply or effect of high dose of alcohol, and drug abuse.
2. **Psychological amnesia:** These types of amnesia occur due to psychiatric diseases where the person has his identity also.
   - Childhood amnesia is due to the differences in the ways young children and older people encode and store information. Defensive amnesia is where people forget their names, where they have come from, who their spouses are, and many other important details of their past lives. It is called defensive because this is usually considered to be a way of protecting oneself from the guilt or anxiety that can result from intense, intolerable life situations and conflicts. It is thus an extreme of repression.
   - Normal ageing has its problems too, but the typical forgetfulness of old age is hardly severe enough to be called amnesia. The memory problem centers largely on the storage of relatively recent events; it is anterograde in nature.

THINKING

People think—that is obvious. During most of our waking hours, and even when we are asleep and dreaming, we are thinking, what are you thinking about right now? To some extent, you are thinking about the words on this page. But perhaps you are also thinking about your breakfast, your classmate's dress, the argument you had with your friend in the morning, your notebook—the list could be endless. At any given moment in time, consciousness contains a rapidly shifting pattern of diverse thoughts and feelings.

What do we do when we think? We might say that thinking consists of the cognitive rearrangement or manipulation of both information from the environment and symbols stored in long-term memory.

Definitions of Thinking

- Thinking is an activity concerning ideas, symbolic in character initiated by a problem or task which the individual is facing, involving some trial and error but under the directing influence of that problem and ultimately leading to a conclusion or solution of the problem.
  —*Warren*
- Thinking is the organization and reorganization of current learning in the present circumstances with the help of learning and past experiences.
  —*Vinacke (1968)*
- Thinking is the perceptual relationship which provides for the solution of the problem.
  —*Maier*

Types of Thinking

1. **Perceptual or concrete thinking:** It is based on perception. Perception is the process of interpretation of sensation according to one's experience. It is called concrete thinking as it is carried over the perception of actual or concrete objects and events.

   It is one-dimensional and literal thinking which has limited use of metaphor without understanding nuances of meaning. Being the simplest form of thinking, small children are mostly benefitted from this type of thinking.

2. **Conceptual or abstract thinking:** It does not require the perception of actual objects or events. It is also called abstract thinking as it makes the use of concepts or abstract ideas. It is superior to perceptual thinking as it economizes efforts in understanding and helps in discovery and invention.

3. **Creative thinking:** It refers to the ability for original thinking, to create or discover something new. It is the ability to integrate the various elements of the situations into

a harmonious whole to create something novel. In other words, cognitive activity directed toward some creative work refers to creative thinking. Creative thinkers are great boons to society as they enrich the knowledge of mankind.

In creative thinking, there is general freedom from rigid thought patterns, i.e., freedom from "the old beaten track." The creative thinker tries to achieve something new, to produce something original and something unique.

There are some common stages of critical thinking such as the following:

a. *Preparation:* This means the whole preparation of a person for creative work. It can be general preparation and specific preparation for specific problems. It involves formulation of a problem, collection of information, survey of relevant work in the area, preliminary knowledge of the subject, and trial and error—all are essential for creative thinking.
b. Incubation occurs when the individual is unable to find a solution in spite of long and concentrated efforts. The ideas which were interfering with the solution of a problem tend to fade away. What he learns and experiences in the meantime may give clues to a solution.
c. *Illumination/inspiration:* The creative idea, the solution of the problem comes to the mind all of a sudden, in a sudden flash. It provides a specific direction toward the goal and it makes the person think in that direction.
d. *Evaluation:* The thinker finds out if the solution which has come to his mind is correct or not.
e. *Verification/revision:* If the solution is found to be correct, it is accepted. If it is wrong or does not suit the assumption of the creative thinker, he has to again start from the beginning. In certain cases, some modification or revision may be necessary.

4. **Logical thinking/reasoning:** It is the cognitive process of looking for beliefs, conclusions, actions, or feelings. It is the process of drawing conclusions based on evidence. It is a form of controlled thinking of a problem.

The reasoning is the highest form of thinking to find out causes and predict effects. An individual tries to solve a problem by incorporating two or more aspects of his past experience. It is classified into the following:

- *Inductive reasoning:* This is a process of reasoning from parts to the whole, from examples to generalizations. It is carried out generally within the field known as informal logic or critical thinking.
- *Deductive reasoning:* This moves from the whole to parts, from generalizations to underlying concepts to examples. Formal logic is described as "the deductive arguments."
- *Abductive reasoning:* It is a cognitive process that often involves both inductive and deductive arguments.

5. **Problem-solving:** It is a tool, skill, and a process. It is a tool because it can help you solve an immediate problem or to achieve a goal. It is a skill because once you have learned it you can use it repeatedly, such as the ability to ride a bicycle, add numbers, or speak a language. It is also a process because it involves taking a number of steps.

You can engage in problem-solving if you want to reach a goal and experience obstacles on the way. At the point at which you come up against a barrier you can engage in a problem-solving process to help you achieve your goal. Every time you use a problem-solving process, you are increasing your problem-solving skills.

Problem-solving cycle

To solve a problem take the following steps, one at a time.

Step 1. Identify the problem: Identify and name the problem so that you can find an appropriate solution.

Step 2. Explore the problem: When you are clear about what the problem is you need to think about it in different ways. Ask yourself the following:
- How is this problem affecting me others?
- How does anybody else experience this problem?
- What do they do about it?

Seeing the problem in different ways is likely to help you find an effective solution.

Step 3. Set goals: Once you have thought about the problem from different angles you can identify your goals. What is that you want to achieve? Do you want to:
- Improve your health?
- Increase your time management?
- Complete the assignments to the best of your ability?
- Finish the assignments as soon as possible?

Step 4. Look at alternatives: After the goal decision, you need to look for possible solutions. You can "brainstorm" for ideas to collect a long list of possibilities. You can seek ideas about possible solutions from others, books, or the internet.

Step 5. Select a possible solution: From the list of possible solutions, you can sort out which are most relevant to your solution and which are realistic and manageable.

Step 6. Implement a possible solution: Once you have selected a possible solution you are ready to put it into action. You will need to have energy and motivation to do this because implementing the solution may take some time and effort.

Step 7. Evaluate: Just because you have worked your way through the problem-solving process, it does not mean that you automatically solve your problem. So you can evaluate the effectiveness of your solution by asking yourself.

- How effective was that solution?
- Did it achieve what I wonder?
- What consequences did it have on my situation?

If you feel dissatisfied with the result, then you can begin the steps again and the cycle goes on.

6. **Convergent versus divergent thinking:** Convergent thinking is the cognitive processing of information around a common point, an attempt to bring thoughts from different directions into a union for a common conclusion.

Divergent thinking starts from a common point and moves outward into a variety of perspectives. For example, teachers use the content as a vehicle to prompt diverse or unique thinking among students rather than a common view.

Levels of Thinking

There are six levels of thinking/learning within a cognitive hierarchy of behaviors.

Level 1. Knowledge: It involves the recall of facts, principles, and terms in the forms in which they are learned.

Keywords: Who, what, when, omit, where, which, choose, find, how, define, label, show, spell, list, match, name, relate, tell, recall, select

Examples: When did ....happen? Which one..................?

Level 2. Comprehension: It represents the lowest form of understanding. The student knows what is being communicated without relating it to other material or seeing it in its fullest meaning. It demonstrates an understanding of facts and ideas by organizing, comparing, translating, interpreting, giving descriptions, and stating main ideas.

Keywords: Compare, contrast, demonstrate, interpret, explain, extend, illustrate, infer, outline, relate, rephrase, translate, summarize, show, classify

Examples: What facts or ideas show..................? Which is the best answer.......................?

Level 3. Application: It involves the use of abstractions in concrete situations such as nursing or nursing or other specific situations. It is solving problems by applying acquired knowledge, facts, techniques, and rules in a different way.
Keywords: Apply, build, choose, construct, develop, interview, make use of, organize, experiment with plan, select, solve, utilize, model, identify
Examples: What would result if ....?
Can you make use of the facts to...............?

Level 4: Analysis: It is examining and breaking information into parts by identifying motives or causes, making inferences, and finding evidence to support generalizations.
Keywords: Analyze, categorize, compare, contrast, discover, dissect, divide, examine, inspect, simplify, survey, take part in, test for, distinguish, list, distinction, theme, relationships, function, motive, inference, assumption, conclusion.
Examples: What are key parts or features of ....?
What motives are there.......................?
What evidence can you find.............?

Level 5: Synthesis: It is compiling information together in a different way by combining elements in a new pattern or proposing alternative solutions.
Keywords: Build, choose, combine, compile, compose, construct, create, design, develop, estimate, formulate, imagine, invent, make up, originate, plan, predict, propose, solve, solution, etc.
Examples: Can you propose an alternative...............?
Can you formulate a theory for...............?
What facts can you compile....................?

Level 6: Evaluation: It is presenting and defending opinions by making judgments about information, validity of ideas, or quality of work based on a set of criteria.
Keywords: Award, choose, conclude, criticize, decide, defend, determine, evaluate, judge, justify, measure, compare, mark, rate, recommend, prioritize, prove, disprove, etc.

Examples: What is your opinion of.............?
Would it be better if...................?
How would you rate the............?

Alterations in Thinking

Thought process is the "how" of the patient's self-expression. A patient's thought process is observed through speech.

- ❖ **Psychosis:** It is a mental disorder in which reality testing is not intact; behavior may violate gross social norms. It is just the opposite to neurosis in which reality testing is intact and behavior may not violate social norms. Many psychiatric disorders such as schizophrenia, mania, depression, etc., come under psychosis. It includes various disturbances in thinking.
- ❖ **Delusion:** It is a false, persistent, irrational belief not shared by persons of the same age, race, education standard which cannot be altered by logical arguments. Delusions are classified into.
  - *Persecutory delusions:* The individuals feel interfered, discriminated against, threatened, or mistreated. For example, the patient says, "My family members want to kill me."
  - *Delusion of reference:* The individual feels that others are talking about him, other's remarks/actions have special significance for him.
  - *Delusion of influence/passivity:* The individual believes that he is influenced by and controlled by others. For example, "The cardiologist puts transmitter near heart that controls my feelings and thoughts."
  - *Delusions of sin and guilt:* The individual has a belief that he has committed unforgivable sin/some wickedness in past leads to calamity to others. So, he is evil and worthless.
  - *Hypochondriacal delusions:* These are delusions of some bodily disease.
  - *Nihilistic delusions:* The individual has a false idea that the self, a part of the self, others, or the world is non-existent.

- *Delusion of grandeur:* The individual has an exaggerated feeling of importance, power, knowledge, or identity, e.g., "I am Prime Minister."

INTELLIGENCE

Human beings differ from each other in their ability to understand, think, and behave cognitively. They have different abilities to understand complex ideas to adapt effectively to the environment, to learn from experience, to engage in various forms of reasoning, etc., so for all this to take place individual needs to use his/her intelligence.

Definitions

Intelligence is the ability to solve problems, or to create products, that are valued within one or more cultural settings. —**H Gardner**

Intelligence is performing an operation on a specific type of content to produce a particular product. —**JP Guilford**

Intelligence is that facet of mind underlying our capacity to think, to solve novel problems, to reason and to have knowledge of the world. —**M Anderson**

Intelligence is the global capacity of an individual to act purposefully, to think rationally and to deal effectively with his environment —**Wechsler**

Characteristics of Intelligence

- Intelligence is an innate natural endowment of the child.
- It helps the child in maximum learning in a minimum period of time.
- The child is able to foresee the future and plan accordingly.
- The child is able to take advantage of his previous experiences.
- The child faces the future with compliance.
- He develops a sense of discrimination between right and wrong.
- The development period of intelligence is from birth to adolescence.
- There is a minor difference in the development of intelligence between boys and girls.
- There are individual differences with regard to the intelligence between boys and girls.
- Intelligence is mostly determined by heredity but a suitable environment is necessary to improve it.
- Intelligence is the ability for adjustment to the environment and the ability to perceive relationship between various objects and methods, solve problems, think independently, learn maximum period of time, and to benefit from one's own experience and the experience of others.
- Intelligence is an inborn ability of an individual, the distribution of intelligence is not equal among all human beings.
- There is a wide individual difference that exists among individuals with regard to intelligence.

Types of Intelligence

Thurstone classifies intelligence in the following ways:
- **Spatial:** It involves moving from one location to another or determining one's orientation in space.
- **Perceptual:** It involves the ways in which people interpret their experiences to distinguish between reality and fantasy.
- **Number or numerical:** It involves solving numerical equations and complex mathematical problems.
- **Verbal:** It is the ability to understand concepts and framing of words such as problem-solving, abstract reasoning.
- **Word-fluency:** It is the ability to list words rapidly in certain designated categories such as words that begin with a particular letter of the alphabet.
- **Reasoning:** It is general process of thinking rationally to find valid conclusions.

According to EL Thorndike

a. **Concrete intelligence:** Concrete intelligence is also known as mechanical intelligence. It is the intelligence that has the relation with concrete materials. It is the ability of an individual to comprehend actual situations and to react to them adequately. Concrete intelligence is evident from various activities in our daily life. This kind of intelligence is measured by performance tests and picture tests in which an individual is asked to manipulate concrete materials.

b. **Abstract intelligence:** Abstract intelligence indicates the ability to respond to words, numbers, formulas, diagrams, letters, etc. This formula is conspicuously absent in animals. An abstractly intelligent person is able to discover relations among symbols and to solve various problems with the help of such aids (symbols, formulas, diagrams, letters, etc.).

c. **Social intelligence:** Social intelligence means the ability of an individual to react to social situations in his or her daily life. Social intelligence is possessed by those people who are able to handle people well and also have the ability to make friends easily and understand human relations. Adequate adjustment in social situations is the index of social intelligence.

The Nine Types of Intelligence: Howard Gardner

1. Naturalist Intelligence
2. Musical Intelligence (Musical Smart)
3. Logical-Mathematical (Number/Reasoning Smart)
4. Existential Intelligence
5. Interpersonal Intelligence (People Smart)
6. Bodily-Kinesthetic Intelligence (Body Smart)
7. Linguistic Intelligence (Word Smart)
8. Interpersonal Intelligence (Self Smart)
9. Spatial Intelligence (Picture Smart)

Emotional Intelligence

Peter Salovey was the pioneer from Yale University who developed the idea of EQ or emotional intelligence. Goleman expanded upon this theory. Goleman includes conscientiousness, self-confidence, optimism, communication, leadership, and initiative. Most intelligence can be grouped into one or three clusters—abstract, concrete, or social intelligence. Social intelligence (Thorndike)—ability to understand and relate to people. Emotional intelligence has its roots in social intelligence.

Emotional intelligence includes:
- Being aware of one's own emotions
- Being able to manage one's own emotions
- Being sensitive to the emotions of others
- Being able to respond to and negotiate with other people's emotionally
- Being able to use one's own emotions to motivate oneself
- Emotionally intelligent individuals are said to be particularly adept at regulating emotions.

Theories of Intelligence

The theories are grouped into mainly two types—factor theories and cognition theories.

1. Factor Theories

a. **Unitary theory or monarchic theory:** Intelligence consists of one factor. It believes in universal fund of intellectual competency which can be used in all aspects. Intelligence can be utilized in any area of life. A child may have good intelligence in mathematics but may be poor in civics. It has some drawbacks such as some situations it does not suit well. The Unitary theory stands rejected.

b. **Anarchic theory or multifactor theory:** Propagated by Thorndike this theory considers intelligence a combination of numerous separate elements or factors. According to him, the mind is a host of highly particularized and independent faculties. The theory maintains that from a man's ability to do one kind of work we can infer absolutely nothing as to his ability to do another kind of work. If a boy is good at literature, we can judge absolutely nothing about his ability to study chemistry. There is certain positive relationship between these factors still.

c. **Spearman's two-factor theory or eclectic theory:** This is a very popular theory. According to Spearman, intelligence is the ability to think constructively. Spearman (1927) proposes that intelligence consists of two abilities, viz. 'G'-general ability and 'S'-special ability. General factor or ability works in conjunction with a special ability. In all intellectual activities of the human being along with general ability, there will also be a special ability that is related to such action.

d. **Thurston's group factor theory:** Louis Thurston came out with the group factor theory (1937) saying that intelligence is a cluster of abilities. These mental operations then constitute a group. He pointed out that there were seven primary mental abilities and later on added two more.
- *Verbal comprehension factor:* Words and ideas
- *Verbal fluency factor:* Rapid producing words, sentences
- *Numerical factor:* Arithmetic ability
- *Perceptual speed factor:* Rapid recognition of words and letters
- *Inductive reasoning factor:* Reasoning from the specific to the general
- *Spatial visualization factor:* It is involved in visualizing shapes, rotations of objects, and how pieces of a puzzle fit together
- *Memory factor:* Ability to recall
- *Deductive reasoning:* Ability to use the generalized results correctly
- Problem-solving ability factor: Ability to solve problem independently

2. Cognition Theories

These theories are otherwise called process-oriented theories. They focus on intellectual processes; the patterns of thinking and reasoning in people used to solve problems. These theories consider intelligence as a process that helps to deal with problems and to find out the answers. They are called cognitive theories because of their focus on fundamental cognitive processes. The important theories are:

a. **Cattell and Horn's theory:** Cattell (1971) and Horn (1978) have proposed this theory in which they have distinguished two types of intelligence.
   1. *Fluid Intelligence:* This is an innate, biologically or genetically determined capacity, and not influenced by education or training. This capacity helps the person in learning and problem-solving. This is the ability that is useful in understanding and adjusting to strange situations. This ability develops fully in people by the end of an individual's adolescence.
   2. *Crystallized intelligence:* It is a learned or acquired capacity. It is influenced by environmental factors such as education, training, culture, knowledge, and learned skills. This ability can be observed in the behavior of a person while dealing within culture, traditions in society, his knowledge in worldly affairs, through the skills in handling machinery, tools, etc. Generally, it continues throughout life. Though both types of intelligence are independent, they are interrelated.

b. **Information processing theory of intelligence**
   - This theory was proposed by American Psychologist Robert Sternberg (1984).

- He distinguished between information processing components and meta-components. Components are the steps to solve a problem and the meta-components are the basics of knowledge that one has to know to solve the problem.
- The information processing is like a process of solving a problem by an individual in which he proceeds to solve a problem which he comes across, gathers the necessary information, and makes use of this information for completing that task.

The steps are:
- Identifying the relevant information (encoding)
- Drawing the necessary inferences (inferring)
- Establishing relationship between past and present experiences (mapping)
- Applying the inferred relationship (application)
- Justifying the correct solution (justification)
- Providing the correct solution (response)

c. **Jensen's theory of mental functioning**
- Arther Jensen (1969) proposed this theory.
- According to him, the functioning of one's mind depends upon the type and degree of intelligence one possesses.
- Jensen splits intelligence into two types of abilities—associative abilities and cognitive abilities.
- Associative ability is the capacity to learn, identify, discriminate, remember, and reproduce the learned information and experiences.
- Cognitive or conceptual ability is concerned with higher-order thinking, reasoning, analyzing, and problem-solving.
- According to Jensen, associative abilities are related to biological maturation and the cognitive is dependent on education and culture, leading to more individual differences.

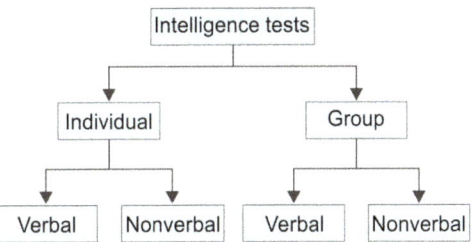

Flowchart 4: Intelligence test.

Measurement of Intelligence

The intelligence test can be classified as follows (**Flowchart 4**):

Individual Verbal Test

The test involves the use of language and is administered to an individual at a time. An example of this is Stanford–Binet scale. French Psychologist Alfred Binet (Father of Intelligence) has constructed this scale.

- This test contains 30 items arranged in order with increasing difficulty. At age 3 point out nose, eyes, and mouth and at age 7 what is missing in the unfinished picture.
- The test is for people from 2 to 20 years. The Indian version is called Samanya Budhi Pariksha. The scores are used to calculate IQ.

Individual Performance Test

In this test, the contents and responses are in the form of performance. Language is not used at all. The performance in these activities is tested. Some of them are Block Building/Cube Construction—asked to make a structure or design by means of blocks or cubes; to fit the blocks in the hole; tracing a maze; picture arrangement. These tests try to emphasize the significance of the performance. It is evaluated by the number of attempts and the duration taken to complete the test.

Another commonly used individual performance test is the Wechsler–Bellevue intelligence test. It has two versions such as WISC (Wechsler adult intelligence scale). This is sometimes referred to as both verbal and performance scales simultaneously. The scale consists of 11 subsets. Six are verbal and 5 are performance. The scores are added to calculate the IQ.

Wechsler–Bellevue Intelligence Test

Verbal Scale:
- Test for general information
- Test for general comprehension
- Test for arithmetic reasoning
- Test for distinction between similarities
- Test for digits span
- Test for vocabulary

Performance Scale:
- Digit symbol test
- Picture completion test
- Block design test
- Picture arrangement test
- Object assembly test

Some questions are:
1. Consider all numbers from 1 to 60 in sequence. If you add any two consecutive numbers, will the result be: **Odd, Even, It depends?**
2. When the letters are rearranged in ANGRIATEN, do you get the name of a: **State, Country, Continent, Planet, Ocean?**
3. If berry weighs 150 pounds, ted weighs 125 pounds, and Matt weighs 175 pounds, any two of them together weigh 300 pounds: **True or False?**

Group Verbal Tests

The tests necessitate the use of language and are applied to a group of individuals.

Some of the common tests are:
- Army alpha test (developed during World War I)
- CIE verbal group test of intelligence (Hindi) developed by Professor Uday Shankar
- The group test of general mental ability constructed by S Jalota

Group Nonverbal Tests

These tests do not use language and are applied to a group. Some of the common tests are Army Beta test, CIE nonverbal group test, etc.

Advantages of group tests:
- Can be administered to very large numbers simultaneously
- Simplified examiner role
- Scoring typically more objective
- Large, representative samples often used leading to better-established norms

Disadvantages of group tests:
- Examiner has less opportunity to obtain cooperation and maintain interest.
- Not readily detected if examinee is tired, anxious, and unwell.
- Evidence that emotionally disturbed children does better on individual than group tests.
- The examinee's responses are more restricted.
- Normally an individual is tested on all items in a group test and may become bored over easy items and frustrated or anxious over difficult items.
- Individual tests typically provide for the examiner to choose items based on the test taker's prior responses—moving onto quite difficult items or back to easier items. So individual tests offer more flexibility.

Verbal versus Nonverbal Test

Advantages of performance test:
- Useful for those without language (illiterate, foreign language, problems with sense organs, etc.)
- Good to understand skills in mechanical jobs, etc.

Disadvantages of performance test:
- Cannot predict scholastic ability
- Very costly
- Less reliable as the chance of success is more

- Good for mental ability but not good enough for abstractions and concepts

Mental Age and Intelligence Quotient

Mental age is a concept related to intelligence. It looks at how a specific child, at a specific age—usually today, now performs intellectually, compared to average intellectual performance for that physical age, measured in years.

The physical age of the child is compared to the intellectual performance of the child, based on performance in tests and live assessments by a psychologist. Scores achieved by the child in question are compared to scores in the middle of a bell curve for children of the same age. An intelligence quotient (IQ) is a total score derived from one of several standardized tests designed to assess human intelligence. This term was initiated by the German psychologist William Stern.

IQ is a score obtained by dividing a person's mental age score, obtained by administering an intelligence test, by the person's chronological age, both expressed in terms of years and months. The resulting fraction is multiplied by 100 to obtain the IQ score.

There are two means of calculating it:
1. According to Stanford–Binet scale:
   IQ = Mental Age (MA)/Chronological Age (CA) × 100M
2. According to Wechsler scale:
   IQ = Attained or Actual Score/Expected mean score for age × 100 (**Table 3**)

Table 3: Wechsler (WAIS-III) 1997 IQ test classification.

IQ range (" deviation IQ)	IQ classification
130 and above	Very superior
120–129	Superior
110–119	Average
80–89	Low average
70–79	Borderline
69 and below	Extermely low

Uses of Intelligence Tests

- **For the purpose of selection:** Admission to a course, decide scholarships, to give specific assignments, selection for co-curricular activities
- **For the purpose of classification:** Classification of students to improve teaching-learning experiences
- **For the purpose of promotion:** Promotion in educational, occupational, and social situations
- **Knowing one's potentiality:** This helps the teacher in the following ways: giving guidance, helping in learning the process, improving the level of aspirations, etc.
- For diagnostic purposes
- Helps in research work

Limitations of Intelligence Tests

- **Intelligence tests and students:** inferiority/Superiority leads to problems and misbehavior.
- **Intelligence test and teachers:** Prejudice on students, lack of support for some students, etc.
- **It also creates segregation and conflicts:** None of the intelligence is non-biased. It is unjust to deny the right of others in admission/promotion etc.

Only cognitive aspects are touched by these facts. Factors such as interests, attitude, and motives are not considered in intelligence tests.

■ APTITUDE

Some people can paint beautifully, but cannot sing; some are good at oral communication, but find it difficult to handle any mechanical device. These basic differences bring satisfaction to the individual. The reason for the differences is mainly due to aptitude.

Aptitude means quickness in learning and understanding. It may be a natural talent or an acquired ability.

It is the special aptness or fitness for a special ability, such as mechanical, musical, artistic, scholastic, or religious.

In everyday life, we usually come across individuals who under similar circumstances surpass other persons to acquire certain knowledge or skills and prove themselves more suitable and efficient in certain specific jobs. Such persons are said to possess certain specific abilities or aptitudes, besides general intellectual abilities or intelligence, which help them in achieving success in some specific occupations or activities.

Definitions

Aptitude refers to those qualities characterizing a person's way of behavior which serves to how well he can learn to meet and solve certain specified kinds of problems.
—*Bingham 1937*

It is a combination of characteristics indicative of an individual's capacity to acquire (with training) some specific knowledge, skill, or set of organized responses, such as the ability to speak a language, to become a musician, to do mechanical work. —*Freeman 1971*

Aptitude is a condition, a quality or a set of qualities in an individual which is indicative of the probable extent to which he will be able to acquire under suitable training, some knowledge, skill or composite of knowledge, understanding and skill. —*Traxler 1957*

Characteristic Concept of Aptitude

- Certain aspects of many aptitudes may be inborn.
- It depends upon heredity and environment.
- Attitude differs from ability and achievement. Ability is present-oriented whereas achievement is past-oriented. But aptitude is future-oriented.
- Aptitude measures specific abilities.
- Aptitude is an innate component of a competency to do a certain kind of work at a certain level.
- Aptitudes are learned potentialities.
- Aptitude is derived from general mental ability and it predicts one's possible success or failure in a vocation.
- Aptitude helps an individual to learn faster and achieve success.
- Aptitude is very helpful in choosing any kind of activity, in which we wish to be successful or enjoy.
- Aptitude is different from skill and proficiency. Skill is the ability to perform a given act with ease and precision, skill is a psychomotor activity, but proficiency has the same meaning, except that it is more comprehensive.

Types of Aptitude

1. Sensory Aptitude

- All those aptitudes which are related to the sensory capacities and abilities of children.
- Aptitude differs with each sense organ, some may have aptitude in sense of sight, others may have either sense of smell or sense of taste.
- It is purely based on sensory capacity.
- Sensory aptitudes are related to the sensory abilities of the children.

2. Mechanical Aptitude

- Some persons have a specific bent of mind for the tasks related to the use of mechanical abilities.
- This aptitude involves the ability to understand and solve problems involving mechanical relationships and arrangements such as those, which occur in the adjustment, repair, and assembly of machinery.

3. Artistic Aptitude

- It is related to the expression of artistic abilities and capacities are included in this category.
- Here, the activities are related to the affective domain.
- The esthetic sense is exhibited in activities.

4. Professional Aptitude
❖ The aptitudes are related to the activities of various professions and occupations are included in this category.
❖ It helps to predict the future success of an individual in the field.
Examples: Clerical aptitude, legal aptitude, teaching aptitude, banking aptitude.

5. Scholastic Aptitude
❖ The aptitudes of the scholastic and academic nature are included in this category.
❖ These aptitudes demonstrate and predict the future success of an individual in the learning of a particular subject.
Examples: Scientific aptitude, engineering aptitude, medical aptitude, linguistic aptitude.

Testing of Aptitude
❖ Aptitude measurements are used to predict success or failure in an activity. Aptitude tests measure the degree or level of one's special flair.
❖ They are chiefly used to estimate the extent to which an individual would profit from a specific course or training or predict the quality of his or her achievement in a given situation.

■ TYPES OF APTITUDE TEST
1. Verbal reasoning
2. Numerical reasoning
3. Abstract/inductive/diagrammatic reasoning
4. Logical reasoning
5. Specialty/technical aptitude test
    ■ Mechanical aptitude tests
    ■ Musical aptitude tests
    ■ Art judgment aptitude tests
    ■ Professional aptitude tests
    ■ Legal, engineering, research aptitude tests
    ■ Scholastic aptitude tests

1. **Verbal reasoning:**
    ■ This test measures the ability to comprehend complex written materials and deduct relevant information and conclusions.
    ■ Verbal reasoning tests also include spelling, grammar, logic, and vocabulary tests.
2. **Numerical reasoning:** Numerical reasoning test includes a wide range of aptitude tests varying from "basic arithmetic tests" through "estimation tests" that measure speed in making educated mathematical estimations to "advanced numerical reasoning tests" that measure the ability to interpret complex data presented in various graphic forms and to deduce information and conclusions.
3. **Abstract/inductive/diagrammatic reasoning:**
    ■ These aptitude tests measure logical reasoning and perceptual reasoning skills.
    ■ These aptitude tests do not rely on acquired linguistic or numeric abilities.
    ■ But these rely on innate abilities and are thus called nonverbal reasoning tests.
4. **Logical reasoning:**
    ■ The logical reasoning test is an aptitude test meant to assess the ability to understand and make comprehensive conclusions from the provided data.
    ■ It is one of the most common aptitude tests and although it may seem like one of the most difficult, with practice it becomes much simpler than it seems to be first.
5. **Mechanical aptitude test:**
    ■ Sensory, motor capacities and perception of spatial relations, the capacity to acquire information about mechanical matters, and the capacity to comprehend mechanical relationships
    ■ Tests include:
        ♦ Minnesota Mechanical assembly test
        ♦ Revised Minnesota paper from board

- Stenquist Mechanical Aptitude test
- Bennet test of Mechanical Aptitude test

6. **Clerical aptitude test:**
   - Perceptual ability of words and numbers with speed and accuracy
   - Intellectual ability to grasp the meaning of words and symbols
   - Motor abilities to use various types of machines and tools

   Examples:
   - Detroit clerical aptitude test
   - Minnesota vocational test for clerical workers
   - The clerical ability test prepared by the University of Mysore
   - Clerical aptitude test Battery

7. **Musical aptitude tests:**
   - The musical talents
   - The components include:
     - Discrimination of pitch
     - Discrimination of intensity of loudness
     - Discrimination of time interval
     - Judgment of rhythm

   Test items in this battery are presented on phonograph records.

8. **Aptitude for graphic art:**
   - The Meier art judgment test
   - Horne art aptitude inventory
   - The Meier art judgment test; there are 100 pairs of representational pictures in black and white.

9. **Tests of scholastic and professional aptitudes:**
   - Stanford scientific aptitude test by DL Zyne
   - Science aptitude test (after higher secondary stage)
   - Moss scholastic aptitude test for medical students
   - Tale legal aptitude test
   - Shah's teaching test

Individual Differences in Intelligence and Aptitude

Individual differences stand for the variation or deviations among individuals in regard to a single characteristic or a number of characteristics.

Classifications
- Physical differences
- Psychological differences

Sub-types
Differences related to:
- Physical growth and development
- Mental growth and development
- Motor skills and abilities
- Emotional make up
- Socialization
- Morality
- Esthetic sense
- Interest
- Attitudes, beliefs, values
- Self-concept
- Psychomotor skills
- Study habits
- Achievements

Causes for the Differences
- Heredity
- Environment
- Individual differences in performance on cognitive tasks are due to differences in working memory capacity, information processing speed, and the breadth of procedural knowledge
- Factors such as age, sex, and environment effect the level of aptitude.

Nursing Implications of Aptitude
- The knowledge of the aptitude will also give optimism to nurses' future success.

- Knowledge of the aptitude will be helpful to the nurse to develop a proper attitude for the profession.
- If a nurse has an aptitude for her profession she is bound to be a successful nurse, whatever the impediments she might meet in her path.

CONCLUSION

Aptitude refers to those qualities or characteristics of a person's way of behavior that serve to indicate how well he can learn to meet and solve certain kinds of problems.

QUESTION BANK

MULTIPLE CHOICE QUESTIONS

1. Which of the following brain areas has been shown to be important for memory?
   a. Cerebellum
   b. Amygdala
   c. Hippocampus
   d. All of the above
2. The most common effortful processing technique where information is repeated is:
   a. Rehearsal
   b. Mnemonic
   c. Recall
   d. Recognition
3. Which step of the perception process tells recalling the present situation by learning through past experiences?
   a. Receptor process
   b. Symbolic process
   c. Affective process
   d. All of the above
4. Events that we perceive are at the focus of:
   a. Perception
   b. Sensation
   c. Experience
   d. Illusion
5. Perception gives meaning to:
   a. Hallucination
   b. Sensation
   c. Illusion
   d. None of the above
6. In sensory memory, the information is lost within:
   a. 1 second
   b. One-fourth of a second
   c. One-third of a second
   d. 2 seconds
7. Reasoning is an example of:
   a. Controlled thinking
   b. Free thinking
   c. Creative thinking
   d. Problem-solving
8. Intelligence is a mental ability
   a. Innate
   b. Acquired
   c. Both a and b
   d. None of the above
9. Items used in group intelligence test are:
   a. Verbal
   b. Nonverbal
   c. Both a and b
   d. None of the above
10. Chronological age is defined as:
    a. Mental age
    b. Mental maturity
    c. Actual age
    d. None of the above

UNIT VI: Coginitive Psychology

11. **Mental age is defined as:**
    a. Mental maturity
    b. Chronological age
    c. Actual age
    d. None of the above
12. **Mental retardation is classified into:**
    a. Mild
    b. Moderate
    c. Severe
    d. Profound
13. **In India popularly used intelligence test is:**
    a. Wechsler-Bellevue test
    b. Bhatia test
    c. Binet test
    d. None of the above
14. **Habits are learned through:**
    a. Repetition
    b. Knowledge
    c. Actions
    d. Behavior
15. **Where does high intelligence come from?**
    a. Genetics
    b. Environment
    c. Both a and b
    d. Neither a nor b
16. **A student with a high aptitude in verbal reasoning and a strong interest in reading is more likely to succeed as a:**
    a. Journalist
    b. Engineer
    c. Athlete
    d. Agriculturalist
17. **Which law of learning deals with satisfaction and dissatisfaction?**
    a. Law of effect
    b. Law of use
    c. Law of exercise
    d. Law of readiness
18. **Which type of learning is slow?**
    a. Trial and error
    b. Conditioning
    c. Insight
    d. Observation
19. **The psychological factor(s) involved in learning is/are:**
    a. Maturation
    b. Motivation and intelligence
    c. Mental health
    d. Physical health
20. **The physiological factor(s) affecting the learning process is/are:**
    a. Motivation
    b. Intelligence
    c. Physical and mental health
    d. Working period

ANSWER KEY
1. b	2. a	3. b	4. c	5. b	6. b	7. c	8. a
9. c	10. c	11. a	12. d	13. c	14. a	15. c	16. a
17. b	18. b	19. b	20. c				

SHORT ANSWER TYPE QUESTIONS
1. What is attention?
2. Explain features of attention?
3. What is distraction? Explain.
4. How will you assess attention of a person?
5. Enlist the disorders of attention.
6. Define the concept and meaning of perception.
7. What is the importance of perception in nursing?
8. Define the term learning.
9. Explain types of learning.

10. What is social learning theory? Explain with its experiment.
11. Explain the learning process.
12. Enlist factors affecting learning.
13. List down study habits of learning.
14. Define memory.
15. Define forgetting.
16. What are the factors responsible for forgetting?
17. What are the ways to improve thinking?
18. Write short note on IQ and Wechsler adult intelligence scale.
19. What are the factors affecting intelligence?
20. How are aptitude tests important in our daily life?

LONG ANSWER TYPE QUESTIONS

1. What are the factors that affect attention?
2. Explain the steps to eliminate distraction.
3. Define perception. Explain its types.
4. What do you mean by the term learning? Explain theories of learning.
5. Enumerate theory by the term learning. Explain theories of learning.
6. Who gave insight theory of learning? Explain.
7. Describe factors affecting learning.
8. Describe the principle of operant conditioning.
9. Explain Pavlov's theory in detail.
10. Write types of memories. Explain according to the type of information.
11. How memory can be improved?
12. Describe the theories of forgetting in detail.
13. Define thinking. What are the types of thinking?
14. What is critical thinking? Explain its stages.
15. What is the difference between illusion and hallucination?
16. Define intelligence and explain its various types.
17. How is intelligence applicable in nursing? How can you assess intelligence?
18. Explain concept of aptitude.
19. How can we measure aptitude?
20. What are aptitudes tests? Classify them.

UNIT VII

Motivation and Emotional Processes

OUTLINE

- Motivation—Meaning, Concept, Types, Theories of Motivation, Motivation Cycle, Biological and Special Motives
- Emotions—Meaning of Emotions, Development of Emotions, Alteration of Emotion, Emotions in Sickness, Handling Emotions in Self and Other
- Stress and Adaptation—Stress, Stressor, Cycle, Effect, Adaptation and Coping
- Attitudes—Meaning of Attitudes, Nature, Factor Affecting Attitude, Attitudinal Change, Role of Attitude in Health and Sickness
- Psychometric Assessment of Emotions and Attitude—Introduction
- Role of Nurse in Caring for Emotionally Sick Client

■ INTRODUCTION

Motivation is a term that refers to a process that elicits, controls, and sustains certain behaviors. Motivation is a group of phenomena that affect the nature of an individual's behavior, the strength of the behavior, and the persistence of the behavior. For instance, an individual has not eaten, he or she feels hungry, as a response he or she eats and diminishes feelings of hunger. There are many approaches to motivation—physiological, behavioral, cognitive, and social. It is the crucial element in setting and attaining goals—and research shows you can influence your own levels of motivation and self-control. According to various theories, motivation may be rooted in a basic need to minimize physical pain and maximize pleasure, or it may include specific needs such as eating and resting, or a desired object, goal, state of being, ideal, or it may be attributed to less-apparent reasons such as altruism, selfishness, morality, or avoiding mortality. Motivation is related to, but distinct from, emotion.

Meaning

Motivation is that internal force that pushes an individual to move toward a goal. Technically, the term motivation can be traced to the Latin word *movere*, which means "to move." Thus, motivation helps the individual to commence some activity. Normally, motivation remains in resting state but once it is aroused, it forces the person to perform the required activity.

Concept of Motivation

Today, virtually all people—lay people and scholars—have their own concept of motivation and they include various terms such as motives, needs, wants, drives, desires, wishes, incentives, etc., in defining motivation.

To understand the concept of motivation, we have to examine three terms—motive,

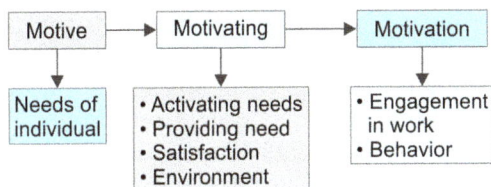

Fig. 1: Relationship between motive, motivating, and motivation.

motivating, and motivation and their relationship **(Fig. 1)**.

Motive

Based on the Latin word *movere*, motive (need) has been defined as follows: "A motive is an inner state that energises, activates, or moves (hence motivation), and that directs behavior towards goals."

Motive has been described as follows:
"A motive is restlessness, alack, a yen, a force. Once in the grip of motive, the organism does something to reduce the restlessness, to remedy the lack, to alleviate the yen, to mitigate the force."

Here we can differentiate between needs and wants. While needs are more comprehensive and include desires—physiological and psychological, wants are expressed in a narrow sense and include only those desires for which a person has money to satisfy the wants.

There are many psychological needs, such as social needs, recognition needs, etc., which do not fall in the category of wants.

Motivating

Motivating is a term that implies that one person (in the organizational context, a manager) includes another (say, employee), to engage in action (work behavior) by ensuring that channel to satisfy the motive becomes available and accessible to the individual.

In addition to channelizing the strong motives in a direction that is satisfying to both the organization and the employees, the manager can also activate the latent motives in individuals and harness them in a manner that would be functional for the organization.

Motivation

While a motive is the energizer of action, motivating is the channelization and activation of motives and motivation is the work behavior itself. Motivation depends on motives and motivating; therefore, it becomes a complex process.

Definitions of Motivation

❖ "Motivation is something that moves the person to action and continues him in the course of action."
❖ "Motivation refers to the way in which urges, drives, desires, aspirations, need direct, control or explain the behavior of human beings." —**Mc. Farland**
❖ "Motivation is the force within the individual that influences strength and direction of behavior." —**Mills**
❖ "Motivation is a predisposition to act in a specific goal directed manner."
—**Hellriegel and Slocum**
❖ "Motivation is the complex force starting and keeping a person at work in an organization. Motivation is something that moves the person to action, and continues him in the course of action already initiated." —**Dubin**
❖ According to Webster's New Collegiate Dictionary, a motive is "something (a need or desire) that causes a person to act." **Motivate**, in turn, means "to provide with a motive," and motivation is defined as "the act or process of motivating."

These definitions have several common denominators to help us characterize

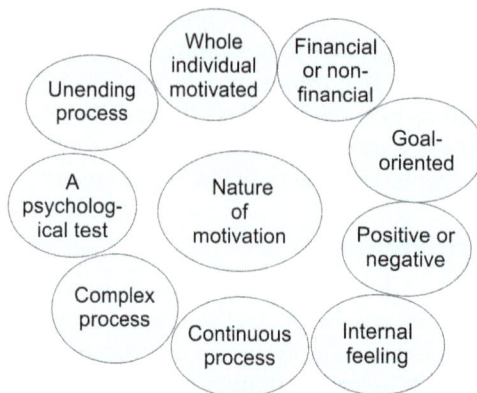

Fig. 2: Nature of motivation.

the motivation phenomenon such as the following:
1. An internal need energizes and activates behavior.
2. Drive is the inner force that propels behavior in a specific direction.
3. Goals are the incentives or payoffs that reinforce private satisfaction, which in turn reinforce the perpetuation of needs.

After defining motive, motivating, and motivation, we can see the relationship among these.

Nature of Motivation (Fig. 2)
- Unending process: Human wants keep changing and increasing.
- A psychological concept deals with the human mind.
- The whole individual is motivated as it is based on the psychology of the individual.
- Motivation may be financial or non-financial: Financial includes increasing wages, allowance, bonus, etc.
- Motivation can be positive or negative: Positive motivation means use of incentives—financial or non-financial, e.g., of positive motivation—confirmation, pay rise, praise, etc. Negative motivation means emphasizing penalties. It is based on the force of fear, e.g., demotion, termination.
- Motivation is goal-oriented behavior.
- Motivation is an internal feeling of an individual. It cannot be observed directly;

we can observe an individual's action and interpret his behavior in terms of underlying motives. This leaves a wide margin of error. Our interpretation may not reveal the individual's true behavior.
- Motivation is a continuous process that produces goal-directed behavior. The individual tries to find alternatives to satisfy his needs.

Motivation is a complex process. Individuals may differ in their motivation even though they are performing the same type of job. For example, if two men are engaged in cutting stones for constructing a temple, one may be motivated by the amount of wages he gets and the other by the satisfaction he gets by performing the job.

Types of Motivation (Fig. 3)
Intrinsic
Intrinsic motivation refers to motivation that is driven by an interest or enjoyment in the task itself and exists within the individual rather than relying on any external pressure. Intrinsic Motivation is based on taking pleasure in an activity rather than working toward an external reward. Students who are intrinsically motivated are more likely to engage in the task willingly as well as work to improve their skills, which will increase their capabilities. Students are likely to be intrinsically motivated if they attribute their educational results to factors under their own control, also known as autonomy, believe that they have the skill that will allow them to be effective agents in reaching desired goals (i.e., the results are not determined by luck), are interested in mastering a topic, rather than just rote-learning to achieve good grades. It is usually associated with high educational achievement and enjoyment by students.

Extrinsic Motivation
Extrinsic motivation refers to the performance of an activity to attain an outcome, which then contradicts intrinsic motivation. Extrinsic motivation comes from outside of the

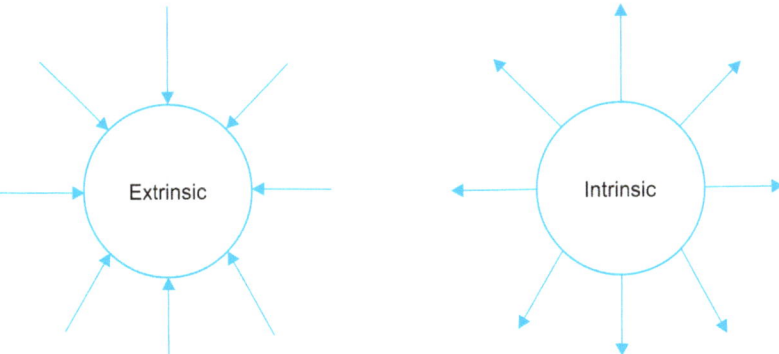

Fig. 3: Types of motivation.

individual. Common extrinsic motivations are rewards such as money and grades, coercion and threat of punishment. Competition is in general extrinsic because it encourages the performer to win and beat others, not to enjoy the intrinsic rewards of the activity. A crowd cheering on the individual and trophies are also extrinsic incentives.

Social psychological research has indicated that extrinsic rewards can lead to overjustification and a subsequent reduction in intrinsic motivation. In one study demonstrating this effect, children who expected to be (and were) rewarded with a ribbon and a gold star for drawing pictures spent less time playing with the drawing materials in subsequent observations than children who were assigned to an unexpected reward condition. For those children who received no extrinsic reward, Self-determination theory proposes that extrinsic motivation can be internalized by the individuals if the task fits with their values and beliefs and therefore helps to fulfill their basic psychological needs. Extrinsic motivation comes from outside of the performer. For example, money, trophies.

Classification of Motives

Psychologists do not totally agree on how to classify various human motives. However, some psychologists tend to classify motives according to whether they are unlearned or learned or whether they are psychologically or physiologically based. The following is the classification:

- **Primary motives** are the ones that are unlearned and are physiologically based. Defined this way the most commonly recognized primary motives include hunger, thrust, sleep, avoidance of pain, sex, etc.
- **General motives** are the ones that are unlearned but not physiologically based. Primary needs seek to reduce the tension and stimulation. Although not all psychologists agree the motives such as curiosity, manipulative activity, and affection fall in this category.
- **Secondary motives** develop as human society develops economically and becomes more complex. Examples of the secondary motives are needs for power, need for affiliation, need for achievement, need for security, need for status, etc.
- **The achievement motive:** David C McClelland is most closely associated with the study of achievement motive. Out of his extensive research has emerged a clear profile of characteristics of high achievers. Achievement motive can be expressed as a desire to perform in terms of a standard of excellence or to be successful in competitive situations. The specific characteristics of a high achiever are: (a) moderate risk-taking, (b) need for

immediate feedback, (c) satisfaction with accomplishment, and (d) preoccupation with the task.

- **The power motive:** According to Alfred Adler power motive is essential to control others and to direct others' behavior. The power attaches to one's personal competence. In an organization because of his competence a person comes to acquire power. It is necessary that he recognizes that the power he has is because of organization.
- **The affiliation motive:** This motive is indicative of the need to belong to and be accepted by others. The consideration of this motive is important in the discussion of group dynamics. The higher the need for affiliation among the members of the group; the higher is the group cohesiveness.

Theories of Motivation

There are many different views as to what motivates workers. The most commonly held views or theories are discussed below and have been developed over the last 100 years or so. Unfortunately, these theories do not all reach the same conclusions! A few important theories and models of motivation are briefly discussed below.

Maslow's Theory of Hierarchy of Needs (Fig. 4)

Abraham Maslow (1908–1970) gave a hierarchical theory of motivation that explains both tension-reducing and tension-increasing action of human behavior. Maslow put forward a theory that there are five levels of human needs which our inborn needs are arranged in a sequence of stages from most primitive to most human.

All of the needs are structured into a hierarchy (see below) and only once a lower level of need has been fully met, would individuals be motivated by the opportunity of having the next need up in the hierarchy satisfied. For example, a person who is dying of hunger will be motivated to achieve a basic wage to buy food before worrying about having a secure job contract or the respect of others.

Self-actualization

It is a need for fulfillment, that is, one becomes everything that he is capable of being.

The person who has achieved this highest-level presses toward full use of his talents, potential, and capabilities.

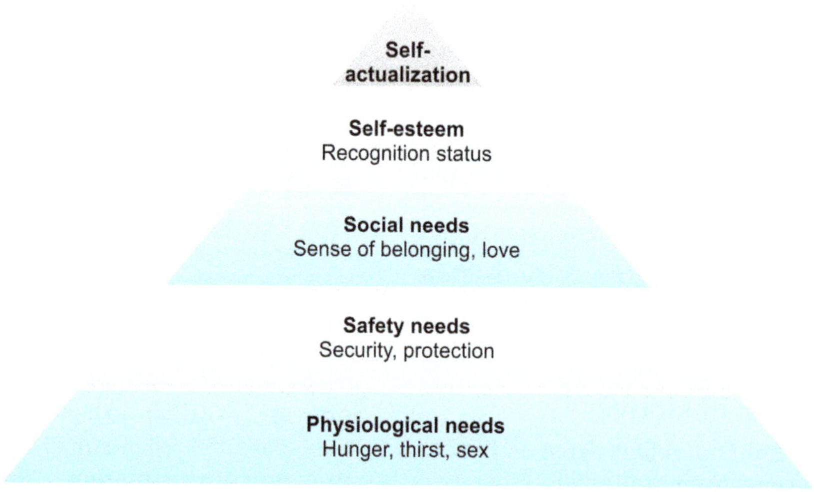

Self-actualization

Self-esteem
Recognition status

Social needs
Sense of belonging, love

Safety needs
Security, protection

Physiological needs
Hunger, thirst, sex

Fig. 4: Maslow's hierarchy of needs.

Characteristics of self-actualized persons:
* They are realistically oriented.
* They accept themselves for what they are.
* Their thought is unconventional and spontaneous.
* They are problem-centered.
* They have a need for privacy.
* They are independent.
* They have spiritual experience.
* They identify with people. They have intimate relationships.
* They are democratic.
* They are creative and have good sense of humor.
* They appreciate the environment.

Herzberg's Two-factor Theory

Frederick Herzberg's two-factor theory, intrinsic/extrinsic motivation, concludes that certain factors in the workplace result in job satisfaction, but if absent, they do not lead to dissatisfaction but no satisfaction. The factors that motivate people can change over their lifetime, but "respect for me as a person" is one of the top motivating factors at any stage of life.

He distinguished between:
* **Motivators** (e.g., challenging work, recognition, responsibility) which give positive satisfaction
* **Hygiene factors** (e.g., status, job security, salary, and fringe benefits) that do not motivate if present, but, if absent, result in demotivation. The name "Hygiene factors" is used because, like hygiene, the presence will not make you healthier, but absence can cause health deterioration. The theory is sometimes called the "Motivator-Hygiene Theory" and/or "The Dual Structure Theory."

Alderfer's ERG Theory

Alderfer, expanding on Maslow's hierarchy of needs, created the *ERG theory*. This theory posits that there are three groups of core needs—existence, relatedness, and growth, hence the label: ERG theory. The existence group is concerned with providing our basic material existence requirements. They include the items that Maslow considered to be physiological and safety needs. The second group of needs is those of relatedness—the desire we have for maintaining important interpersonal relationships. These social and status desires require interaction with others if they are to be satisfied, and they align with Maslow's social need and the external component of Maslow's esteem classification. Finally, Alderfer isolates growth needs' to be an intrinsic desire for personal development. These include the intrinsic component from Maslow's esteem category and the characteristics included under self-actualization.

Expectancy Theory (Fig. 5)

Expectancy theory was developed by Victor Vroom and is a very popular theory of work motivation.

Vroom suggests that motivation will be high when workers feel:

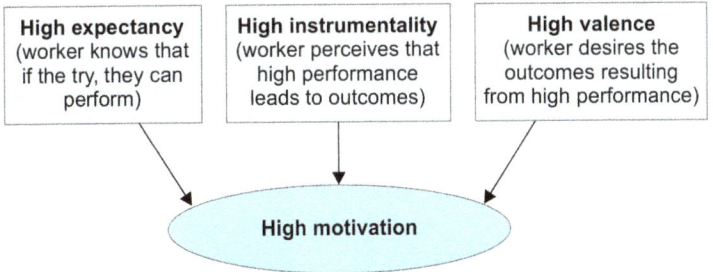

Fig. 5: Expectancy theory of motivation.

- High levels of effort lead to high performance.
- High performance will lead to the attainment of desired outcomes.

This consists of three areas: *expectancy, instrumentality, and valence.*

Incentive Theory

A reward, tangible or intangible, is presented after the occurrence of an action (i.e., behavior) with the intent to cause the behavior to occur again. This is done by associating positive meaning with the behavior. Studies show that if the person receives the reward immediately, the effect is greater, and decreases as duration lengthens. The repetitive action-reward combination can cause the action to become a habit. Motivation comes from two sources—oneself and other people. Reinforcers and reinforcement principles of behavior differ from the hypothetical construct of reward. A reinforcer is any stimulus change following a response that increases the future frequency or magnitude of that response. Positive reinforcement is demonstrated by an increase in the future frequency or magnitude of a response due to the past being followed contingently by a reinforcing stimulus. Negative reinforcement involves stimulus change consisting of the removal of an aversive stimulus following a response.

Applying proper motivational techniques can be much harder than it seems. Steven Kerr notes that when creating a reward system, it can be easy to reward A, while hoping for B, and in the process, reap harmful effects that can jeopardize your goals.

Incentive theory in psychology treats the motivation and behavior of the individual as they are influenced by beliefs, such as engaging in activities that are expected to be profitable. Incentive theory is promoted by behavioral psychologists, such as BF Skinner and literalized by behaviorists, especially by Skinner in his philosophy of radical behaviorism, to mean that a person's actions always have social ramifications; and if actions are positively received people are more likely to act in this manner, or if negatively received people are less likely to act in this manner.

Incentive theory distinguishes itself from other motivation theories, such as drive theory, in the direction of motivation. In incentive theory, stimuli "attract," to use the term above, a person toward them. As opposed to the body seeking to re-establish homeostasis pushing it toward the stimulus. In terms of behaviorism, *incentive theory* involves positive reinforcement; the stimulus has been conditioned to make the person happier. For instance, a person knows that eating food, drinking water, or gaining social capital will make them happier. As opposed to *drive theory*, which involves negative reinforcement, a stimulus has been associated with the removal of the punishment—the lack of homeostasis in the body.

Intrinsic Motivation and the 16 Basic Desires Theory

Starting from studies involving more than 6,000 people, Professor Steven Reiss has proposed a theory that found 16 basic desires that guide nearly all human behavior. The 16 basic desires that motivate our actions and define our personalities as:

1. Acceptance, the need for approval
2. Curiosity, the need to learn
3. Eating, the need for food
4. Family, the need to raise children
5. Honor, the need to be loyal to the traditional values of one's clan/ethnic group
6. Idealism, the need for social justice
7. Independence, the need for individuality
8. Order, the need for organized, stable, and predictable environments
9. Physical activity, the need for exercise
10. Power, the need for influence of the will
11. Romance, the need for sex
12. Saving, the need to collect

13. Social contact, the need for friends (peer relationships)
14. Social status, the need for social standing/importance
15. Tranquility, the need to be safe
16. Vengeance, the need to strike back/to win

In this model, people differ in these basic desires. These basic desires represent intrinsic desires that directly motivate a person's behavior, and are not aimed at indirectly satisfying other desires. People may also be motivated by non-basic desires, but in this case, this does not relate to deep motivation, or only as a means to achieve other basic desires.

Motivation Cycle or Process (Flowchart 1)

In the initiation, a person starts feeling need or desire. There is an arousal of need so urgent that the bearer has to venture in search to satisfy it. This leads to creation of tension, which urges the person to forget everything else and cater to the aroused need first. This tension also creates drives and attitudes regarding the type of satisfaction that is desired. This leads a person to venture into the search for information. This ultimately leads to evaluation of alternatives where the best alternative is chosen. After choosing the alternative, an action is taken. Because of the performance of the activity satisfaction is achieved which then relieves the tension in the individual.

MOTIVES

Biological Motives

Biological motives are called physiological motives. These motives are essential for the survival of the organism. Such motives are triggered when there is imbalance in the body. The body always tends to maintain a state of equilibrium called "Homeostasis" in many of its internal physiological processes.

This balance is very essential for a normal life. Homeostasis helps to maintain internal physiological processes at optimal levels. The nutritional level, fluid level, temperature level, etc., are maintained at a certain optimal level or homeostasis levels. When there is some variation in these levels the individual is motivated for restoring the state of equilibrium.

Physiological Motives

a. **Hunger motive:** We eat to live. The food we take is digested and nutritional substances are absorbed. The biochemical processes get their energy from the food to sustain life. When these substances are exhausted, some imbalance exists. We develop hunger motive to maintain homeostasis. This is indicated by the contraction of stomach muscles causing some pain or discomfort called hunger pangs. Psychologists have demonstrated this phenomenon through experiments.

b. **Thirst motive:** In our daily life, regularly we take fluids in the form of water and other

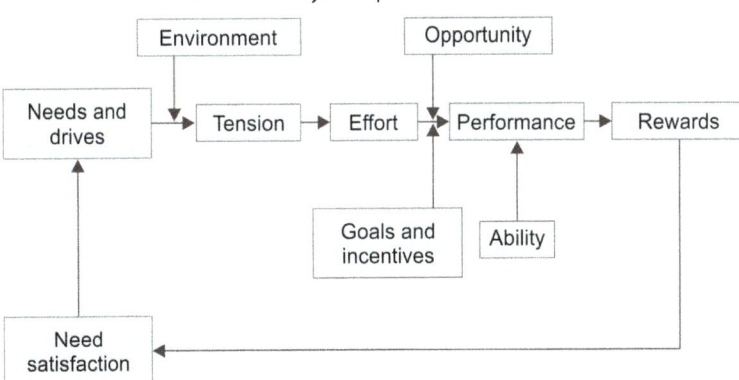

Flowchart 1: Cycle or process of motivation.

beverages. These fluids are essential for our body tissues for normal functioning. When the water level in the body decreases, we develop a motive to drink water. Usually, thirst motive is indicated by dryness of the mouth. Experiments by psychologists have shown that just dried mouth getting wet is not enough. We need to drink a sufficient quantity of water to satiate our thirst.

c. **Need for oxygen:** Our body needs oxygen continuously. We get it through continuous respiration. Oxygen is necessary for the purification of blood. We cannot survive without a regular supply of oxygen. Lack of oxygen supply may lead to serious consequences such as damage to the brain or death.

d. **Motive for regulation of body temperature:** Maintenance of normal body temperature (98.6°F or 37.0°C) is necessary. Rise or fall in the body temperature causes many problems. There are some automatic mechanisms to regulate body temperature, such as sweating when the temperature rises above normal or shivering when it falls below normal.

These changes motivate us to take the necessary steps, e.g., the opening of windows, putting on fans, taking cool drinks, removing clothes, etc., when the temperature increases to above normal level; and closing doors and windows, wearing sweaters, taking hot beverages when the temperature falls. In this way, we try to regulate the body temperature.

e. **Need for sleep:** Sleep is an essential process for the normal functioning of the body and mind. When our body and mind are tired they need rest for rejuvenation of energy. It is observed that there is an excess accumulation of a toxin called "Lactic acid" when tired. After sleep it disappears and the person becomes active. Sleep deprivation also leads to psychological problems such as confusion, inability to concentrate, droopy eyelids, muscle tremors, etc.

f. **Need for avoidance of pain:** No organism can continue to bear the pain. Whenever we experience pain we try to avoid it. We are motivated to escape from painful stimulus. For example, when we are under the hot sun we go to shade. When something is pinching we avoid it.

g. **Drive for elimination of waste:** Our body cannot bear anything excess or anything waste. Excess water is sent out in the form of urine or sweat. So also digested food particles after absorption of nutritional substances are sent out in the form of stools. We experience discomfort until these wastes are eliminated.

h. **Sex motive:** This is a biological motive and this arises in the organism as a result of the secretion of sex hormones such as androgens and estrogens. Sex need is not essential for the survival of the individual, but it is essential for the survival of the species. However, fulfillment of the sex need is not like satisfying hunger or thirst. Society and the law exercise certain codes of conduct. Human being has to adhere to these rules. Usually, this need is fulfilled through marriage.

i. **Maternal drive:** This is an instinct or an inborn tendency. Every normal woman aspires to become a mother. Psychologists have motivation, emotion, and attitudinal processes learned from related studies; this is the most powerful drive. That is why in many cases the women who cannot bear children of their own, will sublimate that motive and satisfy it through socially acceptable ways, such as working in orphan schools, baby sittings, or adopting other's children.

Social Motives

Physiological motives discussed above pertain to both animals as well as human beings, but the social motives are specific only to human beings. These are called social motives because they are learned in social groups as a result of interaction with the family and society. That is why their strength differs from one individual to another. Many social motives are recognized by psychologists. Some of the common social motives are as discussed below.

a. **Achievement motive:** Achievement motivation refers to a desire to achieve some goal. This motive is developed in the individual who has seen some people in the society attaining high success, reaching high positions and standards.

   He/she develops a concern to do better, to improve performance. David C McClelland who conducted a longitudinal study on characteristics of high and low achievers found that the high achievers choose and perform better at challenging tasks, prefer personal responsibility, seek and utilize feedback about the performance standard, have innovative ideas to average standards, and accept failures easily. Parents must try achievement in their future life.

   They must allow children to take decisions independently, and guide them for higher achievement from childhood so that the children develop high achievement motivation.

b. **Aggressive motive:** It is a motive to react aggressively when faced frustrations. Frustration may occur when a person is obstructed from reaching a goal or when he is insulted by others. Even in a fearful and dangerous do-or-die situation the individual may resort to aggressive behavior. An individual expresses such behavior to overcome opposition forcefully, which may be physical or verbal aggression.

c. **Power motive:** People with power motive will be concerned with having an impact on others. They try to influence people by their reputation. They expect people to bow their heads and obey their instructions. Usually, people with high power motives choose jobs, where they can exert their powers. They want people as followers. They expect high prestige and recognition from others. For example, a person may aspire to go for jobs suh as police officer, politician, Deputy Commissioner, etc.

d. **Acquisitive motive:** This motive directs the individual for the acquisition of material property. It may be money or other property. This motive arises as we come across different people who have earned a lot of money and led a good life. It is a human tendency to acquire all those things which appear attractive to him.

e. **Curiosity motive:** This is otherwise called stimulus and exploration motive. Curiosity is a tendency to explore and know new things. We see people indulge in a traveling to look at new places, new things, and new developments taking place outside their environment. People want to extend their knowledge and experiences by exploring new things. Curiosity motive will be very powerful during childhood. That is why they do not accept any toy or other articles unless they examine them from different angles, even at the cost of spoiling or breaking the objects.

f. **Affiliation motive:** It is a tendency to associate oneself with other members of the group or the same species. The individual will be interested in establishing, maintaining, and repairing friendly relationships and will be interested in participating in group activities. The individual will conform to social norms, morals, and other ethical codes of the groups in which he/she is interested. To a greater extent affiliation is developed because many of the needs such as basic needs, safety, and security needs are fulfilled.

g. **Self-esteem motive:** It is a need where the individual wants appraisal, respect, and regard from others. The individual realizes a need to be important and significant in society. But the respect and regard will be given by the others only if the person has some special skills and competencies to contribute to the development of others. For this purpose, he develops expertise in special fields such as education, sports, art, etc. Maslow also gives a higher order to this need in the need hierarchy theory of motivation.

h. **Love and hope motive:** Individuals also feel the need to be related to others. It is closely related to the need for affiliation. But it is little more than that because individual not simply the company of others but also wants to develop some emotional relation with special ones. In this need, individual wants affection and commitment. Hope is another important psychological need that motivates the person in adverse and aversive conditions. The life is not so smooth. It is full of problems and troubles. But every problem leads to experience and exploration of potentials. But the persistent effort is required. The effort need the energy to mobilize the individual for a solution. This energizing pull is a kind of incentive which is based on the hope of outcome. Thus, hope gives incentive, and the individual experiences pull toward the goal.

Measurement of Motives

The methods for the measurement of motives may be classified as direct, indirect, and experimental depending upon the nature of the adopted measures or techniques.

Direct Methods

It includes all methods and techniques that permit the subject to express his motives through verbal or other overt behavior. The major methods may be a questionnaire, inventories, motivation scales, checklists, naturalistic observations, interviews, autobiographies and other self-descriptive measures.

Indirect Method

When the subject is either unaware of his motives or is determined not to reveal his real motives, the use of indirect methods is recommended the most. The material given to the subject consists of fairly ambiguous or unstructured stimulus situations. The subject is expected to provide clues or his hidden or true motives by responding to these unstructured stimuli.

All the projective techniques such as Rorschach inkblot test, thematic apperception test (TAT), child apperception test (CAT), completion tests, word association techniques, role-playing, and socio-drama.

Experimental Method

These consist of measures involving objective observation under controlled conditions. Firstly, the researcher makes some tentative hypotheses and then tests them in laboratory or laboratory-like conditions for arriving at some objective, reliable, and valid conclusions. For example, one may hypothesize that the persons having high achievement motive must differ in many predictable ways from persons with low achievement motive.

■ EMOTIONS

Introduction

Can you imagine life without emotion— without joy, anger, sorrow, or fear? Emotions are very important in the life of an individual. Different emotions such as love, anger, hatred, fear, etc., can be observed in the behavioral reactions of humans. Emotions not only can make life and everything colorful and pleasurable but can also turn the conditions, to hell. Thoughts and decisions do have some reasoning and rationality because of intelligence but these can also be determined by weak or strong feelings of emotionality. However, emotions can be controlled and applied successfully in various situations of life. It is called emotional intelligence.

UNIT VII: Motivation and Emotional Processes

Meaning

The word emotion is derived from a Latin word *Emovere* meaning a stir-up state or excitement. In a simple way, emotion is a state of excitement or disturbance—mental and physiological. Usually, emotions are equated with feeling but there is a difference in feeling and emotions. Feeling is experience at the cognition level which is general in nature and there is no bodily disturbance. But when bodily or physiological disturbances are included with feelings, then it is called emotions.

Definitions

Emotion is an acute disturbance of the individual as a whole. Psychological in origin, conscious experience and visceral functioning.
—*PT Young*

Emotions are episodes in which the individual is moved or excited. —*Gates*

Emotion is a complex state of organism involving bodily and mental changes and marked by strong feeling. —*James Drever*

Emotions resemble the effective response and have special biological significance for the organism. —*Boring and Field*

It is a complex pattern of change in response to a situation perceived as personally significant including physiological arousal, feeling, thoughts, and behaviors.

Feeling: Feeling denotes the pleasure or pain dimension of emotions.

Mood: Mood is an affective state of long duration, but less intense than emotions.

Characteristics of Emotions

- It is a subjective feeling. Experience of emotions varies from person to person.
- Emotion varies in intensity (high, low) and quality (happiness, sadness, fear).
- It helps in verbal and nonverbal communication.
- It also helps us interpret the situations.
- It leads to bodily arousal.

Factors Affecting Emotions

- Subjective factors and situational context influence the experience of emotions.
- These factors are gender, personality, and psychopathology of certain kinds.
- Evidence indicates that women experience all the emotions except anger more intensely than men. Men are prone to experience the high intensity and frequency of anger.
- This gender difference has been attributed to the social roles attached to men (competitiveness) and women (affiliation and caring).

Biological Basis of Emotions

It is also based on the functioning of different parts of the brain such as cortex, hypothalamus, reticular formation amygdala, etc. To develop a complete understanding of emotions, these must be explained.

Cerebral Cortex

The emotion is a state of disturbance or excitement. Although, this disturbance takes place in different physiological changes the individual also consciously experiences the emotion. Individual feels aware that he is in anger, love, jealousy, hatred, fear. An individual can describe his state of emotion. This is possible only with the cerebral cortex. James Lange and Cannon-Bard also described in their respective theories of emotions that conscious experience of emotions develop at cortex when the stimulation about emotional situation reaches the cerebral cortex. Schacter also described in his theory that emotional experience is based on the cognitive appraisal of the situation. The signs and cues in the situation give experience of emotion and it requires the processing of these cues at the cerebral cortex.

It is observed that appraisal of emotional situation involves the working of the right hemisphere. The right cerebral hemisphere plays an important role in emotional functions. In some cases where the right cerebral hemisphere was damaged, individuals were unable to understand the emotionality in voice and scenes. The right hemisphere also seems to be specialized for the expression of emotions. Patients with damaged right hemisphere were unable to express their emotions.

Amygdala

It is an important part of the limbic system. It is involved in the emotions of threat and danger. It plays a key role in the interpretation of emotional information relating to threat and damage. The patients with damaged amygdala were unable to understand these negative and unpleasant emotions. From an evolutionary perspective, thus amygdala is important in reacting quickly to threats and dangers for the survival of the individual. Even the stimulations on amygdala also support its functioning in emotions.

Hypothalamus

It is another important part of the limbic system related to emotions. It lies just below the thalamus and just above the pituitary gland. The hypothalamus is a complex structure involved in regulating a wide variety of emotional and motivational behaviors. According to Cannon-Bard theory, hypothalamus discharges the impulses to cerebral cortex and different parts of the body, and thus a conscious experience of emotions and physiological changes takes place. Bard in his various experiments proved the importance of emotions. When the hypothalamus of cats was electrically stimulated, cats express expression of aggression. In another experiment, when it was removed, cats were not able to express emotions. Only mechanical or rudimentary expression was visible. Thus, the hypothalamus contributes to emotions.

Reticular Formation (RF) or Ascending Reticular Activating System (ARAS)

It is a network-like structure present at the brainstem and also spreads on the cortex. Lindsley in his theory of activation considers reticular formation as important in the experience of emotions. The arousal of the cortex depends upon the stimulation of RF which spreads it on the cortex. As the arousal increases, then at a higher state, it is experienced as emotion. So, emotion is a high state of arousal of the cortex. In this regard, the RF plays an important role in carrying arousal to the higher state.

Lindsley also considered ascending reticular activating system (ARAS). ARAS is spread over gray matter, pons, midbrain, and diencephalons. ARAS receives sensory inputs from various sensory pathways. This structure stimulates higher brain centers to keep the arousal state of the brain. ARAS can also widely stimulate the hypothalamus, so that stimulation can reach any emotion center. Lindsley observed in studies that electrical stimulation of ARAS could develop similar EEG patterns as observed in emotions. Lindsley also observed that neural centers, which control the emotions, are present in brainstem reticular formation (BSRF). Thus, BSRF also plays an important role in emotions.

The major function of ARAS is to keep the brain in awakening state. The more the ARAS is stimulated, the higher will be the arousal or activation in the organism. If ARAS is calm, then cortical functioning will be of the lowest kind and the person will feel sleepy. Sensory inputs pass through ARAS, where these are either inhibited or facilitated. Those sensory inputs, which are inhibited at ARAS, never reach the cortex and the person never gets aware of that information. Sensory inputs, which are facilitated gets spread over the projection areas on the cortex and the person gets aware of that information. ARAS alerts the cortex to receive these outer sensory inputs. This effect is called arousal reaction. However, it is wrong to think that ARAS functioning depends upon the outer sensory inputs. Neural impulses from the cortex itself can stimulate ARAS. Thus, ARAS can be stimulated by external as well as internal stimulation. Thus, the emotional experience at the cortex is regulated by the facilitating and inhibiting control of ARAS.

Adrenal Glands

These are also known as ductless glands which secrete directly into the blood. This secretion is called hormones. The stimulation of endocrine glands is associated with emotions. Especially, the adrenal glands secrete in emergency and emotional situations. The adrenal gland is present near the kidney. It is a pair of glands present on the kidneys. The upper part is called the cortex and the lower is medulla. In an emotional situation, it secretes epinephrine which helps the individual to face stressful and emotional conditions. Whereas the adrenal medulla secretes norepinephrine which brings the body to normal and relaxed state. It is observed that a decrease in the secretion of the adrenal gland lowers the individual resistance to a stressful and emotional situation.

Sympathetic Nervous System

It is a part of the autonomic nervous system. It normally functions in emotional and emergency situations. During the emotional or stressful conditions, it brings various physiological changes in the body that releases a lot of energy and provide strength to the body to cope with the conditions. Various physiological changes associated with its activation are as follows:
* Heartbeat is accelerated.
* Respiration rate increases.
* Hormone level in the blood rises.
* Sugar level in blood increases.
* Slow down the digestive functioning.
* Blood circulation increases.

These are autonomic reactions, and the changes are associated with emotions. In the case of extreme excitement, these changes may get out of control. When the emotional situation is over, then the other part of autonomic nervous system, i.e., the parasympathetic nervous system slows down these changes to a normal level.

Theories of Emotions

James–Lange Theory

One of the earliest physiological theories of emotion was given by James (1884) and supported by Lange, hence, it has been named the James-Lange theory of emotion. The theory suggests that environmental stimuli elicit physiological responses from viscera (the internal organs such as heart and lungs both are associated with muscle movement).

The main implication made by these theories is that particular events or stimuli provoke particular physiological changes, and the individual's perception of these changes results in the emotion being experienced.

James-Lange theory argues that your perception about your bodily change, such as rapid breathing, a pounding heart, and running legs following an event brings forth emotional arousal. However, this theory faces a lot of criticism (**Fig. 6**).

For example: For detail refer **Figure 7**.

Limitation
* From our common sense experience, it looks very odd that individual starts to run on observing a lion and after running some distance experiences fear.
* When physiological changes were developed artificially by injecting certain drugs, subjects respond no experience of emotion. This theory has no explanation for patient.
* Various studies have proved that hypothalamus plays an important role in the origin of emotions.
* Further, various emotions basically have the same physiological changes. How the cortex differentiates different

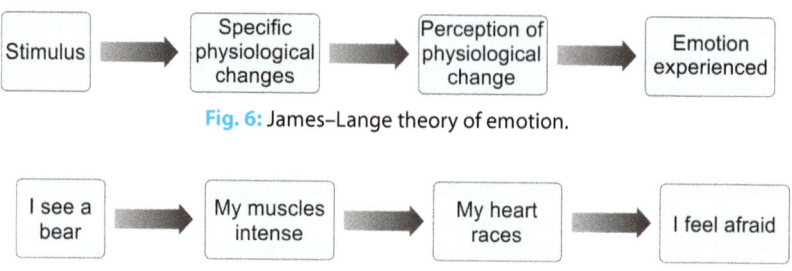

Fig. 6: James–Lange theory of emotion.

Fig. 7: Example of James–Lange theory.

emotions—the theory has no answer to this.

Cannon–Bard

Cannon (1927) proposed this theory and later Bard (1934) also confirmed this theory. It is stated that the entire process of emotion is mediated by the thalamus which after perception of the emotion-provoking stimulus, conveys this information simultaneously to the cerebral cortex providing the feeling of emotion and the sympathetic nervous system causing physiological arousal.

The cerebral cortex then determines the nature of the perceived stimulus by referring to past experience. This determines the subjective experience of the emotion; at the same time the sympathetic nervous system and the muscle provide physiological arousal and prepare the individual to take action (**Fig. 8**).

Limitation

- Thalamus and hypothalamus do play important role in emotions. However, some emotions and their effects are retained for long durations. Sometimes thalamus and hypothalamic do not have this capacity of maintaining an emotion for many years.
- Various studies on cats were cited in the favor of the theory. But the emotional expression of cats was very mechanical, stereotyped, and diffused.
- Emotions also sometimes have a motivational perspective. Emotional behavior is also organized and purposeful. This theory has ignored this perspective of emotions.
- Some other studies prove that besides the thalamus and hypothalamus, other parts of the brain are also found related to emotions such as prefrontal cortex and cerebellum. This theory has given no importance to it.
- In some studies, it has been found that if the cortex is removed and then the thalamus, it does not have any effect on the expression of anger of cats. This theory has no explanation for it.

Schachter–Singer Theory

This theory is also called "two factor theory" or "cognitive labeling theory." This states that for an emotion to occur, there must be physiological arousal and second, there must be an explanation for the arousal.

So, there must be some kind of attention-getter and the reason why it got that specific person's attention. It accounts for subjective interpretation. It does not account for specific physiological states associated with some emotions (**Flowchart 2**).

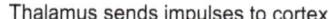
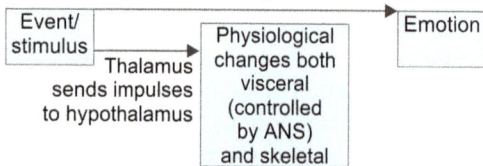

Fig. 8: The Cannon–Bard theory of emotion. (ANS: autonomic nervous system)

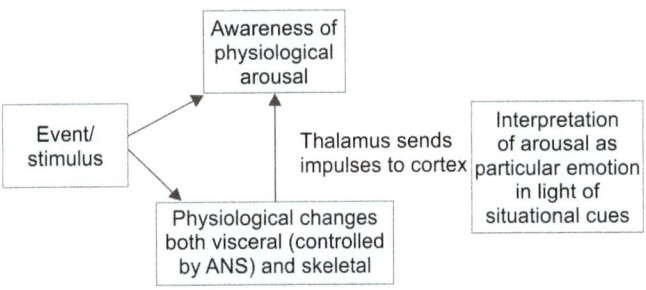

Flowchart 2: Schachter–Singer theory of emotion.

(ANS: autonomic nervous system)

Lazarus Theory

It most heavily emphasizes the cognitive aspect. This theory explains that an emotion-evoking stimulus or event triggers a cognitive appraisal, which is followed by emotion and physiological arousal.

Activation Theory of Emotions

This theory was given by Lindsley (1951). Lindsley tried to explain the emotion with the arousal level. The arousal of the cortex of a person depends upon the stimulation of reticular formation (RF). RF is a structure that makes an organism alert about particular stimuli and produces general arousal. But it also starts the behavior and maintains it till the satisfaction of the goal. RF on the brainstem has excitatory and inhibitory connections with the motor neurons of the spinal cord, through which it controls the activities of muscles. Projections from RF to cerebrum are very important as these maintain the stimulation for cortical functions. Studies also show that if cortical areas are stimulated, changes in the function of RF or brainstem are also observed. It is also found that RF can also develop changes in sensory inputs. Thus, Lindsley concluded that RF has a control on muscular activities, cortical functioning, and also sensory inputs, through which it controls different behavior of the organism.

Motivation and emotions are considered as higher arousal states. Lindsley also considered ascending reticular activation system (ARAS). ARAS is spread over gray matter, pons, midbrain, and diencephalon. ARAS receives sensory inputs from various sensory pathways. This structure stimulates higher than brain centers to keep the arousal state of the brain. ARAS can also widely stimulate the hypothalamus. Lindsley also observed that neural centers, which control emotions, are present in brainstem reticular formation (BSRF). Thus, BSRF also plays an important role in emotions.

Limitation

- This theory does explain strong emotions such as aggression very well but is unable to describe soft emotions which are not based on a higher arousal state.
- Lindsley described emotional and no-emotional behaviors as the same, it does not differentiate between these different behaviors.
- It does not differentiate between emotion and motivation, however, it develops confusion.
- Perception also plays important role in emotions. The same situation can be reacted differently by two individuals. This theory has given no significance to perception in emotions.
- Perception also plays important role in emotions. The same situation can be reacted differently by two individuals. This theory has given no significance to perception in emotions.

Arnold's Theory of Emotion

Arnold believes that the cognitive process of an individual interprets this feeling and controls the behavior toward these feelings. Individual first perceives the stimulus situation. This perception is categorized as bad, indifferent, and good. If the stimulus is good, it will be received, bad is rejected, and indifferent ignored. Evaluation of a stimulus is not simply based on memory and past experiences but also on whether it is bad or good. This evaluation is immediate, and it takes place before physiological changes and emotional experiences. For example, if a person is having panic time at some place and suddenly saw a bull coming toward him, he will move away from the place. So, perception of situation is very important step in emotions. Arnold believes that physiological change and emotional experience both are determined by the cortex.

Lazarus et al. (1970) progressed this work. Lazarus pointed out that the evaluation of emotional stimulus controls the emotional reaction of a person. This evaluation differs for different emotions. Social conditions and cultural background also play important role in the evaluation of a stimulus.

However, this theory is also having certain limitations; like other theories, it does not explain different parts of the brain participating in emotional and physiological mechanisms.

Physiological Changes in Emotions

Emotions are always accompanied by strong physiological changes as follows:

1. **Heartbeat:** Emotional reactions result in fluctuations in heart rate. It may rise or fall. These can be measured by **ECG (electrocardiogram)**.
2. **Blood pressure:** Constriction and expansions in blood vessels in emotion can vary the blood pressure. Constriction raises the blood pressure whereas expansion leads to lowering of blood pressure. It can be measured by a sphygmomanometer.
3. **Respiratory rate:** Variation in the rate of breathing develops during emotion. It may rise or fall.
4. **Pulse rate:** Emotions also change the pulse rate of a person. Pulse rate can be measured by a sphygmomanometer.
5. **Hormonal changes:** Hormonal secretion takes place during emotions. The level of certain hormones may rise in emotions.
6. **Brain waves:** Alertness of the brain is observed in the form of waves. In daytime alert stage that requires deep thinking leads to fast waves. Relaxed wakefulness is accompanied by waves. Speed waves also decrease in emotional reaction, such variations in wave speed have been observed. It can be measured by **EEG (electroencephalogram)**.
7. **Digestive system:** Emotional reactions can result in changes in secretions in the digestive tract; that is why some people report digestive troubles during emotions.
8. **White blood corpuscles:** These are important components of our immunity system. Any changes in the numbering of these can expose the body to various diseases. During strong emotional reactions, it is the strength of these cells that decreases.
9. **Galvanic skin response:** It refers to bioelectric conductance in the skin. Emotions are also accompanied by variation in bioelectric potential in the skin which can be measured by bio-feedback apparatus for **Galvanic skin response (GSR)**.

Measurement of Emotions

Before measuring emotions, one must be able to characterize emotions and distinguish them from other states. Now, emotions are best treated as a multifaceted phenomenon consisting of the following components— behavioral reactions, expressive reactions, physiological reactions, and subjective feeling.
1. **Nonverbal instruments to measure emotions:** It consists of instruments

that measure either the expressive or physiological component of emotion.

a. *For expressive reactions:* It is the facial, vocal, and postural expression that accompanies the emotion. For example, anger comes with a fixed stare, contracted eyebrows, compressed lips, vigorous movements, raised voices, almost shouting.
- Facial expression instruments are facial expression analysis tool (FEAT) and Facial Electromyography (EMG) for facial muscle activity.
- Vocal expression instruments measure the effects of emotion in multiple vocal cues, e.g., average pitch, pitch changes, speaking rate, voice quality, and articulation.

b. *For physiologic reactions:* Emotions show a variety of physiological manifestations that can be measured with a diverse array of techniques. Examples are the instruments that measure blood pressure, skin responses, heart rate, adrenaline levels, brain waves, papillary responses, tears, and perspiration. Some ANS instruments such as IBM's emotion mouse and variety of wearable sensors can help the computers to gather multiple physiological signals while experiencing an emotion and polygraph-lie detector.

2. **Verbal instruments to measure emotions:** These assess the subjective feeling component of emotions, i.e., thoughts which are observed indirectly through:
- Spoken and written words on rating scales
- Answers to open-ended questions on surveys and during interviews
- Responses to projective instruments, sentence stems, etc.
- Self-assessment or perceptions regarding the behavior and intentions of others
- Other cognitive function such as rational/logical thinking

Verbal instruments used are self-reports, rating scales, pictogram (e.g., self-assessment manikin or SAM), and PREMO (product emotion).

Emotions in Nursing

1. **Help the patient feel comfortable:** Give a warm welcome to the patient. Let him feel that he is an important guest. Do not show judgmental attitude toward the patient. Orient the client with unit and ward staff to provide the feeling of security and assurance of personal safety.

2. **Interact with the patient and relatives:** Introduce yourself to the patient. Stay with the patient. Communicate with him for expression of feeling and release of anxiety.

3. **Alert with basic needs of the patient:** Help the patient to determine the unmet needs. A nurse should be an expert to understand the link of emotions with unmet needs, e.g., need for acceptance when the patient is rejected. When physiological needs are met, then comes the next higher need in the hierarchy and to meet them.

4. **Understand negative emotions:** Understand the use of defenses by the patient. Find out the problem, the patient is facing and its cause. Clarify the problem that he is facing by comparing the perception of the patient's problem with her own perception of that same problem. Acknowledge feelings of anger, guilt, helplessness, and powerlessness while taking care of them.

5. **Promote positive feeling:** Deal with the emotions and take a more concrete problem-solving approach to emotional reactions. Encourage explorations of feeling. Develop alternative strategies for creating changes that are realistically possible. Promote relaxation techniques. Promote healthy interpersonal relationships.

6. **Develop empathy:** Understand the patient's situation, feelings, and motives. Accept the patient as he is.
7. **Prevent psychosomatic illness:** Help the patient to relax. Arrange for professional help if severe emotional reactions.

Alteration in Emotion

Up to this point, it is discussed how the mechanism of emotion works. But now some questions are still to answer about the occurrence of emotions. Some of these are as follows:

- What is the sequence of occurrence of a variety of emotions?
- What is the duration of emotion?
- How does the emotion change?

With reference to these questions, an attempt is made to understand the alteration in emotions. It is not that one emotion occupies the mind and body of a person forever but the emotion keeps on varying in different situations. In certain situation, individual may feel happy and excited but the change in the situation may result in anger or aggression. For example, an individual is happy with friends but as soon as reach at working place may experience depression and sadness. Even in the same situations, some alteration in emotion can be experienced because of external or internal factors. For example, a person is enjoying a lovely party but suddenly becomes frustrated and angry because of recall of some unpleasant memories associated with a person coming in party. So, the mind cannot remain occupied with a single emotion, but it undergoes alteration in emotions. Further, there is no permanent sequence of alteration of emotions. However, in some cases, some predictions can be possible. For example, in the case of bipolar depression, alteration between excited and depressive mode can be predicted with a specific pattern. Alteration of emotions is also related to the duration of an emotion. In some cases, a particular emotion such as anger or excitement can stay for many hours to many days whereas in other cases it may be a short duration although, prediction is difficult; but in some cases, it is possible if the nature and personality experience different emotions for short duration only whereas sensitive people to experience one particular emotion for long duration, for example, patient suffering with depression can remain depressed for more than 6 months.

Another aspect should be felt here that it is not that emotions always occur alternatively. In some cases, an individual can experience a mixture of more than one emotion in one particular situation. For example, unpleasant feelings, frustration, anger, depression, and pain can occur together.

It can be said that alteration in emotion is a natural process that is experienced universally by every individual. This alteration cannot be predicted but if the conditions and situation are known along with the nature of the person some possibility of prediction is available.

Emotion in Health and Sickness

Emotion has great significance in sickness. Emotion is accompanied by strong physiological disturbances, if the patient is already suffering from physiological disorders. It may exaggerate the condition. An emotional state can further deteriorate the health of a patient, for example, for a patient suffering from blood pressure or heart attack, any excitement can be dangerous. On the other side emotion in sickness can create various behavioral problems in patients, which further aggravates the health problems. For example, severe anxiety and fear can make patients irritating in behavior and non-cooperative in treatment. Reluctance, as taking any advice or medicine, makes the patient trouble for doctors and nurses.

Depression is another emotional reaction that is categorized as mood disorder. It is itself a sickness. It is a feeling of sadness and dejection. Patients feel a loss of energy and show no interest in the social and routine type of activities. Sleep problems also develop during depression. The problem becomes further when the patient stop talking, and food and continuous weight loss is serious concern.

Anxiety is another emotional reaction that a patient can feel during sickness. Anxiety is a feeling of apprehensiveness about pending danger in the environment. Anxiety itself develops certain psychological troubles if it becomes severe.

Various anxiety disorders can be developing such as phobias, obsessive-compulsive disorder, hysteria, etc. These psychological problems require special attention other than the patient already suffering. Sickness, hospital environment and break from routine life increase the anxiety level of the patient.

Irritation also develops and a patient quarrel with other on petty matters and unnecessary emotional turmoil becomes troubles for the health of the patient. Anger develops because of frustration. The patient feels annoyed with the things happening to him.

▌ STRESS AND ADAPTATION

Stress

Stress is part of being human, and it can help motivate you to get things done. Even high stress from serious illness, job loss, a death in the family, or a painful life event can be a natural part of life. You may feel down or anxious and that is normal too for a while.

Stress is a universal phenomenon. All people experience it. Stress is a pattern of specific and nonspecific responses an organism makes to stimulus events that disturb its equilibrium. The stimulus events include a huge variety of external and internal conditions that collectively are called stressors.

Definition of Stress

"Stress is the nonspecific response of the body to any demand."
—Hans Selye

Stress can be defined as any type of change that causes physical, emotional, or psychological strain. Stress is your body's response to anything that requires attention or action.

Stress is the feeling of being overwhelmed or unable to cope with mental or emotional pressure.

Stressors

A stressor can be defined as an internal or external event or situation that creates the potential for any event, force, or condition that results in physical or emotional stress.

Sources of Stress-Stressors

Physiologic: Trauma, surgery, radiation, body chemistry alterations, infectious processes.

Environmental: Pollutants, sensory overload, loss of privacy, unpleasant noises, odors, untidy surroundings.

Psychological: Fear, anxiety, psychological distress.

Sociocultural: Financial status, vocational pressures, family dysfunction, child-rearing, ageing, retirement, religious beliefs.

Workplace: Workload, demanding boss, job design, working conditions, physical work layout.

Individual: Family issues, personal economic problems, and individual's personality, broken families and marriages.

Day-to-day stressors: Common occurrences such as getting caught in a traffic jam, arguments with a spouse/roommate.

Stress Cycle (Fig. 9)

❖ Stress has both acute and chronic effects on the physiology as well as the psychology of an individual. If a person is not able to successfully adapt to changing situation, it may result in distress whereas successfully adapting to changing situation leads to wellness.

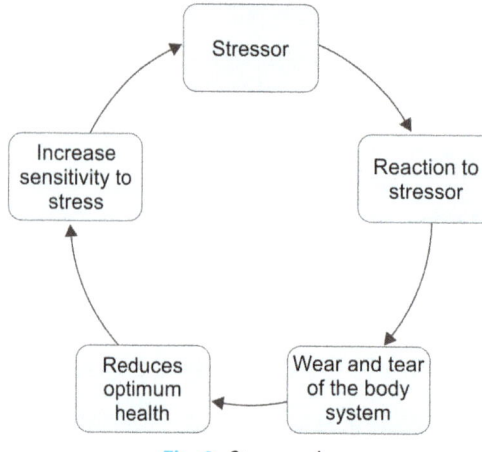

Fig. 9 : Stress cycle.

- **Stressors:** It is the stimuli that proceed or precipitate stress which causes bodily and mental tension. Stress has two types—internal stressor includes stressors that exist within an individual, e.g., illness, fever, etc. External stressor includes stimuli that occur from the external environment and result in stress, e.g., noise, death, etc.
- **Reaction to stress:** Upon encountering a stressor, the body reacts with a "fight-or-flight" response and the sympathetic nervous system is activated. Hormones such as cortisol and adrenaline are released into the bloodstream to meet threats or danger.
- **Wear and tear of the body systems:** Human body tries to cope with the existing stress by activating the sympathetic nervous system. Long-term activation of this system may lead to fatigue, restlessness, and excessive alertness and gradually the body system goes through the wear and tear process.
- **Reduce optimum health:** If stressors sustain beyond the body's capacity, the health of the person deteriorates and leads to many health problems such as hypertension, somatic problems, diabetes, and many other psychosomatic problems.
- **Increase sensitivity to stress:** If stress is not resolved adaptively, it may increase the person's sensitivity to a subsequent stressor. In such conditions a person may re-experience the traumatic events more severely.

Effect of Stress

- Physical
- Emotional
- Psychological

1. Physical Response

- Muscle aches, stiffness, profuse sweating, or facial flushing
- Cold, clammy hands
- Facial tics: rapid eye blinking, etc.
- Tapping feet or drumming fingers
- Headaches
- Sleep problems
- Dizziness
- Fatigue
- GI symptoms: nausea, etc.
- Skin disorders: rashes, hives, acne
- Back pain
- Change in appetite
- Palpitations

2. Emotional Response

- Anger
- Anxiety
- Depression
- Memory loss
- Lack of concentration
- Apathy
- Lack of self-esteem
- The feeling of hopelessness, helplessness, etc.
- Less idealism or passion

3. Psychological Response

- Stress for a longer period of time may cause psychological problems in some individuals
- Symptoms are:
  - Social isolation phobias
  - Compulsive behavior
  - Eating disorders
  - Night terrors

Types of Stress

While there are many different kinds of stress, based on research studies about the types of stress in psychology, stress can be divided into three primary types.

1. Acute Stress

Acute stress results from your body's reaction to a new or challenging situation. It is that feeling you get from an approaching deadline or when you narrowly avoid being hit by a car. We can even experience it as a result of something we enjoy. Like an exhilarating ride on a roller coaster or an outstanding personal achievement.

Acute stress is classified as short-term. Usually, emotions and the body return to their normal state relatively soon.

2. Episodic Acute Stress

Episodic acute stress is when acute stresses happen frequently. This can be because of repeatedly tight work deadlines. It can also be because of the frequent high-stress situations experienced by some professionals, such as healthcare workers. With this type of stress, we do not get time to return to a relaxed and calm state. And the effects of the high-frequency acute stresses accumulate. It often leaves us feeling like we are moving from one crisis to another.

3. Chronic Stress

Chronic stress is the result of stressors that continue for a long period of time. Examples include living in a high-crime neighborhood or constantly fighting with your life partner.

This type of stress feels never-ending. We often have difficulty seeing any way to improve or change the situation that is the cause of our chronic stress.

Stress Adaptation

According to Hans Selye (1907–1982), the doctor who pioneered stress research, stress is the nonspecific response of the body to any demand on it. As Selye noted, stress occurs as a response to a range of circumstances. Biologically, stress reactions evolved as an emergency response intended to prepare an individual for fight-or-flight, that is, either to defend oneself or try to run away from a threat. In psychological terms, stress is a response of the body to whatever is perceived as an emergency situation.

General Adaptation Syndrome

General adaptation syndrome (GAS) is a theory that describes the physiological changes the body experiences when under stress. The syndrome includes three stages—the alarm stage, the resistance stage, and the exhaustion stage.

- **The alarm stage:** The first GAS stage contains two substages:
  - In the **shock phase**, body temperature and blood pressure both decrease. Loss of fluid from body tissues also occurs.
  - In the **countershock phase**, the body's fight-or-flight response is triggered. Heart rate and blood pressure increase as stress hormones and adrenaline are released.
- **The resistance stage:** Following the alarm stage, the body begins to repair itself. If the stressful situation is resolved, the body continues to repair itself until it returns to its pre-stress state. If the stressful situation is not resolved, the body remains on high alert, eventually adapting to the higher stress level. Stress hormones and blood pressure remain elevated. This can lead to hypertension and heart problems as well as irritability, frustration, and poor concentration.
- **The exhaustion stage:** This stage occurs during prolonged or chronic stress when the body's adaptation to higher stress levels starts to break down. The body no longer has the strength or resources to fight stress. Signs of the exhaustion stage include, but are not limited to, the following:
  - Trouble sleeping
  - Severe loss of concentration

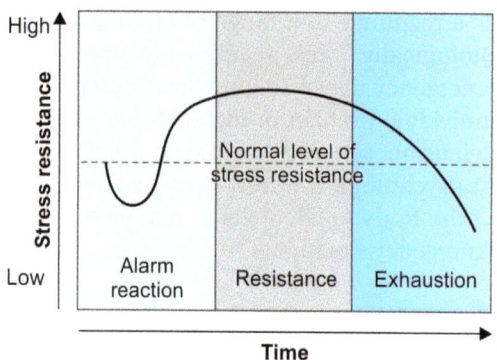

Fig. 10: General adaptation syndrome (GAS).

- Fatigue
- Depressed mood
- Trembling or jumpiness
- Anxiety attacks
- Crying spells
- Stress-related illnesses

For short-term or mild stressors, the alarm stage is not harmful. It is a natural mechanism that is designed to protect the body from danger. However, when prolonged or chronic stress is experienced, the body may not be able to repair itself in a timely manner, which can lead to the exhaustion stage.

Understanding the stages of GAS can help with the identification of personal stress signals, which can help with the reduction of stress levels (**Fig. 10**).

Local Adaptation Syndrome

The local adaptation syndrome (LAS) is a physiological response to a stressor (e.g., trauma, illness) on a specific part of the body. For example, if the person cuts a hand, the LAS initiated inducing localized information. The classic symptoms (inflammation, redness, swelling, and warmth) occur at the injured site. If the inflammation does not resolve with LAS the individual then experiences the GAS as the entire body becomes effected.

Stress Management

Physical Techniques

- Exercise
- Rest
- Nutrition
- Yoga

Mental Techniques

- Meditation
- Guided imagery
- Brain programming

Stress-Adaptation Coping Strategies to Help with Physical Well-being

- **Relaxation techniques**: Relaxation techniques can help us gain more control over the stress we encounter. This is because it is a technique that helps bring about the opposite bodily changes of the stress response or can reduce muscle tension.
- **Eat regular well-balanced meals and get plenty of rest**. When your body is run down, things can look worse than they really are and your ability to cope with them is also reduced. Limit your coffee to three cups per day and remember that chocolate and cola drinks also contain caffeine.
- **Exercise:** A physical workout is a great tension releaser. Find something that you enjoy and do it on a regular basis. It can be as simple as walking or as demanding as racquetball. Exercise can reduce anxiety and depression, reduce muscle tension and temporarily distract us from our stressors.

Techniques to Help with Academic Well-being

- **Learn to pace yourself**: No matter how hard you try, you cannot be in high gear all the time. Take rests while working. Set realistic goals and then take time out to reward yourself once you have reached them.
- **Realize your limits and plan around them**: Do not take on more than you can handle. If you have a number of must-do

Flowchart 3: Physiological changes as per stages of GAS.

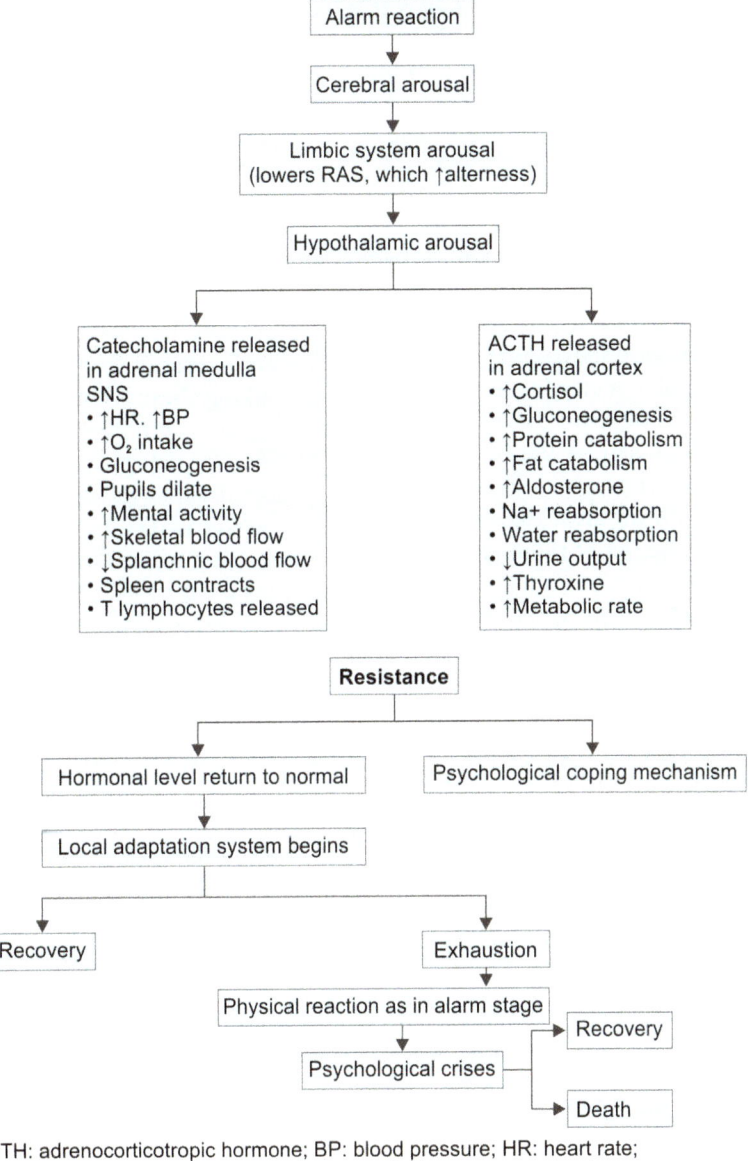

(ACTH: adrenocorticotropic hormone; BP: blood pressure; HR: heart rate; RAS: reticular activating system; SNS: symapthetic nervous system)

tasks, tackle them one at a time, in the order of their urgency. It is probably better to turn tasks away than to leave work unfinished. Unfinished business is a major source of stress.

* **Make the most of your time:** Try to work as efficiently as you can in blocks of time by utilizing a realistic time schedule.

Counseling services staff can help you develop more effective time management skills.

* **Streamline your assignments:** Break complex assignments down into manageable components.
* **Plan for change:** Some changes can be predicted and by predicting change, you

can reduce the shock of being unprepared. If you are a prospective student, talk with other students to learn about the changes they experienced. This information may lead you to prepare ahead of time for the inevitable changes. For example, learn a word-processing computer program before you have to type an assignment for class. Develop effective study skills. Go to class prepared with your readings and homework completed. Ask the professor questions either in class or after class when you do not understand something. Get in the habit of reviewing lecture notes immediately after the lecture to help reinforce the learning which just took place. Also, review notes and readings weekly. By following these suggestions, you will probably be better prepared to study for examinations.

- **Take time out for yourself away from your responsibilities:** For at least a short period each day to sort out your thoughts and feelings. How much time you need will depend on a number of factors. However, even 15 minutes devoted to yourself can help. Also, use this time to relax.
- **Have fun**: Plan to do something that you enjoy on a regular basis.

Techniques to Help with Psychological Well-being

- **Identify and deal with the cause**: It is important to determine what is causing your distress. Otherwise, you may only superficially deal with your distress so that little relief is experienced. Without this step, stress will build and continue. You may ask yourself: What has changed? When did I start feeling distressed? How are my beliefs or thoughts contributing to how I see the stressful situation? Am I expecting too much? Do I not believe I can handle the situation? By identifying the cause, we can more accurately select ways of coping such as revising our expectations, improving study techniques, or gaining support from others.
- **Be aware of negative self-talk** and negative attitudes.
- **Thought stopping:** Monitor your negative thinking and when it starts say aloud to yourself, "STOP!" The thoughts can come back, and probably will, but when they do, you can use the same technique to stop them again. It will take time and practice to break the habit of negative thinking. However, do not use the technique to stop reasonable worries and appropriate thinking about what you need to do.
- **Engage in positive self-talk:** Encourage yourself with phrases that are positive rather than negative.
- **Restrict worrying:** If you find yourself engaging in catastrophic thinking (i.e., imagining all of the terrible scenarios or possibilities) try to restrict your worrying to specific times and places. Find a chair in a place at home and at school that you do not particularly like to sit in. Make at least two appointments to go to your worry chair every day and worry for about 20 minutes. Do not do anything else in that chair. This will help get your worrying under control.
- **However, to only worry will not lead to an improved outcome:** It is, therefore, important to recognize when you are only worrying and move beyond worrying into problem-solving. You may ask yourself "What is the cause of my worrying?" and "Is there anything that can be done to modify the situation?" It may be helpful to speak with a counselor to help you with this process.
- **Talk out your troubles:** Learn to talk things over with someone you trust. It releases pressure, makes you feel better, and sometimes can help you see a new side to your problem. If you find yourself getting preoccupied with emotional difficulty, resist letting it get in your way. Counseling

Services staff are available to listen to you. Learn to distance yourself. When you find yourself in a heated argument, stop and ask yourself "Is this something really worth fighting for?"
* **Do not fight the inevitable:** Accept what you cannot change.
* **Humor:** Laughter is a great stress-reducer.
* **Stress diary:** Keeping a stress diary allows us to monitor stress reactions and the events that precede them. This will help to identify the stressors that trigger stress reactions. For example, you may find that you experience a headache whenever you find yourself running late. Eliminating the stressor (i.e., running late) may allow you to eliminate the stress reaction (i.e., a headache).
* **Alter the view:** The way in which we view stressors and our ability to handle them has a profound effect on our ability to cope. Often, it is not the original stressor (e.g., an examination) but our reaction to it (e.g., excessive worrying) that causes the greatest amount of stress. Can you view the stressor in a more favorable light? Could things be worse? Can any good come out of dealing with the stressor?
* **Reassess:** Underestimating our ability to cope (e.g., negating previous successes, good study habits, or intelligence) or overestimating our ability (e.g., I can learn in a few nights what most students take an entire semester to learn) can also contribute to stress.

Stress in Relation to Sickness

* It can leave its impact at both psychological and physiological levels.
* At the physiological level, stress puts heavy pressure on various physiological mechanisms and its continuous pressure can develop different physiological disorders in the body.
* It causes some non-repairable damage to the body. It can lead to cardiovascular troubles such as hypertension and heart attack, migraine, headache, asthma, etc.
* Continuous stress produces catecholamine hormone in the body which puts pressure on the heart.
* Stress increases the proneness to accidents or injuries.
* To reduce the stress individual may apply defense mechanisms and excessive use can disturb the mental health of the person.
* The irritation, anxiety, and restlessness may be some of its results. But continuous use of defense mechanisms can lead to different delusions.
* If the stress continuous hallucinations can also develop. Continuous stress can also lead to the death of a person.

Stress in Nursing

There is no doubt that the nursing profession is very stressful. It is stressful in various ways. Managing the demands of a job, the responsibility of patients, tight schedule, and emergency situations at the hospital are a few things that reflect the intensity of stress involved in the nursing profession. As most nurses are women in the profession, responsibilities at home and at the hospital may develop conflict. Living under such continuous stress can become a cause of her own health problems—both mental and physical. So, it is necessary for a nurse to remember some important strategies or programs to reduce her stress on the job without disturbing her work efficiency. A few points are given below:
1. Avoid unnecessary arguments with others.
2. Take rest whenever it is possible.
3. Always take care of food and health.
4. Should learn some yoga exercises which can relax
5. Can listen to music or TV programs which relax and entertain
6. Avoid noisy conditions if it is possible.
7. Compromise with the hectic conditions of the nursing profession.

ATTITUDE

Meaning of Attitude

The term "attitude" refers to a tendency to evaluate a person, object, or idea with some degree of approval or disapproval.

Attitudes are evaluative statements indicating one's feeling either favorably or unfavorably toward persons, objects, events, or situations. Attitude is a very complex cognitive process just like the personality of an individual.

Definition

Attitude is defined as "a learned predisposition to respond in a consistently favorable or unfavorable manner with respect to a given object." That is, attitudes affect behavior at a different level than do values.

It is the evaluation expressed by terms such as liking-disliking, pro-anti, favoring-not favoring, and positive-negative. They are the feeling tone aroused by any attitude object.

Attitude is a little thing that makes a big difference (Winston Churchill).

Components of Attitude

- **Affective component:** The opinion or belief segment of an attitude. It includes liking or disliking of the person. This consists of the emotional feeling of the person. For example, one person likes the nursing profession, or others may or may not.
- **Behavioral component:** An intention to behave in a certain way toward someone or something. Thus, expressed attitudes usually have a consistent relationship to behavior. But again this depends upon the kind of attitudes and the kind of circumstances. For example, the agenda of the political parties and the actual outcome of an election.
- **Cognitive component:** It is made up of thoughts and beliefs the people hold about the object of the attitude. It is, therefore, what we have learned about something. It is what we believe to be true about it. For example, wear a protective mask for the prevention of corona.

Nature/Features of Attitude

Attitude can be characterized in different ways:
- Aspects of valence—the degree of favorableness or unfavorableness toward the event
- Aspects of multiplexity—number of the elements constituting the attitude
- Relation to need aspect—vary in relation to needs they serve
- Centrality aspect—the importance of attitude object to someone.
- Need and problem—it is totally based upon a person's need and problem
- Not innate—it is learned behavior not innate.
- Change with time and situation—time and situation effect the individual attitude
- Learned through experience—positive and negative attitude of the person toward anything makes the person's experience.
- Related to feelings and beliefs of people
- Effects one's behavior positively or negatively
- May be unconsciously held

Functions of Attitude

- **The adjustment function:** Attitudes often help people to adjust to their work environment.
- **Ego-defensive function:** Attitudes help people to retain their dignity and self-image.
- **The value-expressive function:** Attitudes provide individuals with a basis for expressing their values.
- **The knowledge function:** Attitudes provide standards and frames of reference that allow people to understand and perceive the world around them.

Formation of Attitude

- **Experience with object:** Attitude can develop from a personally rewarding or punishing experience with an object.
- **Classical conditioning:** It involves involuntary responses and is acquired through the pairing of two stimuli.
- **Operant conditioning:** It is based on the "Law of Effect" and involves voluntary responses, behaviors.
- **Vicarious learning:** Formation of attitude by observing the behavior of others and consequences of that behavior.
- **Family and peer groups:** A person may learn attitudes through imitation of parents.
- **Neighborhood:** Involves being told what attitudes to have by parents, schools, community organizations, religious doctrine, friends, etc.
- **Economic status:** Our economical and occupational positions also contribute to attitude formation.
- **Mass communication:** Television, radio, newspaper, and magazine feed their audiences large quantities of information.

Factors Affecting Attitude

There is a multitude of factors that cause attitude changes which are as follows:

Family: Family is a primordial institution, it is a basic unit of society. It acts as a powerful source for the formation of attitudes. Attitudes developed by an individual, whether positive or negative, are the result of family influence. As these attitudes are acquired from the primary stages of development it is very difficult to undo.

Peers: Peer groups refer to same-age people. They include same-age friends, neighbors, classmates, etc. The child easily internalizes these attitudes from them. Especially in the adolescent stage peer group plays a vital role.

Conditioning: When we are conditioned or adjusted to a certain setup of people, situation, etc. Acceptance of these conditions leads to both positive and negative attitudes. Negative reinforcements such as punishment, teasing, criticizing, and troubling may lead to developing a negative attitude.

Social adjustment functions: As most people prefer to lead a peaceful life they keep away from conflicts and unnecessary friction with others. This paves way for a positive attitude toward other beings. Our attitudes facilitate and maintain our relationships with members of positively valued groups. Usually, we want to go with significant others to us, and rebel against those unwanted.

Direct instruction: Sometimes direct instruction can influence attitude formation. This is in the case of commercials and advertisements in the media. For example, somebody gives information about a product or a recent trend in the diet we tend to have an attitudinal change toward that product which may be positive or negative.

Modeling: Modern society is shaped by media and consumerism. If we see a role model, a hero, or a celebrity we try to imitate their habits such as smoking, drinking, and dressing too.

Satisfaction of wants: It is the nature of man that he tries to have a positive attitude toward those people and objects which satisfy his wants and unfavorable attitudes toward those who do not satisfy his wants.

Prejudices: Prejudices are preconceived ideas or judgments where one develops some attitudes on other people, objects, etc., without the proper information. For example, disliking a teacher or a co-worker without knowing their abilities just because of their caste, religion, nationality, etc.

Attitudinal Change

Change is the nature of man—is a common proverb. But well-established attitudes tend to be resistant to change, whereas others may be more flexible to change. Attitude can be changed in a variety of ways. Some of the ways of attitude change are as follows:
- By obtaining new information from other people and mass media
- Direct experiences and incidents that occur daily, lead to a change in attitude.
- Attitudes may change through legislation and laws passed by a country.
- As every person is a member of a group or a reference group influence of one another modifies attitudes also.
- Situation and consequences of situation lead to attitudinal change.

Factor Affecting Attitude Change

Carl Hovland gave a model of attitude-change showing important factors at each stage (**Flowchart 4**). There must be a communicator who holds a particular position on some issue and is trying to convince others to hold this position. To do so, he produces a communication designed to persuade people that his position is correct and to induce them to change their own positions in the direction of his.

1. Source of Communication

a. **Prestige of the communicator:** Prestige to how expert the communicator is perceived to be in the area of concern and how much he is respected by the individual receiving the communication. For example, the necessity of receiving polio drops given by superstar "Amitabh Bachchan" is found more influential than any other low-prestige person on television.

b. **Intentions:** A major problem for a communicator is how to convince the audience that he is a disinterested observer. One way is when he argues against his self-interest.

   For example, when a nurse supervisor argues in favor of greater power for law enforcement agencies, she virtually produces no attitude change. But when she argues for greater protection of the nurses' rights and against strengthening law-enforcement agencies, change occurs.

c. **Similarity:** People tend to be influenced more by people who are similar to them than by people who are different. For example, someone is similar to us in terms of national, economic, racial, and religious background, and we also share many ideological values.

d. **Liking:** A communicator who is trusted, is more difficult to reject, and his message should produce more attitude change.

e. **Reference group:** It is a group to which an individual belongs. For example, we belong to nursing and we are much interested in nurses' group and activities run by nurses.

f. **The sleeper effect:** It appears that the effect of the source of a communication is strongest immediately after exposure to the communication and is much less important

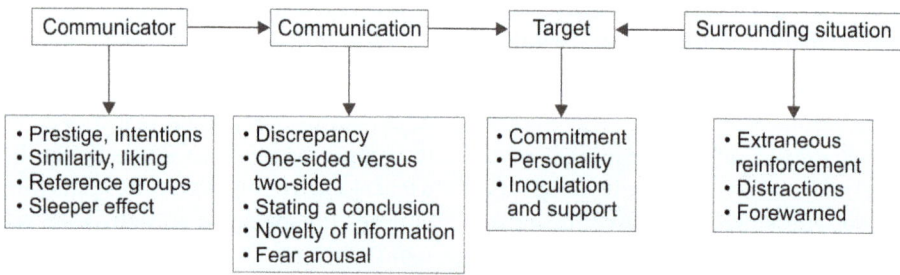

Flowchart 4: Factors affecting attitude change.

some time later. The immediate effect of the positive communicator is greater than that of the negative communicator. After 3 weeks, however, when the subjects are not reminded of the source of the communications, the effect of the positive communicator has declined while that of the negative communicator has increased. This is called the sleeper effect because the influence of the negative communicator is greater than it appears at first.

2. The Communication

a. **Discrepancy:** As mentioned earlier, the major source of stress in any influence situation comes from the discrepancy between the target's initial attitude and the attitude advocated by the communication. The greater the discrepancy, the greater the stress. If a smoker is told that smoking may cause his teeth to turn yellow, there is less stress than if he is told that smoking causes cancer. There is more attitude change with greater discrepancy.

b. **One-sided versus two-sided communications:** To produce the maximum effect, it appears that two-sided communication produces more attitude change when making the speaker appear better informed, more dispassionate, more objective, and less obviously attempting to persuade the listener.

c. **Stating a conclusion:** It helps to avoid the possibility that anyone in the audience could misinterpret it. On the other hand, the speaker may appear less intent on convincing the audience of a particular issue and the audience is encouraged to reach the conclusion without help, which may increase its effectiveness.

d. **Novelty of the information:** A communication that contains new information on an issue should be more effective than one that simply contains information with which the audience is already familiar. Thus, it is desirable to make it seem something new.

e. **Fear arousal:** Arousing fear is one of the most natural ways of trying to convince someone of something. A student nurse is emphasizing the importance of brushing one's teeth three times a day, after every meal. She explains the dangers of not doing so and explains the advantages of good dental care.

3. Characteristics of the Target

a. **Commitment:** It is the extent to which he feels reluctant to give up his initial position. Greater the strength of commitment to his own attitude, it is harder for the individual to change his attitude.

b. **Inoculation and support:** Another source of resistance to change in the target comes from an individual's past experience with the issue. We can strengthen his body generally, by giving him vitamins, exercises, and so on, and we can strengthen his defenses against that particular disease by building up antibodies.

c. **Personality factor:** A number of characteristics such as self-esteem, sex differences, defensive styles, etc.

4. Situational Factors

a. **Forewarned:** If someone is told ahead of time that he is going to be exposed to persuasive communication, he is better able to resist persuasion by that message.

b. **Distraction:** Too much distraction prevents the persuasive message from being heard at all and reduces its effectiveness to zero.

c. **The arousal of aggression:** People under an annoying, frustrating experience are more likely to accept the punitive communication and nonaggressive people would likely to accept lenient communication.

d. **The effect of reinforcement:** The reinforcement or incentive approach produces an attitude change situation. It consists of an interplay of forces as a result of which it pushes the individual to change his attitude. When a nurse is rewarded with "Best

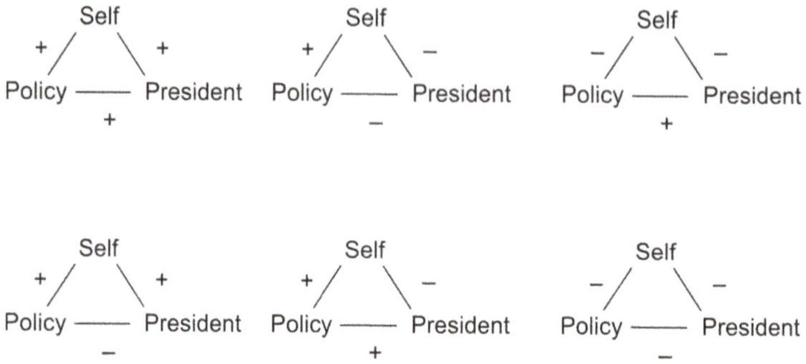

Bedside Nurse" she herself and also others are influenced to show such an attitude in the future.

Theories of Attitude Formation

1. Balance Theory—by Heider (1946–1958)

The theory is concerned with consistency in the judgment of people and issues that are linked by some form of relationship. People seek balance in their cognitive structure and attitude change comes when the system is not balanced. It emphasized the positive and negative valence of attitudes toward objects or persons which might not agree with one another.

These theory statements are shown by plus or minus signs. It predicts that when all the signs are positive, a state of balance exists. If there is one negative sign or three negative signs, the outcome is negative leading to an imbalanced state (just like multiplication of two minuses yield a plus). Therefore, the balance occurs when there are either no negative signs or two negative signs (**Figs. 11A and B**).

2. Congruity Theory

Osgood and Tannenbaum (1955) postulate that the imbalance between attitudes is resolved by summing the amount of their positive or negative quality. There is a pair of attitudes on which one has a positive sign and one has a negative sign. The greater the amount of the positive or negative quality of an attitude, the less likely it is to change when paired with something of an opposite sign. While congruity is a stable state, incongruity is an unstable one. Focus on changes in the evaluation of source and concept linked by associative or dissociative assertion. Change in attitude to resolve incongruity (**Fig. 12**).

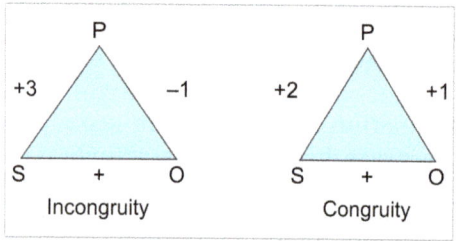

Fig. 12: Osgood and Tannenbaum congruity theory.

The valence goes from +3 to –3 on the usual attitude scale. Suppose you like a public figure at the highest scale value of +3 and then learn that he favors a policy that you dislike at the relatively moderate level of –1. The prediction is that you are more likely to alter the attitude toward the policy, in a more favorable or positive direction rather than the attitude toward the political figure in an unfavorable direction. However, the actual result may be a less negative or neutral attitude, rather than a positive one.

3. Cognitive Dissonance Theory (Festiner, 1957)

When related cognitions, feeling, or behaviors are inconsistent or contradictory, it creates an unpleasant state of tension that motivates people to reduce their dissonance by changing their

Figs. 11A and B: (A) Three balanced states; (B) Three imbalanced states.

UNIT VII: Motivation and Emotional Processes

Flowchart 5: Attitude-behavior process model.

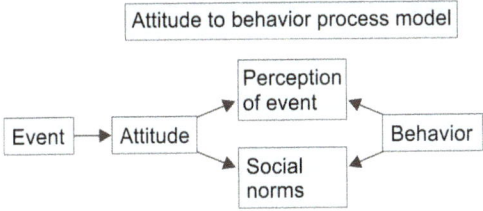

cognitions, feeling, or behaviors. For instance, a person who starts with a negative attitude toward marijuana will experience cognitive dissonance if they start smoking marijuana and find themselves enjoying the experience. The dissonance they experience is thus likely to motivate them to change their attitude toward marijuana, or to stop using marijuana.

Attitude-Behavior Process Model (Fazio and Powell, 1989) (Flowchart 5)

"Attitudes can guide a person's behavior even when the person does not actively reflect and deliberate about the attitude."

Types of Attitude (Table 1)

Positive Attitude

- Positive attitude helps you cope more easily with the daily affairs of life. It brings optimism into your life and makes it easier to avoid worry and negative thinking. If you adopt it as a way of life, it will bring constructive changes into your life, and makes you happier, brighter, and more successful.
- With a positive attitude, you see the bright side of life, become optimistic, and expect the best to happen. It is certainly a state of mind that is well worth developing.

Negative Attitude

- A negative attitude is characterized by a great disdain for everything; someone who constantly points out the negative in everything.
- A negative attitude is contagious and therefore avoiding people with one is the best way of prevention. Once you have a negative attitude, you will unlikely be able to recover and a self-fulfilling prophecy takes hold.

Measurement of Attitude (Box 1)

Thurstone scale: In this method first the data is collected from the respondent and next the data is collected from the others and then the whole process is compared to find out the attitude.

Likert scale: It provides five parameters for the attitude measurement to measure the attitude very clearly:
1. Strongly approved
2. Approved
3. Undecided
4. Disapproved
5. Strongly disapproved

Table 1: Characteristics of positive and negative attitude.

Positive	Negative
• Smile easily	• Rarely smiles
• Willing to change ideas and behavior	• Unwilling to change
• Can see another person's point of view	• Cannot see another person's point of view
• Rarely complains	• Blames others for own mistakes
• Accepts responsibility for mistakes	• Very critical of others
• Seldom criticizes others	• Thinks only of self
• Is considerate of others	• Does not look other people in the eyes
• Look other people in eyes when talking with them	• Forces own opinions on others
• Respects opinion of others	• Often makes excuses
• Never make excuse	• Has few interests
• Has a variety of interest	

UNIT VII: Motivation and Emotional Processes

Box 1: Different direct scales for assessing attitudes toward the church.

1. **Thurstone scale (adapted from Thurstone and Chave, 1929)**
   Check the statements with which you agree:
   a. I enjoy the church because there is a spirit of friendliness there
   b. I respect any church members' beliefs, but I think it is all "bunk"
   c. I think the organized church is an enemy of science and truth
   d. I believe in what the church teaches but with mental reservations
   e. I feel that church services give me inspiration and help me to live up to my best during the following week
   f. I feel the need for religion but do not find what I want in any one church

2. **Likert scale**
   For each statement, check the extent to which you agree.
   a. I believe that the church is the greatest institution in America today.
   (+2) _____ Strongly agree
   (+1) _____ Moderately agree
   (0) _____ Netural
   (−1) _____ Moderately disagree
   (−2) _____ Strongly disagree
   b. The church represents shallowness, hypocrisy, and prejudice.
   (−2) _____ Strongly agree
   (−1) _____ Moderately agree
   (0) _____ Neutral
   (+1) _____ Moderately disagree
   (+2) _____ Strongly disagree

3. **Semantic differential scale**
   Rate how you feel about the church on each of the scales below:

   Good ___ ___ ___ ___ ___ Bed
       (+2) (+1) 0 (−1) (−2)

   Unfavorable ___ ___ ___ ___ ___ Favorable
       (−2) (−1) 0 (+1) (+2)

   Pleasant ___ ___ ___ ___ ___ Unpleasant
       (+2) (+1) 0 (−1) (−2)

4. **One-item rating scale**
   How much do you like the church?
   Not at all ___ ___ ___ ___ ___ ___ ___ Very much
        1   2   3   4   5   6   7

Guttman scale: This scale measure how much positive or negative attitude towards particular thing, object, organization, or a person. It was developed by Louis Guttman in 1940s. Widely used in the measurement of attitudes and public opinion.

Bogardus scale: Seven-point scale raising from most favorable picture.

Opinion survey: By giving questionnaires to individual and groups to find out the result and measure the attitude accordingly.

Interview: By asking a person yes and no questions about a particular objective to understand the attitude.

Projective survey: By providing a person a particular situation and asking him to handle it alone to understand the attitude.

Role of Attitude in Health and Sickness

- Positive attitude is good for mental health.
- A positive mental attitude benefits health, longevity, and quality of life.

UNIT VII: Motivation and Emotional Processes

- Positive thinking reduces stress by eliminating negative self-talk.
- A person's attitude toward his illness has a huge impact. A positive attitude has a curative effect. Attitude helps in the management of chronic diseases.
- The nurse must promote a positive attitude toward rehabilitation.
- Nurses should try to understand the attitude of patients and inculcate positive attitude in patients regarding hospital, staff, and treatment to ensure quality care.
- Nurses should try to analyze the nature of attitude which determines patients' behavior and should change them into a favorable one.
- Patients often develop negative attitudes toward their illness, therefore, the nurse must determine to make the patient comfortable by giving attention to small details that will create therapeutic environment around the patient and the patient may feel at home.

QUESTION BANK

MULTIPLE CHOICE QUESTIONS

1. **What type of factor motivation is?**
   a. Physical
   b. Social
   c. Psychological
   d. Cultural
2. **The factor that directs to energize the behavior of humans and other organisms is called:**
   a. Instincts
   b. Leadership
   c. Motivation
   d. Competition
3. **The process of arousing, sustaining, and regulating activity is known as:**
   a. Learning
   b. Motivation
   c. Habit
   d. Maturation
4. **Perception about your bodily changes, following an event, brings forth emotion is:**
   a. Activation theory
   b. Hypothalamic theory
   c. Cannon–Bard theory
   d. James–Lange theory
5. **Both drive and incentives are factors in mobilizing one's:**
   a. Resources
   b. Ability
   c. Need
   d. Aspirations
6. **Who had given the hierarchy of human need?**
   a. Thorndike
   b. Maslow
   c. Guilford
   d. Koffka
7. **Which one of the following is an emotion?**
   a. Amusement
   b. Attention
   c. Stimulus
   d. Memory
8. **Which of the following motives are considered as primary motives?**
   a. Social motives
   b. Physiological motives
   c. Educational motives
   d. Psychological motives
9. **A student works hard to get the first rank in the class. The type of motivation behind his hard work is:**
   a. Intrinsic motivation
   b. Extrinsic motivation
   c. Zero motivation
   d. None of the above

UNIT VII: Motivation and Emotional Processes

10. **Which theory of emotion deals with the idea "Emotional experience depends upon emotional behavior?"**
    a. James–Lange theory
    b. Hypothalamic theory
    c. Activation theory
    d. Motivational theory
11. **Which one of the following is an emotion?**
    a. Memory
    b. Fear
    c. Attention
    d. Stimulus
12. **Which gland in your body starts the stress responses?**
    a. Lymph gland
    b. Pituitary gland
    c. Thyroid gland
    d. All of the above
13. **Which is a helpful way to deal with stress?**
    a. Meditation
    b. Exercise
    c. Talking with others
    d. All of the above
14. **Who was given the adaptation model?**
    a. Hans Selye
    b. Boring and Field
    c. Gates
    d. James–Lange
15. **Cognitive component of attitude is related to:**
    a. Thinking
    b. Behavior
    c. Affect
    d. Perception

ANSWER KEY

| 1. c | 2. c | 3. b | 4. d | 5. c | 6. b | 7. a | 8. b |
| 9. b | 10. a | 11. b | 12. b | 13. d | 14. a | 15. a | |

SHORT ANSWER TYPE QUESTIONS

1. Explain the cycle of motivation.
2. Give the concept of motivation.
3. How will you measure motives?
4. What is meant by the term "emotion?"
5. What is the role of the nurse to control emotion in a patient?
6. What is the role of emotion in health and sickness?
7. Write about the coping strategies of stress.
8. What are the types of stress?
9. Classify the stressors.
10. What are the sources responsible for stress?
11. Explain the cycle of stress.
12. What are the factors that affect the attitude?
13. What are the components of attitude?
14. What do you mean by attitudinal change?

LONG ANSWER TYPE QUESTIONS

1. Define motivation. What do you mean by biological and social motives?
2. What are the types of motivation?
3. Explain the theories of motivation.
4. Explain the hierarchical theory of motivation with diagram.
5. Which parts of our body control emotion?

UNIT VII: Motivation and Emotional Processes

6. Describe theories of emotion.
7. How will you measure emotions?
8. Define stress. Explain different types of stressor.
9. What are the effects of stress?
10. What is stress adaptation?
11. Define attitude. Explain the role of attitude in health and sickness.
12. Explain the theories of attitudes.
13. Explain balance theory in detail.
14. Explain the psychometric assessment of attitude.

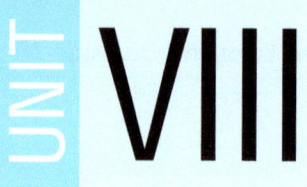

Psychological Assessment and Tests

OUTLINE

- Introduction
- Types, Development, Characteristics, Principles, Uses, Interpretation
- Role of Nurse in Psychological Assessment

■ INTRODUCTION

Psychosocial or psychological assessment is an evaluation of an individual's mental health and social well-being. It helps to assess the behavior, perception, thought process, and various other mental processes and an individual's ability to function in the community. The assessment consists of a series of questions asked by the health professional to get insight into people's psychological problems.

The psychosocial assessment of a patient is an extremely important part of nursing care. Nurses use various assessment techniques such as history taking, mental status examination (MSE), mini-mental status examination, and psychological tests. These assessment techniques help nursing professionals to identify if the individual is mentally ill or mentally healthy.

Psychometric assessment is a specialized assessment procedure for determining such characteristics of an individual as intellectual capacity, motive pattern, self-concept, perception of the environment, roles to be taken up, anxiety or depression, coping pattern, and general personality integration.

■ METHODS USED FOR PSYCHOSOCIAL ASSESSMENT

1. **History taking**: It involves details about the individual including his personal history and premorbid personality. The main purpose of the history collection is the formulation of diagnosis and identification of a patient's problem. It consists of the following:
   a. Biodata of the patient
   b. Chief complaints
   c. History of present illness
   d. History of past illness—psychiatric, medical, and surgical history
   e. Family history: Family socioeconomic status, family tree, any illness in family members (hereditary)
   f. Personal history: Prenatal, birth and infancy, childhood, adolescence, educational history
   g. Occupational history
   h. Marital and sexual history
   i. Menstrual and obstetrical history: In case of females
   j. Addiction history: Alcohol or drug abuse
   k. Premorbid personality: Attitude toward religion, work, people, personal habits, hobbies, etc.

2. **Mental status examination**: Mental status examination (in the USA) and mental state examination (rest of the world) are detailed assessment of all the mental processes of an individual. The main purpose of the MSE is to find out the disorder of a specific mental process and to relate it to the symptomatology of the patient. It is

the on-the-spot assessment of a patient's behavior.

Outline of MSE
a. **General appearance and attitude:** Facial expressions, mannerism, attitude toward examiner, gait and body posture, comprehension, dress and grooming, physical parameters, and any deformity.
b. **Disorder of motor activity:** Overactivity or underactivity, motor retardation, echopraxia, stupor, stereotyped, waxy flexibility, compulsion, automatic obedience, negativism, autism, and ambitendency
c. **Disorders of thought**
   i. **Disorder of form of thought:** Spontaneity, productivity, poverty of contents, thought block, clang association, incoherence, irrelevance, circumstantiality, tangentiality, perseveration, rate, and quantity of speech (spontaneous, productivity, speed, pitch, rate, reaction time, pressure of speech, tone, or intensity).
   ii. **Disorder of content of thought:** Obsessions, delusions (grandeur, persecution, infidelity, nihilistic, hypochondrias, sin and guilt, etc.), phobia, neologism, word salad, thought insertion, thought broadcasting
   iii. **Disorder of speech:** Echolalia, mutism, aphonia, loose association, flight of ideas, rate of speech, formal or informal speech
e. **Disorder of perception:** Illusions, hallucinations (auditory, visual, olfactory), derealization, depersonalization
e. **Disorders of mood and affect:** Appropriate or inappropriate mood, labile affect or blunt affect, dysthymia, depression, anxiety, elevated mood (euphoria, elation, exaltation, exhilaration, or ecstasy), anhedonia
f. Level of consciousness
g. **Disorders of memory:** Recent, remote, and immediate memory, amnesia, paramnesia, Deja Vu, James Vu, retrograde amnesia, confabulation
h. Attention and concentration
i. Orientation to time, place, and person
j. **Intelligence:** Ability to understand, recall, problem-solving, and decision-making
k. **Abstract thinking:** Similarities and dissimilarities
l. **Insight:** About the problem and self
m. **Judgment:** Social judgment and test judgment

These were the areas by which we can comprehend the mental status of an individual. Especially in the psychiatric settings, this is the most widely used assessment method by nursing professionals.

3. **Mini-mental status examination (MMSE):** It is the short version of the previously explained mental status examination. It was developed by Folstein et al., in 1975. The main purpose of MMSE was quick administration for use by clinicians, especially for non-cooperative patients. It is a brief psychiatric instrument grossly designed to assess cognitive functioning. It consists of five assessment areas.

Mini-Mental State Examination (MMSE)

Patient's Name: _____   Date: _____

Instructions: Score 1 point for each correct response within each question or activity.

Maximum Score	Patient's Score	Questions
5		"What is the year? Season? Date? Day? Month?"
5		"Where are we now? State? County? Town/city? Hospital? Floor?"
3		The examiner names three unrelated objects clearly and slowly; then the instructor asks the patient to name all three of them. The patient's response is used for scoring. The examiner repeats them until the patient learns all of them, if possible.
5		"I would like you to count backward from 100 by sevens." (93, 86, 79, 72, 65, …) Alternative: "Spell WORLD backward." (D-L-R-O-W)
3		"Earlier I told you the names of three things. Can you tell me what those were?"
2		Show the patient two simple objects, such as a wristwatch and a pencil, and ask the patient to name them.
1		"Repeat the phrase: 'No ifs, ands, or buts.'"
3		"Take the paper in your right hand, fold it in half, and put it on the floor." (The examiner gives the patient a piece of blank paper.)
1		"Please read this and do what it says." (Written instruction is "Close your eyes.")
1		"Make up and write a sentence about anything." (This sentence must contain a noun and a verb.)
1		"Please copy this picture." (The examiner gives the patient a blank piece of paper and asks him/her to draw the symbol below. All 10 angles must be present and two must intersect.)
30		TOTAL

Interpretation of the MMSE:

Method	Score	Interpretation
Single cut-off	<24	Abnormal
Range	<21 >25	Increased odds of dementia Decreased odds of dementia
Education	21 <23 <24	Abnormal for 8th-grade education Abnormal for high school education Abnormal for college education
Severity	24–30 18–23 0–17	No cognitive impairment Mild cognitive impairment Severe cognitive impairment

Interpretation of MMSE Scores:

Score	Degree of impairment	Formal psychometric assessment	Day-to-day functioning
25–30	Questionably significant	If clinical signs of cognitive impairment are present, a formal assessment of cognition may be valuable	May have clinically significant but mild deficits. Likely to affect only the most demanding activities of daily living
20–25	Mild	Formal assessment may be helpful to better determine the pattern and extent of deficits	Significant effect. May require some supervision, support, and assistance
10–20	Moderate	Formal assessment may be helpful if there are specific clinical indications	Clear impairment. May require 24-hour supervision
0–10	Severe	Patient not likely to be testable	Marked impairment. Likely to require 24-hour supervision and assistance with ADL

(ADL: activities of daily living)

What is a Psychological Test?

A psychological test is a structured technique to generate a carefully selected sample of behavior. It is used to derive inference about someone's behavior on basis of the results of the tests. We can judge the level of attributes such as intelligence, self-esteem, and aptitude in an individual.

A structured technique is used to generate a carefully selected sample of behavior to make inferences about the psychological attributes of the people who have been tested.

Psychological testing: A field characterized by the use of sample of behavior to infer generalizations about a given individual.

It is a structured technique used to generate a carefully selected sample of behavior to make inferences about the psychological attributes of people who have been tested.

Psychometric testing or psychological testing is the use of a standardized test to quantify psychophysical behavior, mental functioning, abilities, aptitudes, and problem-solving and to generalize about the individual behavior.

Definition

Psychometrics is the field of study concerned with the theory and techniques of educational and psychological measurement which include the measurement of knowledge, abilities, attitudes, and personality traits.

Psychometrics tests are written, visual, or verbal evaluations administered to assess the cognitive and emotional functioning of children and adults.

—*American Psychological Associations*

A psychological test is any procedure on the basis of which inferences are made concerning a person's capacity or liability to act, react, experience, or to structure or order thought or behavior in particular ways.

The Birtish Psychological Society

Why is Psychological Testing Important?

1. Psychological tests help to make important decisions about people. For example, early school placement, college entrance decisions, military job selections.
2. It also helps us to describe and understand the behavior.
3. It helps to measure personal attributes such as personality, emotions, and attitudes of individuals.
4. It helps to measure performance in various fields such as career development, job interviews, etc.
5. These are specific and measure-specific abilities, so these help to save time and energy.
6. Being most economical can be used in any setting such as, psychiatric hospitals, guidance, counseling centers, and any other therapeutic settings.

History of Test Development

Circa 1000 BC: Chinese introduced written tests to help fill civil service positions in civil laws, military affairs, agriculture, and geography.

1850: The United States begins civil service examinations.

1885: Germans tested people for brain damage.

1890: James Cattell develops a "mental test" to assess college students. The test includes measures of strength, resistance to pain, and reaction time.

1905: Binet-Simon scale of mental development was used to classify mentally retarded children in France.

1914: World War I produces the need in the US to quickly classify incoming recruits. Army Alpha test and Army Beta test were developed. Looked at psychopathology.

1916: Terman develops Stanford-Binet test and develops the idea of the intelligence quotient.

1920–1940: Factor analysis, projective tests, and personality inventories first appear.

1941–1960: Vocational interest measures developed.

1961–1980: Item response theory and neuropsychological testing developed.

1980–Present: Wide-spread adaptation of computerized testing. "Smart" tests which can give each individual different test items developed.

Developing/Selecting Appropriate Tests

- Define what each test measures and what the test should be used for.
- Describe the population(s) for which the test is appropriate.
- Accurately represent the characteristics, usefulness, and limitations of tests for their intended purposes.
- Describe the process of test development.

UNIT VIII: Psychological Assessment and Tests

- Provide evidence that the test meets its intended purpose(s).
- Provide either representative samples or complete copies of test questions, directions, answer sheets, manuals, and score reports to qualified users.
- Indicate the nature of the evidence obtained concerning the appropriateness of each test for groups of different racial, ethnic, or linguistic backgrounds who are likely to be tested.
- Describe the population(s) represented by any norms or comparison group(s), the dates the data were gathered, and the process used to select the samples of test-takers.
- When feasible, make appropriately modified forms of tests or administration procedures available for test-takers with handicapping conditions. Warn test users of potential problems in using standard norms with modified tests or administration procedures that result in non-comparable scores.
- When a test is optional, provide test-takers or their parents/guardians with information to help them judge whether the test should be taken, or if an available alternative to the test should be used.
- Provide test-takers the information they need to be familiar with the coverage of the test, the types of question formats, the directions, and appropriate test-taking strategies. Strive to make such information equally available to all test-takers.
- Provide test-takers or their parents/guardians with information about rights test-takers may have to obtain copies of tests and completed answer sheets, retake tests, have tests rescored, or cancel scores.
- Tell test-takers or their parents/guardians how long scores will be kept on file and indicate to whom and under what circumstances test scores will or will not be released.

Characteristics of Psychological Tests

- Measure attributes.
- Give systematic inferences about other person's attitudes, behavior, and intelligence
- A standard way of generating samples of people's behavior
- Test performance of different people can be compared directly.
- Rules are given to reducing subjectivity and improving objectivity.
- Tests can be interpreted easily giving/generating data about the people's characteristics.

Principles of Psychological Tests

- **Validity:** It is the extent to which the test measures what it intends to measure.
- **Reliability:** An extent to which the results obtained are consistent when the test is administered more than once with X reasonable time gap.
- **Practicability:** It can be measured in terms of economy, convenience, and interpretability. Economy considers the affordability of the test; convenience refers to the simplicity and understandability of the test; and interpretability refers to the result obtained from the test, which will be objectively measurable and interpreted.
- **Uniformity:** All tests should have uniformity as different testers will follow the same test steps anywhere.
- **Standardized:** For all types of psychological tests norms are set to work with and should be standardized. There should be consistency in testing and should be done under a controlled environment so that bias due to personal reasons is reduced.

Uses of Psychological Testing

- *Traits*, i.e., introversion and extroversion
- *Certain conditions*, i.e., depression and anxiety

- *Intelligence, aptitude, and achievement,* i.e., verbal intelligence and reading achievement
- *Attitudes and feelings,* i.e., how individuals feel about the treatment that they received from their therapists
- *Interest,* i.e., the careers and activities that a person is interested in
- *Specific abilities, knowledge, or skills,* i.e., cognitive ability, memory, and problem-solving skills
- *Education*—various intelligence tests are used to predict the success chances of students. Tests also help the students to select the right course and subjects with the help of aptitude testing.
- *Career and occupation*—every individual has his/her own capability and talent to do a particular job. Different jobs require different types of skills and personality temperaments and abilities. The psychological test can help individuals to decide for a suitable job which can help them to have success in particular career.
- *Research*—various psychological tests have been widely used to discover and explore new types of relationships among various variables and apply various theoretical perspectives to them. These psychological tests are used to measure various attributes and variables and after statistical interpretation, relationships can be analyzed.

Types of psychological tests are as follows:
1. **Depending upon time limit:** Speed test and power test, e.g., Kaufman assessment battery for children (intelligence test to find fast learners)
2. **Depending upon the number of individuals:** Group tests and individual test
3. **Depending upon language:** Verbal and Non-verbal tests
4. **Depending upon method:** Paper-pencil and performance test
5. Depending upon what is measured: Intelligence tests, aptitude tests, achievement tests, personality tests

Intelligence Tests (Table 1)

Evolution of Intelligence Testing

Alfred Binet and Theodore Simon (1905): Binet-Simon intelligence scale: First intelligence test; measured abstract reasoning skills rather than sensory skills (Galton).

Mental age: Displayed the mental ability typical of a child of that chronological (actual) age.

Lewis Terman (1916): Stanford-Binet intelligence scale—revised Binet scale.
Intelligence quotient (IQ) = (MA/CA) × 100; child's mental age divided by chronological age multiplied by 100. Can compare children of different ages—everyone uses the same scale.

David Wechsler (1955): Wechsler adult intelligence scale is less dependent on verbal ability.

1. **Stanford-Binet test:** Alfred Binet and Theodore Simon (French scientists) devised a new way to test intelligence called the Binet-Simon scale in 1909. Alfred Binet was commissioned by the French government to separate children into vocational versus academic schooling. This intelligence test measured someone's intelligence using the performance method, which involved testing intelligence based on someone's ability to give correct answers to a series of questions.
    To help compare intelligence between different types of people, the Binet-Simon scale used a measure called mental age. For example, if on average a group of 9-year olds scores 20 correct questions, and then a child who is 7 years old scores the same, then that 7-year-old child is said to have a mental age of 9 **(Fig. 1)**.
    In general, mental age should rise as a person grows older. So the older they are, the better they will do on the test. **Between 2 and 23 years of age.**
2. **Army Alpha and Beta tests (Fig. 2)**
   - Army Alpha/Beta IQ test (1917)— designed for World War I recruits.

UNIT VIII: Psychological Assessment and Tests

Table 1: Different types of infant development scales.

Test	Type	Assesses	Age	Method	Administration
Alexander's performance scale	Intelligence and motor	Cognitive function	Below 10 years	Performance on 3 subtests	Individual
Bayley scales of infant development	Infant development	Cognitive and motor function	1–30 months	Performance on subtests measuring	Individual
Beck depression inventory	Personality	Measures depression	Adult	Performance on self-report	Individual
Bender visual-motor gestalt test	Visual motor development	Organic brain damage, ego functions	5–adult	Reproduction of geometric figures	Individual
Bhatia's performance scale	Intelligence	Cognitive and motor development	Boys 11–16 years	Performance on 5 subjects	Individual
Brief psychiatric rating scale	Symptomatology	Symptomatology adult and global pathology	Adult	18-dimensions	Individual
Catell's infant intelligence scale	Infant development	General motor and cognitive	1–18 months	17 scales	Individual
Catell's 16 PF	Personality inventory	Personality conflicts	Adults	Self-reports	Individual
CAT	Projective	Personality conflicts	Child	Makes up stories after viewing pictures	Individual

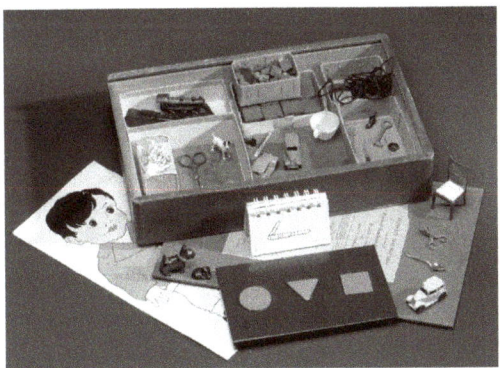

Fig. 1: Test material form M Revised Stanford-Binet scales.

Assumed to be testing native intelligence. Alpha for literates; Beta for illiterates and non-English speakers
- Alpha subtests: Oral directions; arithmetic; practical judgment; analogies; disarranged sentences; number series; information
- Beta subtests: Memory; matching; picture completion; geometric construction

3. **Wechsler Intelligence test (David Wechsler, 1939–1981)**

This contains verbal and performance subtests **(Fig. 3).**
Performance compared to same-age peers—raw score has different interpretation depending on age. Designed widely used test for adults (WAIS), children (WISC), and preschoolers (WPPSI)
WAIS-R testing kit: Testing booklet, story cards, puzzle pieces, block design

Verbal Intelligence test

Information: A person's level of general knowledge

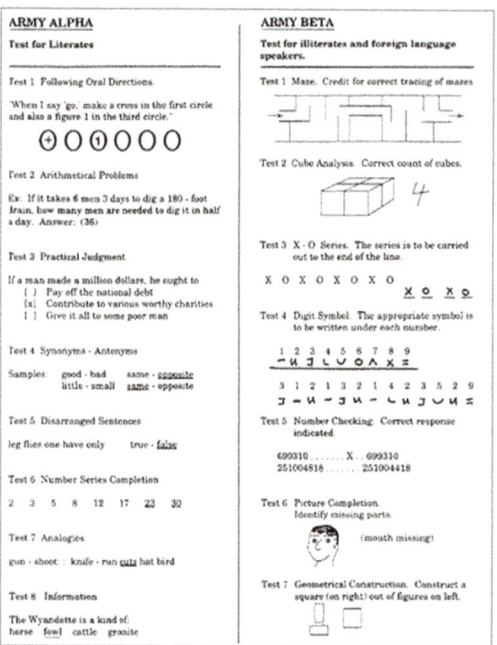

Fig. 2: Alpha/beta testing.

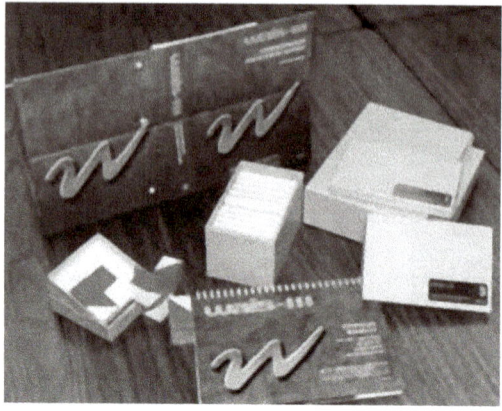

Fig. 3: Wechsler intelligence scale for children.

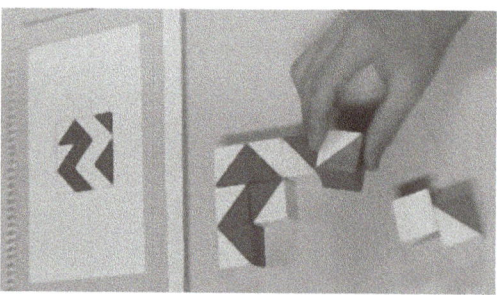

Fig. 4: Picture arrangement.

Comprehension: How well you can understand questions and grasp concepts

Arithmetic: A person's mathematical abilities

Similarities: Measures abstract thought

Digit span: Measures attention span

Vocabulary: How many word meanings you know

Performance Intelligence Test

Digit symbol: Mental flexibility with random symbols

Picture completion: Ability to notice differences between two similar pictures

Block design: Mentally construct printed designs in your head.

Picture arrangement: Arrange pictures in a logical order **(Fig. 4)**.

Object assembly: Place the correct part in relation to a whole.

4. **Raven's progressive matrices (Figs. 5A to C):**
The test consists of 50 designs each of which has a cut-out segment. The subject is shown the 6-8 cut-out alternative pieces and is asked to indicate what to put in the matrix.

There are children progressive matrices, standard progressive matrices, and advanced matrices.

Uses of the Intelligence Tests

1. Predicts to some extent how well we will do in life
2. Many occupations are available only to persons with college or graduate degrees.
3. It takes less time to train persons with higher intelligence to a high level of job knowledge and skill.
4. Persons with higher intelligence tend to perform better in complex jobs.
5. For guidance and counseling
6. Helps to place vocationally
7. Select the right person for promotion.

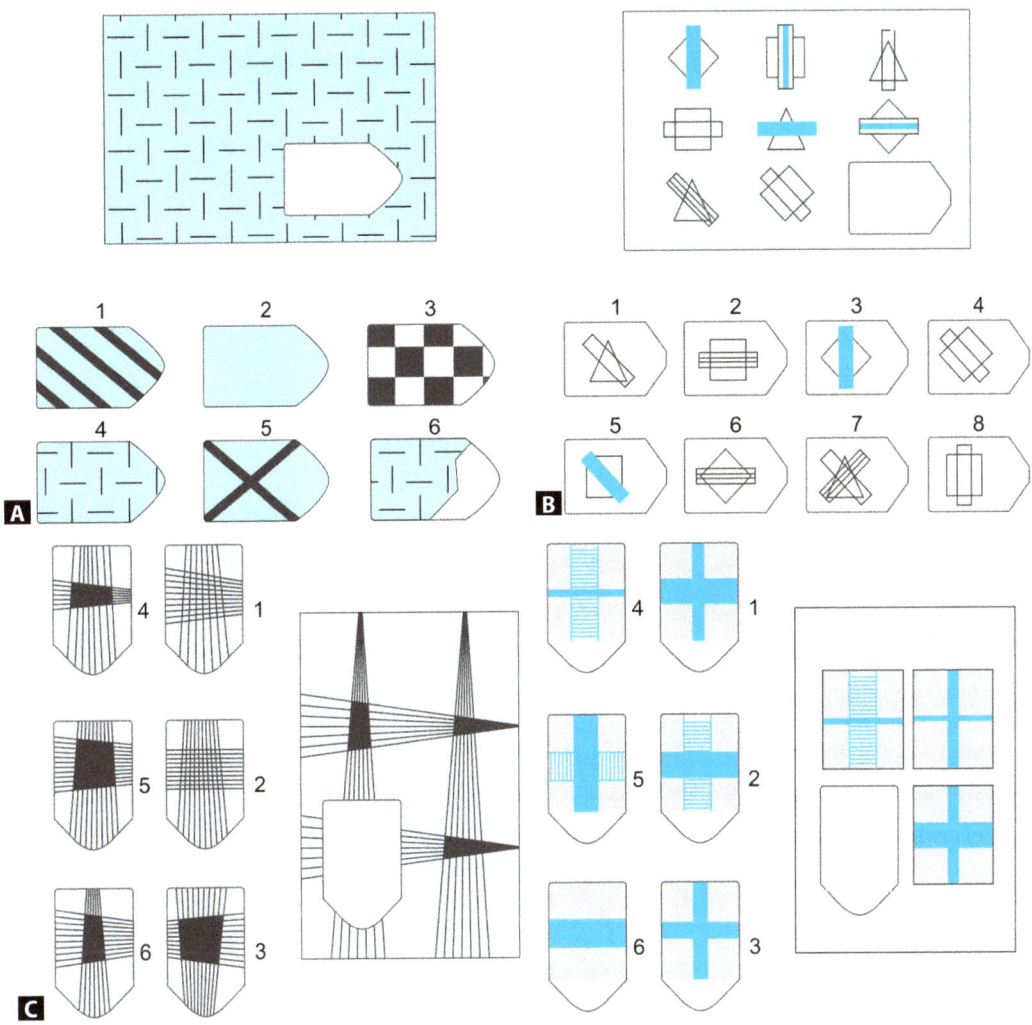

Figs. 5A to C: Raven's progressive matrices.

8. Job selection, diagnosis of mental states, and treatment
9. Helps to measure intellectual functions of memory problem-solving and verbal fluency.
10. Diagnose the differences between two individuals on basis of their intellectual differences and leading to the development of the knowledge about the individual differences.

Personality Testing

Personality is derived from the word persona or the mask. A personality that enables a person to stand out as distinct from others. The term personality can be interpreted in many ways, it includes temperament or character, but is not restricted to those.

Methods of Personality Testing

The following are some methods used:
- The interview
- Observation method
- Rating scales
- Personality inventories
- Case study
- Projection techniques

The personality test is discussed in detail in the unit on personality.

Aptitude Test

There is no clear dividing line between intelligence tests and aptitude tests. Intelligence tests are used to give a broad assessment of intellectual capacity. Aptitude tests are used to measure the more specialized abilities in specific occupations and activities.

Aptitude tests are structured systematic ways of evaluating how people perform on tasks or react to different situations. These have standardized methods of administration and scoring with the results qualified and compared with how others have done on the same tests.

Types of Aptitude Test

General aptitude battery test: These are the most common types of tests majorly conducted for checking different reasoning abilities, numerical abilities, language, spelling, etc.

Differential aptitude test
- It is developed by the psychological corporation of the USA. It consists of some tests.
- This test measures the ability to perform mathematical reasoning tasks.

Attitude Testing

The word attitude has been derived from Latin word aptus which means ability. Attitude is an established way of thinking or feeling reflected in a person's behavior toward others. Attitude is normally defined as a perceptual orientation and response readiness in relation to a particular object or class of objects.

Thurstone attitude scale
- It is the first formal method designed to measure attitude.
- It was developed by Louis Leon Thurstone in 1928.
- Consist of statements that have a range of weights from high to low

Likert scale
- The most popular attitude scale type
- It is also known as a summated rating scale.
- Respondents indicate the extent to which they endorse the statement (agree or disagree)

Forensic Psychiatric Test

- Physical assessment
- Forensic mental health assessment (FMHA)
- Interviews
- Minnesota multiphasic personality inventory
- Wechsler scale for intellectual measurement
- Hamilton anxiety rating scale (HAM-A)
- Hamilton depression rating scale (HDRS)

Performance Testing

Performance testing covers a broad range of engineering or functional evaluations. Testing can be a qualitative or quantitative procedure. Performance testing can refer to the assessment of the performance of a human examinee.

Advantages
- Easy
- Economical
- Higher interrater reliability
- Less response bias

Disadvantages
- Rely on clients which could lead to a response bias
- Tells little about the unconscious process
- Limited to high functioning individuals
- Interpretation not objective
- Interpretation not consistent
- Lack of standard scoring

Neuropsychological Assessment

* Assessment of the neurological deficit predicts the possible organic psychopathology.
* Identification of intact neurological functioning helps in the process of neurorehabilitation (cognitive retraining).
* Evaluation and comparison of various treatment options and their perceived efficacy
* Progressive evaluation and formulation of differential diagnosis
* Among children: Developmental progression of the milestones
* Tackling the mental developmental delay, and taking necessary actions on time

Common areas of assessment include:
* Attention
* Perception
* Intelligence
* Judgment
* Concentration
* Memory
* Earning and thought process

Test of attention and concentration: The capacity to arouse and sustain attention varies with individual time. Most of the illness attention becomes poor and fluctuate. Common tests include:
* Eysenck's Digit Test of Concentration
* Color Cancellation Tasks
* Digit Symbol Subtraction
* Letter Cancellation
* Knox Cube Imitation

Test for Mental Alertness and Retention

Assessing the degree of psychomotor retardation, e.g., differentiating mild to severe. Common tests include Minnesota block reversal test.

Check for reaction time, response time, and productivity/unit time.

Test for Memory

Many of neuropsychiatric illnesses present with complaints of memory loss or forgetfulness. Common verbal tests include Wechsler memory scale. It is the commonly used memory test battery for adults. It is a composite of verbal paired-associate, paragraph retention, visual memory for design, orientation, digit span, reverse recall of the alphabet and counting backward. This test is appropriate for the age group of 16–74.

Postgraduate Institute (PGI) memory scale has been standardized for the Indian population.

Verbal memory is assessed through the presentation of stimuli such as these that must then be recalled: Words, digits, nonsense syllables, and sentences.

Performance tests on memory assessment are:
* Benton Test of Visual Retention—Revised
* Memory for Designs Test

Comprehensive Neuropsychiatric Batteries

* **Luria-Nebraska-neuropsychological battery:** Motor functions, rhythm, tactile functions, visual functions, receptive speech, expressive speech, writing, reading, arithmetic, memory, intellectual processes, pathognomonic, left hemisphere, and right hemisphere
* **Mini-mental state examination (Folstein test):** This is a brief 30-point questionnaire test that is used to screen for cognitive impairment.

The Situational Judgement Test

* The situational judgment test (SJT) assesses the judgment required for solving problems in work-related situations. Hypothetical and challenging situations that one might encounter at work, and that involve working with others as part of a

team, interacting with others, and dealing with workplace dilemmas. In response to each situation, you are presented with five possible actions that one might take in dealing with the problem described. Your task on the test will be to select the one response alternative that is the *most effective* and the one response alternative that is the *least effective* in dealing with the problem described.

- The SJT consists of 50 short descriptions of problem situations. Each of them is followed by two questions (asking you to select the most effective response and the least effective response alternatives). There are thus a total of 100 questions to be answered. Each question is worth 1 mark. Your score will be the total number of correct answers. No specialized training, knowledge, or experience is required to write this test. You will be given 90 minutes to complete this test. Including the time for administrative purposes, a test session takes about 2 hours.

Advantages of Psychometric Assessment

- They lead to judgments that are more valid than judgments made by other means. This is the most important advantage of psychometric assessment.
- They are relatively cheap and easy to administer.
- They are likely to have considerable cost-benefits in long term.
- They help in understanding how people will behave at work.
- Accurately testing the general intelligence of candidates.
- Interpreting candidates' emotions and their ability to maintain relationships.

Disadvantages of Psychometric Assessment

- The tests may not always be accurate.
- Tell little about unconscious response.
- It is a time-consuming process.
- Test anxiety can create a false-negative result.
- Human mind is beyond any assessment and limit. At a time one can behave completely different from the original state.

ROLE OF NURSE IN PSYCHOLOGICAL TESTING

1. It is very important for the nurses to know what a psychological test is, how tests are constructed and used, what the uses of these tests are, and how to interpret the results of tests.
2. The nurses who go for higher studies and research in psychology definitely need this knowledge.
3. Nurse can assess any abnormality in the behavior of the patient.
4. The nurse can assess the mental functioning or capacity of patients to make appropriate diagnoses.
5. She can assess various aspects of the individual such as individual differences, personality, and behavior.
6. When a report is presented to the nurse she must be in a position to understand and interpret the results. By interpreting the result, conclusions can be made to decide what therapies or treatments can be planned.
7. Nurses pursuing higher education and research scholars must be well aware of these tests as they utilize them in their research projects.
8. Nurses can plan care to assist in fulfilling tasks according to the developmental age of individuals.
9. Nurses can counsel and provide guidance to children and their parents to develop realistic expectations.
10. Nurses clarify the patients' and relatives' doubts regarding the psychological tests they have to undergo. Nurses should have a good rapport with the patients and family members.

11. The nurses should reassure the patients about the safety of the tests and the confidentiality of the observations of the psychologist.
12. The nurse observes the patient's behavior and the changes, which occur once the therapy is commenced. The nurse observes, informs, and records these changes in the patient's chart.

QUESTION BANK

MULTIPLE CHOICE QUESTIONS

1. Which of the following tests is used to measure the aptitude of individual?
   a. Personality test
   b. Mental ability
   c. Intelligence test
   d. Emotional test
2. Which of the following criteria of test determines the set of score of test?
   a. Reliability
   b. Norms
   c. Validity
   d. Practicality
3. Which of the following is not a projective technique?
   a. TAT
   b. CAT
   c. Rorschach Ink-Blot test
   d. MMPI
4. Bayley scales of infant development are used to assess which attribute of development?
   a. Cognitive and motor function
   b. Perception
   c. Memory development
   d. Emotional development

ANSWER KEY
1. b   2. b   3. d   4. a

SHORT ANSWER TYPE QUESTIONS

1. What is a psychometric assessment of personality?
2. What is the role of a nurse in psychological assessment?
3. What are the steps of psychological test construction?
4. What are the uses of psychological testing?

LONG ANSWER TYPE QUESTIONS

1. Explain various intelligence tests.
2. Discuss various uses of psychological test.
3. Discuss various methods of psychosocial assessment.

UNIT IX

Application of Soft Skills

OUTLINE

- Types of Soft Skill/Communication
- Communication Process
- Building Relationship with Client and Society
- Interpersonal Relationship (IPR). Definition, Types, and Purposes, Interpersonal Skills
- Barriers, Strategies to Overcome Barriers
- Survival Strategies—Managing Time, Coping Stress, Resilience, Work-Life Balance
- Applying Soft Skill to Workplace and Society—Presentation Skills, Social Etiquette, Telephone
- Etiquette, Motivational Skills, Teamwork, etc.
- Use of Soft Skill in Nursing

■ INTRODUCTION

We need to communicate with others effectively. In fact, effective communication is one of the keys to success. By successfully getting our message across, we convey our thoughts and ideas effectively. The message is the information that we want to communicate. It is essential to be technically sound, but we should also have the ability to express and communicate our ideas clearly and effectively to others in the simplest possible manner. Effective communication and soft skills not only improve our relationships with others, but they also improve our efficiency.

Soft skills play a vital role in academic and professional success. They help us excel in the workplace and their importance cannot be denied in the emerging information or knowledge society. Soft skills are needed to deal with the external world and to work in a collaborative manner with one's colleagues. Soft skills, also known as common skills or core skills, interpersonal skills, social skills, life skills, and emotional intelligence quotients are skills that are desirable in all professions.

Definition of Soft Skills

Soft skills are defined as life skills that are behaviors used appropriately and responsibly in the management of personal affairs. They are a set of human skills acquired via teaching or direct experience that are used to handle problems and questions commonly encountered in daily human life.

It is defined as "abilities for adaptive and positive behavior that enable individuals to deal effectively with the demands and challenges of everyday life."

—*World Health Organization (WHO)*

Soft skills include any skill that can be classified as a personality trait or habit. Interpersonal skills and communication skills are more specific categories of soft skills that many employers look for in job candidates.

Why Soft Skills?

- **Self**: An awareness of the characteristics that define the person one is and wants to become

UNIT IX: Application of Soft Skills

Table 1: Types of soft skills (Canney and Byrne, 2006).

Skill Set	Used for	Examples
Foundation skills	Basic social interaction	Ability to maintain eye contact, maintain appropriate personal space, understand gestures and facial expressions
Interaction skills	Skills needed to interact with others	Resolving conflicts, taking turns, learning how to begin and end conversations, determining appropriate topics for conversation, interacting with authority figures
Affective skills	Skills needed for understanding oneself and others	Identifying one's feelings, recognizing the feelings of others, demonstrating empathy, decoding body language and facial expressions, determining whether someone is trustworthy
Cognitive skills	Skills needed to maintain more complex social interactions	Social perception, making choices, self-monitoring, understanding community norms, determining appropriate behavior for different social situation

❖ **Opportunity**: An awareness of the possibilities that exist, the demands they make, and the rewards and satisfaction they offer
❖ **Aspirations**: The ability to make realistic choices and plans based on sound information and self-opportunity alignment
❖ **Results**: The ability to review outcomes, plan and take action to implement decisions and aspirations, especially at points of transition (Kumar A, 2007).

To SOAR students, need two things:
1. **Academic roots**: Discipline-based knowledge and understanding
2. **Academic wings**: The ability to enhance that knowledge and understanding with awareness (self and others), critical thinking, reflective practice

Types of skills according to Canney and Byrne are depicted in **Table 1**.

TYPES OF SOFT SKILL/COMMUNICATION (FIG. 1)

❖ Effective communication skills
❖ Teamwork
❖ Adaptability
❖ Conflict resolution
❖ Flexibility

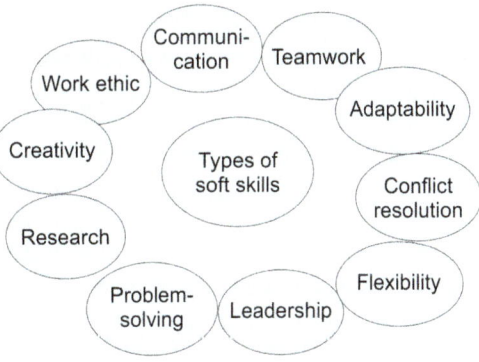

Fig. 1: Types of soft skills.

❖ Leadership
❖ Problem-solving
❖ Research
❖ Creativity
❖ Work ethic

Communication: Communication skills have always been at the top of the list of "essential" skills. There are five ways to communicate at work: (1) **Verbal communication** refers to your ability to speak clearly and concisely. (2) **Nonverbal communication** includes the capacity to project positive body language and facial expressions. (3) **Aural communication** is the ability to listen to and actually hear what others are saying. (4) **Written communication** refers to your skillfulness in composing text messages, reports, and other types of documents. (5) **Visual communication** involves your ability to relay information using pictures and other visual aids.

Teamwork: Different professions or jobs have different requirements and some require constantly working and communicating with other team members. This makes teamwork to be one of the most important soft skills for professional careers which require employees to do team projects and attend frequent meetings, quality patient care, etc.

Adaptability: How easily do you adapt to changes? If you are working in a technology-driven field or start-up, adaptability is especially important. Changes in processes, tools, or clients you work with can happen quickly. Employees who are capable of adapting to new situations and ways of working are valuable in many jobs and industries.\

Conflict resolution: It can be defined as the informal or formal process that two or more parties use to find a peaceful solution to their dispute. A number of common cognitive and emotional traps, many of them unconscious, can exacerbate conflict and contribute to the need for conflict resolution.

Flexibility: Flexibility is an important soft skill since it demonstrates an ability and willingness to embrace new tasks and new challenges calmly and without fuss. Flexible employees are willing to help out where needed, take on extra responsibilities, and can adapt quickly when plans change.

Leadership: Soft skills are important for leadership because skills such as effective communication with team members, making decisions about processes, and maintaining an organized team are essential to productivity and performance. Successful leadership commonly encompasses strong soft skills that enable leaders to motivate and inspire their teams. Additionally, the ability to lead successfully often depends on a leader's ability to strategize, listen to feedback, and incorporate their team's ideas and contributions.

Research: To establish a reputation in academia, today's researchers must also be able to lead project teams, moderate discussions, and communicate their knowledge clearly and persuasively. That is why soft skills such as communication, leadership, and moderation are more important than ever before in scientific professions.

Problem-solving: Employers highly value people who can resolve issues quickly and effectively. That may involve calling on industry knowledge to fix an issue immediately, as it occurs, or taking time to research and consult with colleagues to find a scalable, long-term solution.

Creativity: Creativity is a broad ability incorporating many different skill sets including other soft skills and technical skills. Employees with creativity can find new ways to perform tasks, improve processes or even develop new and exciting avenues for the business to explore. Creativity can be used in any role at any level.

Work ethic: Work ethic is the ability to follow through on tasks and duties in a timely and quality manner. A strong work ethic will help ensure you develop a positive relationship with your employer and colleagues even when you are still developing technical skills in a new job. Many employers would rather work with someone who has a strong work ethic and is eager to learn than a skilled worker who seems unmotivated.

▌HOW TO DEVELOP SOFT SKILLS?

Developing soft skills needs practice. These are acquired and experienced on the spot. Soft skills cannot be acquired by merely reading textbooks. The soft skills we gain equip us to excel in our academic/professional life and our personal life.

It is a continuous learning process. The development of soft skills has two parts. One part involves developing attitudes and attributes, and the other part involves fine-tuning communication skills to express attitudes, ideas, and thoughts.

Perfect integration of ideas and attitudes with appropriate communication skills in oral, written, and nonverbal areas is necessary for successful work.

Attitudes and skills are integral to soft skills. Each one influences and complements the other.

Communication

Introduction

Communication is the process in which people affect one another through the exchange of information, ideas, and feelings. Interpersonal communication is basic to human interaction and essential for nursing practice.

Communication and education are interwoven. Communication strategies can enhance learning. The ultimate goal of all communication is to bring about a change in the desired direction of the person who receives the communication.

Meaning

The word communication is derived from the Latin word "communis," meaning "common." Communication is an interaction between two or more persons that involves an exchange of information between a sender and receiver. Communication is a process of change. To achieve the desired result, the communication necessarily is effective and purposive.

Definition

- "Communication is a process through which individuals mutually exchange their ideas, values, thoughts, feelings and actions between one or more people."
- "Communication is the transfer of information from sender to receiver so that it is understood in its right context."
- Communication is the sum of all the things one person does when he wants to create understanding in the mind of another. It involves a systematic and continuous process of telling, listening and understanding.   —*Louis A. Allen*
- Communication is a process in which a message is transferred from one person to another person through suitable media and the intended message is received and understood by the receiver.

Importance of Communication

1. **Promotes motivation:** Communication promotes motivation by informing and clarifying the employees about the task to be done, the manner they are performing the task, and how to improve their performance if it is not up to the mark.
2. **Source of information:** Communication is a source of information to the organizational members for the decision-making process as it helps identify and assess the alternative course of action.
3. **Altering individual's attitudes:** Communication also plays a crucial role in altering an individual's attitudes, i.e., a well-informed individual will have better attitude than a less-informed individual. Organizational magazines, journals, meetings, and various other forms of oral and written communication help in molding employees' attitudes.
4. **Helps in socializing:** Communication also helps in socializing. In today's life, the only presence of another individual fosters communication. It is also said that one cannot survive without communication.
5. **Controlling process:** Communication also assists in controlling process. It helps controlling organizational member's behavior in various ways. There are various levels of hierarchy and certain principles and guidelines that employees must follow in an organization. They must comply with organizational policies, perform their job role efficiently, and communicate any work

problem and grievance to their superiors. Thus, communication helps in controlling the function of management.

Understanding Communication

A famous quote says "The way we communicate with others and with ourselves ultimately determines the quality of our lives."

"Communication is the means of making the transfer of information productive and goal oriented."

The process of passing any information from one person to the other person with the aid of some medium is termed communication. The first party who sends the information is called the sender and the second party who receives the information, decodes the information, and accordingly responds is called the receiver or the recipient. Thus, in simpler terms, communication is simply a process where the sender sends the information to the receiver for him to respond.

Elements/Process of Communication

There are seven elements of communication (Fig. 2):

1. **Source idea:** The source idea is the process by which one formulates an idea to communicate to others. This process can be influenced by external stimuli such as books or radio, or it can come about internally by thinking about a particular subject. The source idea is the basis for the communication.
2. **Message:** The message is what will be communicated to others. It is based on the source idea, but the message is crafted to meet the needs of the audience. For example, if the message is between two friends, the message will take a different form from communicating with a superior.
3. **Encoding:** Encoding is how the message is transmitted to others. The message is converted into a suitable form for transmission. The medium of transmission will determine the form of the communication. For example, the message will take a different form if the communication will be spoken or written.
4. **Channel:** The channel is the medium of communication. The channel must be able to transmit the message from one party to another without changing the content of the message. The channel can be a piece of paper, a communication medium such as radio, or it can be an email. The channel is the path of the communication from the sender to the receiver. An email can use the Internet as a channel.
5. **Receiver:** The receiver is the party receiving the communication. The party

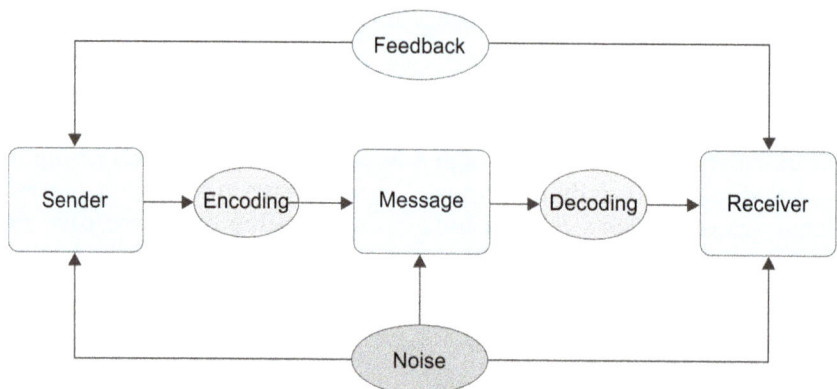

Fig. 2: Process of communication.

uses the channel to get the communication from the transmitter. A receiver can be a television set, a computer, or a piece of paper depending on the channel used for the communication.

6. **Decoding:** Decoding is the process where the message is interpreted for its content. It also means the receiver thinks about the message content and internalizes the message. This step of the process is where the receiver compares the message to prior experiences or external stimuli.

7. **Feedback:** Feedback is the final step in the communication process. This step conveys to the transmitter that the message is understood by the receiver. The receiver formats an appropriate reply to the first communication based on the channel and sends it to the transmitter of the original message.

Characteristics of Communication

- **Clarity:** One of the most essential characteristics of impressive communication is "Clarity." Use simple and sound words, so that listeners can grab them easily. Be clear in your thoughts; jumbled and confused mind cannot deliver a good and clear saying. Avoid using any technical term; try to explain in laymen's language. Use examples to explain and support complex scenarios. Work a little bit on your accent and pronunciation.
- **Aim or goal**: At every stage of your talk/communication, do not forget your "Aim or Goal." Try to deduce acceptable stuff by judging pros and cons impartially. Communicate with a broad and practical mind. Know and analyze the audience.
- **Precision:** Be precise and exact in your approach. Neither be too deep nor be too short. Include some good facts acknowledging your topic. Avoid repeatability, unless required so.
- **Linkage:** Try to maintain a logical link between your sayings. Do not put two opposite faces of coin at the same time. Deliver in a structured and planned way.
- **Globalization and localization:** Try to explain the broader aspects based on the latest trends in globalization and modernization.
- **Style of expressing:** Various speech parameters such as pitch, tone, intensity, etc., should be controlled. Do not be too fast or too slow. Look straight forward and use light humor. Do not be arrogant and make faces. Be natural and practical. Do good homework.
- **Dress properly:** 25% confidence and 25% respect from audiences come automatically if you have dressed up well. Be neat, clean, ironed, and polished irrespective of the fact that you have dressed up formally or informally. Do good hairstyling; avoid any casual or unethical looks.

Principles of Communication

- Communication should be a conviction, i.e., belief or opinion
- Communication should be appropriate to the situation
- Communication should have objectives and purposes
- Communication should promote the total achievement of purposes
- Communication should represent the personality and individuality of the communication
- Communication involves special preparation
- Communication should be oriented to the interest and needs of the receiver
- Communication through personal contact
- Communication should seek attention
- Communication should be familiar

Types of Communication

1. **One-way communication:** The flow of communication is one way from the communicator to the audience. It has certain limitations like knowledge is

imposed and learning is authoritative with very little audience participation with no feedback. Therefore, it does influence human behavior.

2. **Two-way communication:** In this, both the communicators and the audience take part. The process of communication is active and democratic. It is more likely to influence behavior than one-way communication

3. **Formal communication:** It is an officially organized channel of communication and it is delayed communication. It is generally used for all practice purposes. This is authoritative, specific, and accurate and reaches everybody. The medium of formal communication may be department meetings, conferences, telephone calls, interviews, circulars, etc.

4. **Informal network:** This includes gossip circles such as friend's internet group such as minded people, and casual groups. Communication is very fast here. The informal channels may be more active. It follows the grapevine route. Informal communications are quite fast and spontaneous.

5. **Physiological communication:** It is a stimulus received by the body; immediately the brain receives the information and transmits it to the respective organs through the nervous system, where it has to be passed.

6. **Psychic communication:** Extrasensory perception occurs, i.e., something which will occur in the future. The person pertains and predicts that in advance is called psychic communication.

7. **Serial communication:** Person to person the message will be passed like a chain. The sender passes the message to one person, then that receiver passes information to another, and so on.

8. **Symbolic communication:** Good communication requires awareness of symbolic communication, the verbal and nonverbal symbolism used by others to convey meaning.

9. **Visual communication:** The visual form of communication comprises charts and graphs, pictograms, tables, maps, posters, etc.

10. **Verbal communication:** The traditional way of communication has been by word of mouth; language is the chief vehicle of communication. Direct verbal communication by word of mouth may be loaded with hidden meanings.

11. **Oral communication:** Oral communication is transmitting messages orally by meeting the person through artificial media of communication such as telephone and intercom systems.

12. **Written communication:** It is transmitting a message in writing. Written communication can be followed when a record of communication is necessary.

13. **Mechanical communication:** By using mechanical devices the communication will be sent, e.g., internet, radio, TV, etc.

14. **Nonverbal communication:** Communication can occur even without a word. Nonverbal communication is message transmission through body language without using words. It includes bodily movements, positive, facial expressions **(Fig. 3)**. Silence is nonverbal communication. It can speak louder than words.

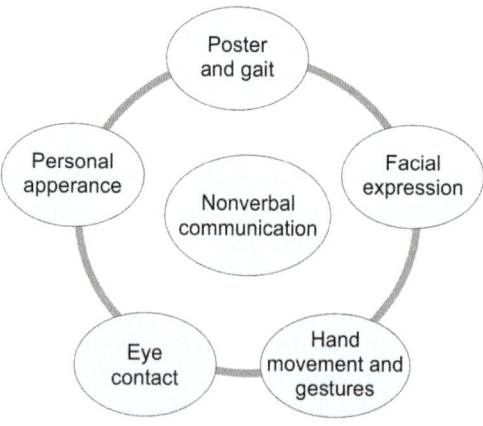

Fig. 3: Factors to consider in nonverbal communication.

Assertive Communication

Assertive communication is communication widely accepted in organizations and assertiveness focus on the difference between successfully closing a deal or losing it. The concept was first introduced by Alberti and Emmons (1990). Assertiveness is used as one of the soft skills in public speaking.

Assertive communication is the ability to express positive and negative ideas and feelings in an open, honest, and direct way. It allows us to take responsibility for ourselves and our actions, without judging, hurting, or blaming other people.

Assertive communication helps to constructively confront, decision-making, and resolve conflict. It is an honest, direct, and appropriate expression of one's feelings, thoughts, and beliefs.

Based on assertive communication assertiveness training or soft skill training is widely used by organizations for their employees.

Assertiveness training was introduced in the 1970s to stand up for their rights and is used in various settings such as social skill training, vocational programs, and others.

Purposes of Assertiveness Training
- To teach strategies for identifying and acting on their desires
- Remaining respectful to others
- To communicate in a clear and honest fashion
- Conflict resolution
- For realistic goal settings
- In case of risky harassment situations at the workplace

Techniques for Assertiveness Training
1. **Information gathering exercise:** In this, the person will list areas of life in which they find difficulty asserting them and work on those areas. Role-plays are designed to help participants practice a clearer and more direct form of communication.
2. Feedback is provided to improve the response and role-plays are repeated.
3. Practice assertive techniques outside training settings. Specific techniques used are self-observation skills, awareness of personal preference, and assuming personal responsibility.

Tips for Becoming Assertive
- Start with small matters and be specific
- Make manageable requests
- Narrow your goals
- Hold your ground
- Choose your moment
- Do not be a competitive complainer
- Stand up for one's basic human rights
- Assume responsibility for your own words
- Do not argue and put on further discussion if the other person gets angry.
- Persistently repeat in a calm voice what is needed.

Advantages of Communication

Oral Communication
- Since it is face-to-face system and hence can be clarified.
- There is an opportunity to ask questions, exchange ideas, and clarify meaning.
- It develops a friendly and cooperative spirit.
- It is easy, quick, and flexible, and hence effective.

Written Communication
- It has permanent record for future reference.
- It will have adequate coverage and accuracy.
- Suitable for communicating lengthy messages.
- It is an authoritative communication.

Assertive Communication
- For growth and development, it is very effective.
- It helps to prevent energy leakage.
- Make individuals aware of their rights.

- It helps to create responsible proactive environment.

Disadvantages of Communication

Oral Communication
- The spoken words may be misunderstood.
- The facial expression and tone of voice of the communicator may mislead the receiver.
- Not suitable for lengthy communication
- It requires the art of effective specificity.
- It has no record for future reference.

Written Communication
- It requires skill and education for understanding.
- It is also one-way communication and hence may not be effective.
- There is no opportunity for the subordinates to ask questions and exchange ideas.
- It may not communicate all aspects.

Assertive Communication
- Overdoing can be harmful.
- It is not equivalent to martial arts training/physical self-defense technique.

How to Improve Soft Skills Using Strategies of Communication

1. **Think before you speak:** Think about the purpose of your communication. What do you hope to accomplish with your words or actions? "Before you speak, ask yourself: Is it kind? Is it necessary? Is it true? Does it improve on the silence?". Also, think about the structure of your communication.
2. **Listening:** The most effective nurse leaders know when to stop talking and start listening. This is especially important in three particular situations. Extreme emotions, such as anger, resentment, and excitement, warrant attention from a personal and a business standpoint. On a personal level, people feel acknowledged when others validate their feelings. Nurses who ignore feelings can create distance between themselves and their colleagues and patients, eroding the relationship and ultimately affecting the working environment.
3. **Questioning:** Many nurses need information but are not sure how to get it. Similarly, their colleagues and patients may have information but do not know how to impart it. Nurses can open the lines of communication by asking good questions. Note that different kinds of questions yield different kinds of results. For example, has the report been completed? Do you know what to do? These are examples of closed questions that are perfectly appropriate in the right situations. Open questions are those that elicit longer responses. They are useful almost any time a nurse wants more than a yes/no answer, for instance, when seeking input from others, looking for information about a particular topic, or exploring a problem.

   Personal questions have a special role in communication. Inappropriate personal questions can alienate patients. Appropriate personal questions, however, can create a sense of camaraderie between patient and nurse.
4. **Using discretion:** Good nurses adopt a policy of discretion, if not confidentiality, with their patients. Only then can they develop the trust that is so vital to productivity. Confidential situations may arise in a number of areas, personal and professional.
5. **Directing:** Notice that directing comes last on the list of communication strategies. It may not be the least important, but it is definitely one to use less often. Directing means giving directions clearly and unequivocally, such that people know exactly what to do and when. It is best used in times of confusion, or when efficiency is the most important goal.

Methods to overcome barriers of communication are explained in **Box 1**.

Box 1: Methods of overcoming barriers of communication.
- Have a positive attitude about communication. Defensiveness interferes with communication.
- Work at improving communication skills. It takes knowledge and work. The increased awareness of the potential for improving communication is the first step to better communication.
- Include communication as a skill to be evaluated along with all other skills. Help other people to improve their communication skills by helping them to understand their communication problems.
- Make communication goal-oriented. When the sender and receiver have a good relationship, they are much more likely to accomplish their communication goals.
- Approach communication as a creative process rather than simply part of chore of working with people. What works with one person may not work with other person such as different channels of communication, listening techniques, and feedback techniques.
- Accept the reality of miscommunication. The best communication fails to have perfect communication. They accept miscommunication and work to minimize its negative impact.
- Warmth and friendliness maintain the quality of communication process.
- An attitude of acceptance, frankness, respect, and lack of prejudice helps to improve communication.
- Empathy is identifying with the way another person feels. An empathetic nurse is sensitive to the patient's feelings and problems but remains objective enough to help toward positive outcomes.
- Comfortable environment is that in which the communication takes place and should be trustable and safe.

Role of Nurse in Good Communication

1. Initiating discussion of goals at the unit and individual levels with the start that the manager directly supervises and involves in the work.
2. Bringing pertinent directives, regulations, accreditation standards, or other factors needing consideration to the discussion
3. Recording written goals and action plans for achieving them
4. Maintaining momentum of progress toward goals, giving positive and constructive feedback to promote progress toward meeting deadlines
5. Communicating to staff the progress toward goals through the use of visual tools
6. Communicate the "why" behind the "what."
7. Realize that effective communication takes time.
8. Accept negative news as information and do not take it personally.
9. Respond non-defensively when people express differing or contradictory ideas and views.
10. Report situations as accurately as possible and avoid downplaying negative factors.
11. Send important organizational messages by at least two methods (for example, e-mail and a written memo or verbally and written).
12. Do not rely so much on written communication as people often do not read it.
13. Use active listening in all conversations.
14. Select the location for discussing sensitive issues carefully.
15. Say what you mean; avoid assumptions and ensure that the receiver has less need to turn to assumptions.
16. State information clearly backed up with research to get to the facts.
17. Think before speaking.
18. If you do not have the answer, state this and that you will look for the information and follow up.
19. Summarize at the end of a lengthy conversation and ask for confirmation from the other party.
20. "I" statements are more effective than "you" statements, which tend to put the other person on the offensive.
21. Thank others for their feedback and suggestions as this recognizes that they have been heard and support further communication.

22. Credibility is critical; trust can make or break how a message is received and interpreted.
23. When difficult questions must be asked or there is a difficult discussion, it is important to select the time when the other person (receiver) might be more receptive.
24. To effectively communicate, we must realize that we are all different in the way we perceive the world and use this understanding as a guide to our communication with others.

COMMUNICATION AND INTERPERSONAL RELATIONSHIPS

At the core of nursing are relationships formed between the nurse and those affected by the nurse's practice. Communication is the means to establish these helping healing relationships. The caring nurse communicates with others in a manner that expresses awareness and respect for persons as an individual. Nurses with expertise in communication can express caring by becoming sensitive to self and others, promoting, and accepting the expression of positive and negative feelings, and developing helping-trust relationships. Nurses who have developed good critical thinking skills make the best communicators. They are able to draw upon theoretical knowledge about communication and integrate this knowledge with what has been learned through personal experience. They can interpret messages received from others, analyze them, make inferences about their meaning, evaluate their effects, explain the rationale for communication techniques used, and self-examine personal communication skills.

Definitions

Relationship

A relationship is an interpersonal process where two or more people interact with each other. "A healthy IPR is one in which individuals involved, experience intimacy with each other while maintaining separate identities."

Intimacy

It is characterized by sensitivity to the needs of the personnel and mutual validation of personnel warmth.

Interpersonal Relationship

Interpersonal relationships are the social associations or connections or affiliations between two or more people.

Phases of Interpersonal Relationship

Hildegard Paplau (1952) gave the interpersonal relationship model. Her model describes the phases in a nurse-patient relationship in terms of the interpersonal process used in psychodynamic nursing **(Fig. 4)**.

Four Phases of the Therapeutic Nurse-Patient Relationship

1. **Orientation phase:** The nurse's orientation phase involves engaging the client in treatment, providing explanations and information, and answering questions.
   - Problem defining phase
   - It starts when the client meets the nurse as a stranger.
   - Defining the problem and deciding the type of service needed

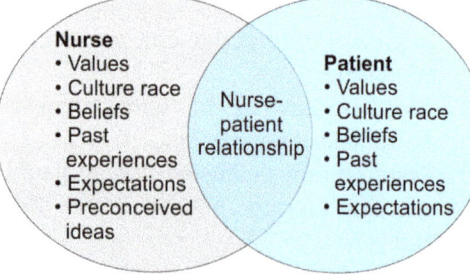

Fig. 4: Peplau's theory of interpersonal relationships.

- The client seeks assistance, conveys needs, asks questions, shares preconceptions and expectations of past experiences.

  The nurse responds, explains roles to the client, identifies problems, and uses available resources and services.

2. **Identification phase:** The identification phase begins when the client works interdependently with the nurse, expresses feelings, and begins to feel stronger.
   - Selection of appropriate professional assistance
   - The patient begins to have a feeling of belonging and a capability of dealing with the problem, which decreases the feeling of helplessness and hopelessness.

3. **Exploitation phase:** In the exploitation phase, the client makes full use of the services offered.
   - In the exploitation phase, the client makes full use of the services offered.
   - Use of professional assistance for problem-solving alternatives
   - Advantages of services are used based on the needs and interests of the patients.
   - The individual feels like an integral part of the helping environment.
   - They may make minor requests or attention-getting techniques.
   - The principles of interview techniques must be used to explore, understand, and adequately deal with the underlying problem.
   - The patient may fluctuate on independence.
   - The nurse must be aware of the various phases of communication.
   - The nurse aids the patient in exploiting all avenues of help, and progress is made toward the final step.

4. **Resolution phase:** In the resolution phase, the client no longer needs professional services and gives up dependent behavior. The relationship ends.

- In the resolution phase, the client no longer needs professional services and gives up dependent behavior. The relationship ends.
- Termination of professional relationship
- The patient's needs have already been met by the collaborative effect of patient and nurse.
- Now they need to terminate their therapeutic relationship and dissolve the links between them.
- Sometimes it may be difficult for both as psychological dependence persists.
- The patient drifts away and breaks the nurse's bond, and a healthier emotional balance is demonstrated, and both become mature individuals.

Factors Enhancing IPR

1. Listen patiently
2. Talk meaningfully
3. Avoid judgment
4. Interpret properly
5. Respect for each other
6. Accept construct criticism
7. Behave genuinely
8. Be sensitive to the needs of the patient
9. Give smile as it makes others feel warm inside and toward you
10. Avoid arguments
11. Try to understand others' view
12. Make others feel important
13. Approach person calmly
14. Admit mistake if committed

Role of Nurse in Improving IPR

1. Willingness to give and take
2. **Acceptance of others:** Nurse comes in contact with others who may be unattractive, aged or young, rich or poor. Keeping in mind professional commitment and ethics the nurse accepts the fact that she needs to give excellent care regardless of her own feelings. Acceptance and cooperation lead to a healthy and

conducive environment for productive working conditions.
3. **Self-acceptance:** If we know or understand why we behave as we do in certain situations will help us to understand the behavior of others and adjust accordingly
4. Keeping the tone of voice and laughter under control.
5. Get along well with all kinds of people.
6. Try to overcome annoying habits of yours, e.g., sniffing, whistling.
7. Be careful with others' possessions.
8. Share appreciation with colleagues and other members of the health team.
9. Try to clear up the misunderstanding at the earliest.

Tips to Improve Interpersonal Relationship at Workplace

- Do not treat the office as your home. There is a certain way of behaving in the workplace. It is essential to be professional at work. Never misbehave with any of your colleagues. Leg pulling, criticism, backbiting are strictly prohibited. It is better to avoid someone you do not like rather than fighting or arguing with him/her. Your office colleagues can be your friends as well but one must know where to draw the line. Too much friendship is harmful and spoils relationships among employees.
- An individual should not interfere in his colleague's work. Superiors must formulate specific rules for all the employees and make sure job responsibilities do not overlap. Overlapping of job responsibility leads to employees interfering in each other's tasks and eventually fighting over small issues. One should be concerned only with his work rather than trying to find out what the other employee is up to.
- Leave your ego behind. Do not bring your personal tensions to work. Think before you speak. Making fun of colleagues is something that is not at all expected out of a professional.
- A team leader should not scold any of his team members in front of others. It might insult him/her. Call the individual concerned either to your cabin or conference room. Avoid comparisons among team members. The employees must be strictly judged according to their work and nothing else. Employees doing well should be suitably rewarded.
- Stay away from nasty politics at the workplace. Do not try to harm anyone. It is absolutely okay to appreciate someone who has done something exceptionally well. Avoid being jealous. It will harm you in the long run. There should be healthy competition among the employees for a healthy environment at the workplace.

RESILIENCE

Resilience is not the absence of distress or difficulty. Resilience is the ability to adapt and grow following adversity. Adaptability, agility, in the face of adversity (difficulties). Flexibility in coping with newer demands and challenges. Not all are equally resilient—resilience can be developed as a skill. Currently, a quarter of all employees view their jobs as the number one stressor in their lives. The World Health Organization describes stress as the "global health epidemic of the 21st century." Many of us now work in constantly connected, always-on, and highly demanding work cultures where stress and the risk of burnout are widespread. Since the pace and intensity of contemporary work culture are not likely to change, it is more important than ever to build resilience skills to effectively navigate your work-life.

Definition

Resilience building is defined as the ability to adapt well to adversity, trauma, tragedy, threats, or even significant sources of stress which can help to manage stress and feelings of anxiety and uncertainty as per the American Psychological Association (APA).

Nurse resilience is defined as the ability to face adverse situations, remain focused, and

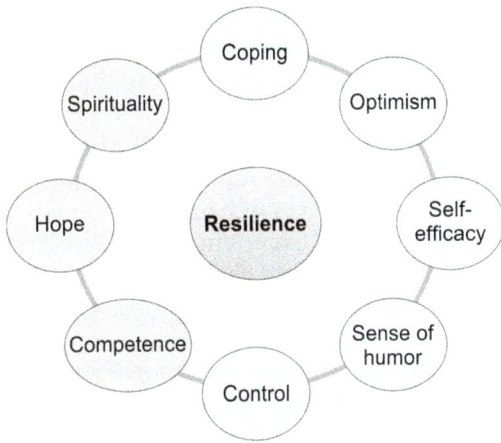

Fig. 5: Qualities of resilient nurse.

continue to be optimistic for the future **(Fig. 5)**. Resilience is a vital characteristic for nurses in today's complex healthcare system.

Importance of Resilience in Workplace

* Occupational stress affects personal and performance outcomes. Workplace stress is correlated with high levels of depression and anxiety, and burnout.
* Burnout has a heavy toll on workplaces, both productively and economically. Burnout is associated with increased rates of absenteeism and reduced productivity—not to mention the negative impact it has on employees. Psychologically resilient employees are better able to cope with stress, and less likely to suffer from "burnout."
* Resilience has been associated with various positive states, including optimism, zest, curiosity, energy, and openness to experience. These positive emotional states are of tremendous value to the workplace.
* Positive emotions build through resilience and lead to "thought-action repertoires" which then result in an urge to think/act in a certain direction.
* The experience of positive emotions (fostered by resilience) can expand activity, open an employee's eyes to a range of possibilities, and increase the likelihood of more creative solutions for workplace behaviors.
* The workers who experience positive affect are more likely to use problem-focused coping which is of great benefit in the work environment. When individuals feel more positive, they tend to also interpret seemingly ordinary events and experiences as positive. Thus, positive emotions foster positivity in the workplace.
* Resilience is not only important for its impact on psychosocial factors such as burnout, adaptive workplace behaviors, and buffering against workplace stress, it has also been implicated in physical well-being. Tugade and Fredrickson (2004) found that "the psychological mindset involved with resilience is reflected in the body as well."
* Therefore, if employees have better physical well-being, they will have a greater capacity to undertake their work, and, in turn, be better placed to further adapt to adversity! It is a win-win situation.

Ways to Build Resilience

1. **Exercise mindfulness**: Social psychologists Laura Kiken and Natalie Shook, for example, have found that mindfulness predicts judgment accuracy and insight-related problem-solving, and cognitive neuroscientists Peter Malinowski and Adam Moore found that mindfulness enhances cognitive flexibility. Strategies can be implemented including a combination of mobile learning, onsite training, webinars, and peer-to-peer learning networks which promotes the greatest chance for mindfulness to become a core competency within an organization. Finally, a number of books and apps also offer structured approaches to

mindfulness, including the book—Fully Present: The Art, Science and Practice of Mindfulness and Mindfulness.

2. **Compartmentalize your cognitive load:** One practical way to think about this is that though we cannot decrease the amount of information we receive, we can compartmentalize our cognitive tasks to optimize the way we process that information. Be deliberate about compartmentalizing different types of work activities such as e-mailing, strategy or brainstorming sessions, and business-as-usual meetings. Compartmentalizing work is useful when you consider that switching from one type of task to another makes it difficult to tune out distractions and reduces productivity by as much as 40%. Nurses must organize their routine work into small sessions and involve cognition in dealing with problems related to day-to-day activities.

3. **Take detachment breaks:** Throughout the workday, it is important to pay attention to the peaks and valleys of energy and productivity that we all experience, what health psychologists call our ultradian (hourly) as opposed to our circadian (daily) rhythms. Mental focus, clarity, and energy cycles are typically 90–120 minutes long, so it is useful to step away from our work for even a few minutes to reset energy and attention. Research suggests that balancing work activity with even a brief time for detaching from those activities can promote greater energy, mental clarity, creativity, and focus, ultimately growing our capacity for resilience throughout the course of the workday. The long-term payoff is that we preserve energy and prevent burnout over the course of days, weeks, and months.

4. **Develop mental agility: It is possible.** Without too much effort—to literally switch the neural networks with which we process the experience of stress to respond to rather than react to any difficult situation or person. This quality of mental agility hinges on the ability to mentally "decenter" stressors to effectively manage them. "Decentering" stress is not denying or suppressing the fact that we feel stressed—rather, it is the process of being able to pause, observe the experience from a neutral standpoint, and then try to solve the problem. When we are able to cognitively take a step back from our experience and label our thoughts and emotions, we are effectively pivoting attention from the narrative network in our brains to the more observational parts of our brains. Being mentally agile and decentering stress when it occurs, enables the core resilience skill of "response flexibility," which renowned psychologist Linda Graham describes as "the ability to pause, step back, reflect, shift perspectives, create options and choose wisely." We often tell our children who are upset to "use your words," for example, and it turns out that stopping and labeling emotions has the effect of activating the thinking center of our brains, rather than the emotional center—a valuable skill in demanding and high-performance workplaces everywhere.

5. **Cultivate compassion**: One of the most overlooked aspects of the resilience skill set is the ability to cultivate compassion—both self-compassion and compassion for others. Compassion increases positive emotions, creates positive work relationships, and increases cooperation and collaboration. Compassion training programs such as the one offered by Stanford University's Center for Compassion, Altruism and Research in Education (CCARE) have demonstrated that compassion cultivation practices increase happiness and well-being and decrease stress. Compassion and business effectiveness are not mutually exclusive. Rather, individual, team,

and organizational success rely on compassionate work culture.

6. **Positivity:** By taking a positive stance at work, employees are more able to adapt to adversity and also hold on to a sense of control over their work environment, putting energy and motivation into work, or, having "vigor." It is also associated with building personal resilience. It is the "opposite" of burnout, which is characterized by emotional exhaustion, physical tiredness, and cognitive fatigue or "weariness."

7. **Emotional insight:** Another example of building personal resilience at work is by developing and strengthening emotional insight. Insight is closely related to emotional intelligence. Individuals with a level of insight have a level of awareness about the full range of emotions they experience, from "negative" through to "positive." They will also consider the ramifications of their own reactions and behavior and the effects their own actions have on others. Psychologically resilient individuals can be described as emotionally intelligent.

8. **Balance:** Individuals can build personal resilience at work by achieving a healthy work-life balance. This is especially challenging in the world we are living in. Technology can mean that employees may have access to work 24 hours a day, 7 days a week. To be able to bounce back from stressful situations, i.e., to be resilient, workers need to have the energy that can be easily depleted if a healthy work-life balance is not in place. Workers need time to relax, unwind, and recuperate.

9. **Spirituality:** Having a sense of spirituality has been linked to developing resilience at work. This may be related to reducing vulnerability and the impact that adversity in the workplace has on the individual. Finding meaning in work and feeling that this work is contributing to a greater good, can buffer against the effect of stress. It may also be because spirituality may lead employees to view even stressful situations as having positive aspects, or "purpose," and appreciating potential benefits.

10. **Reflection:** Becoming more reflective is another way individuals can build resilience at work. In other words, being in tune with one's emotions and emotional reactions can serve to buffer against the effect of stress. Being aware of possible "triggers" to stress can provide individuals with the opportunity to prepare and gather resources so they are better able to "bounce back." If an employee knows that a particular circumstance will be especially challenging, they can then implement coping strategies, such as seeking support. The ability to build resilience is a skill that will serve you well in an increasingly stressful work world. And companies stand to benefit from a more resilient workforce. Building an organizational culture that encourages and supports resilience training just makes good business.

STRESS MANAGEMENT

Stress has been defined in different ways over the years. Originally, it was conceived of as pressure from the environment, then as strain within the person. The generally accepted definition today is one of interaction between the situation and the individual. It is the psychological and physical state that results when the resources of the individual are not sufficient to cope with the demands and pressures of the situation. Thus, stress is more likely in some situations than others and in some individuals than others. Stress can undermine the achievement of goals, both for individuals and organizations. Work-related stress is the response people may have when presented with work demands and pressures that are not matched to their knowledge and abilities and which challenge their ability to cope. Stress occurs in a wide range of work circumstances but is often made worse when employees feel they have little support from supervisors and colleagues, as well as little control over work processes. There is often confusion between pressure or challenge and stress, and sometimes this is used to excuse bad management practice. Pressure at the workplace is unavoidable due to the demands of the contemporary work environment. Pressure perceived as acceptable by an individual may even keep workers alert, motivated, and able to work and learn, depending on the available resources and personal characteristics. However, when that pressure becomes excessive or otherwise unmanageable it leads to stress. Stress can damage an employee's health and business performance.

Definition

Stress term was first introduced by the endocrinologist Hans Seyle in 1949. Stress was described by him as the body's adjustment to new circumstances, and the body's stereotypical and nonspecific response to environmental stimuli that disrupts a personal balance and is described also as a psychosomatic mechanism to regulate and balance the tensions.

Stress is defined as any change that one must adapt to in one's ever-changing world. In particular, stress is any demand (force, pressure, and strain) placed on the body and the body's reaction to it.

Stress is a state manifested by a specific syndrome which consists of all the non-specifically induced changes within biological system. —*Hans Selye*

Stress is defined as a stimulus, life event, or set of circumstances causing a disrupted response that increases the individual's vulnerability to illness. Stress may also be defined as a response, the disruption caused by a noxious stimulus or stressor.

Therefore, stress is a state produced by a change in the environment that is perceived as challenging, threatening, or damaging to the person's dynamic balance or equilibrium. Stress is experienced by everyone who is living, working, and breathing at the very moment.

Workplace Stress

Work stress or job stress is defined as the harmful, physical, and emotional responses that occur when the requirements of the job do not match the capabilities, resources, or needs of the workers.

Work-related stress can be caused by poor work organization (the way we design jobs and work systems, and the way we manage them), by poor work design (for example, lack of control over work processes), poor management, unsatisfactory working conditions, and lack of support from colleagues and supervisors.

The stress response can be an asset for raising levels of performance during critical events such as a sports activity, an important meeting, or in situations of actual danger or crisis. However, if stress becomes persistent, all parts of the body's stress management system (the brain, heart, lungs, vessels, adrenals, and muscles) become chronically over-activated. Over time, this produces physical and/or psychological damage.

Many nurses "accept" health problems that come from the physical and emotional stress of caring for others by not giving equal care to themselves. This is not necessary when we practice holistic self-care. Causes of stress are categorized as external or internal and acute or chronic.

Types of Stressors

- External stressors are adverse physical, mental, emotional, or spiritual conditions around you, such as high-pressure working conditions, noise, or abuse.
- Internal stressors are adverse physical, mental, emotional, or spiritual conditions around you, such as your attitudes, beliefs, and illnesses. Studies show that internal

psychological stressors are rare or absent in most animals except humans.

Types of Stress

- Acute stress is the reaction to an immediate threat commonly known as the fight, flight, or freeze response. The threat can be any situation that is experienced as a threat or danger, even subconsciously or falsely. Common acute stressors include noise, crowding, isolation, hunger, infection, and imagining or recalling threatening events.
- Chronic stress happens when the acute stressors continue without resolution. The instinct to fight, flee, or freeze becomes suppressed and/or exhausted.

Effect of Stress

The psychological effects of stress include:
- The onset of depression or anxiety
- Diminished quality of life
- Difficulty in sleeping
- Emotional instability
- Disruption of social and family life
- Increased use of cigarettes, alcohol, and drugs
- Poor attitude toward work
- Difficulties in communicating with patients
- Difficulty maintaining pleasant relations with coworkers
- Difficulty judging the seriousness of a potential emergency

The physical effects of stress include:
- Over-stimulation of the nervous system
- Heart disease
- Stroke
- Susceptibility to infections
- Immune disorders
- Gastrointestinal problems
- Irritable bowel syndrome
- Peptic ulcers
- Inflammatory bowel disease
- Weight gain
- Weight loss
- Eating disorders
- Diabetes
- Chronic pain
- Muscular and joint pain
- Headaches
- Sleep disturbances
- Sexual and reproductive dysfunction
- Premenstrual syndrome
- Fertility issues
- Effects on pregnancy
- Memory concentration and learning problems
- Allergies
- Skin disorders
- Unexplained hair loss (alopecia areata)
- Teeth and gums (an increased risk for periodontal disease)

Stress Management Strategies

1. **Relaxation techniques**: These are the widely accepted strategies and are used as a complementary method to reduce stress. There are various relaxation techniques such as meditation, deep breathing, progressive muscle relaxation, biofeedback, guided imagery, etc. These techniques can be taught to the employees by organizing workshops, and trained personnel can teach on one-to-one basis depending upon the stress load on the employees.
2. **Coping skill intervention:** This intervention focused on developing the skills in employees how to restructure their work technically and intellectually, using less energy and coping with demands of the workload effectively. Positive reinforcement, cognitive restructuring techniques, problem-solving techniques are some of the coping interventions.
3. **Employee aide programs (EAP)**: In this, employees are given brief treatment therapy for stress reduction for a period of few days. The therapy comprises of behavior therapy and individual therapy.
4. **Staff development program**: Various strategies are inculcated in staff development programs to reduce the stress of the employees—problem-solving,

stress reduction, creating an active stress management program that formalizes staff stress management strategies and activities that are integrated throughout the life of the disaster response program, creating a comprehensive training plan that adequately prepares counselors for their work. Include these components:

- The use of modeling, role play, and simulation exercises to give staff an opportunity to practice crisis counseling, and especially responses to highly distraught people
- Practice on how to conclude a counseling relationship
- Examples of signals that indicate whether talking about problems is bringing relief to the survivor or agitating him/her
- Examples of calming techniques and basic coping skills
- Examples of how to employ the buddy system

5. **Skills training:** Stress can be reduced in some cases through better job-related skills training procedures, where employees are taught how to do their jobs more effectively with less stress and strain. For instance, an employee might be taught how to reduce overload by taking shortcuts or by using new or expanded skills. These techniques would only be successful, however, if management did not follow this increased effectiveness by raising work quotas. Along with this could go greater effort by managers to specify and clarify job duties to reduce ambiguity and conflict. Employees could also be trained in human relations skills to improve their interpersonal abilities so that they might encounter less interpersonal and intergroup conflict.

TIME MANAGEMENT

Time management is more than just managing the work, it also is doing work efficiently in a given period of time. It is using time productively and efficiently and getting the things done and therefore it is very necessary to think about time management.

People who are good at time management are good at getting things done in an organized manner. Prioritizing the needs and work is the best possible way of doing things at right time.

Time management is the process of planning and controlling how much time to spend on specific activities. Good time management enables an individual to complete more in a shorter period of time, lowers stress, and leads to career success.

Implications of Poor Time Management

Let us also consider the consequences of poor time management.

1. **Poor workflow:** The inability to plan ahead and stick to goals means poor efficiency. For example, if there are several important tasks to complete, an effective plan would be to complete related tasks together or sequentially. However, if you do not plan ahead, you could end up having to jump back and forth or backtrack, in doing your work. That translates to reduced efficiency and lower productivity.
2. **Wasted time:** Poor time management results in wasted time. For example, by talking to friends on social media while doing an assignment, you are distracting yourself and wasting time.
3. **Loss of control:** By not knowing what the next task is, you suffer from a loss of control of your life. That can contribute to higher stress levels and anxiety.
4. **Poor quality of work:** Poor time management typically makes the quality of your work suffer. For example, having to rush to complete tasks at the last minute usually compromises quality.
5. **Poor reputation:** If clients or your employer cannot rely on you to complete tasks in a timely manner, their expectations

and perceptions of you are adversely affected. If a client cannot rely on you to get something done on time, they will likely take their business elsewhere.

How to Make Good Time Management

1. **Set smart objective:** You need to accomplish many things in your time. You must be able to determine what is your objective and make sure your objective is always directed toward their achievement.
2. **Determine your priorities:** it is wise to periodically make a list of the tasks that confront you and prioritize them. A good nurse leader knows when to concentrate on the important and eliminate the rest.
3. **Planning:** Planning is very essential to complete the task. You should plan the work and complete that with your full efforts.
4. **Learn to say no:** One crucial element of learning how to improve time management is getting comfortable with saying "No" to things that do not help you reach your goals. When you say "no" to something that is not really adding value to your life or supporting your core values or goals, you are saying yes to something else that is—time to be with family, exercise, or even much-needed sleep.
5. **Minimize distractions:** Think of minimizing distractions as another way of saying "no." So what is distracting you? E-mail? Texts? Social media? Whatever it is, say "no." Eliminate the distraction and the stress that comes with it. Block websites if you have to. Put up an "Away" or "Do Not Disturb" notice on your accounts. Your time is *yours*, so take control of your workspace and time so you can be productive.

■ WORK-LIFE BALANCE

A state of equilibrium in which the demands of both a person's job and personal life are equal. It can be difficult to get the right work-life balance. Experts say success lies not only in carefully defining how you want to spend your time but in making sure you adjust your life and work as your needs change.

Work-life balance is defined as the amount of time you spend doing your job compared with the amount of time you spend with your family and doing things you enjoy.

Follow routines with regular work, hobbies, rest, and exercise; taking breaks/relaxation time, spending quality time with family, friends, and pets; if not possible, video calling to loved ones; taking help from other family members for house chores; humor, listening to music, singing, or watching movies (hobbies); reduce screen time; prayer/meditation.

Sometimes even small changes can make a difference. An unmanageable schedule and out-of-control home life can lead to depression, poor performance at work, conflict with family, and a feeling of burnout that can lead physicians to question whether to stay in medicine at all.

Work-life balance is a comfortable state of equilibrium achieved between an employee's primary priorities of employment position and private lifestyle.

Most psychologists would agree that the demands of an employee's career should not overwhelm the individual's ability to enjoy a satisfying personal life outside of the business environment.

Role of Nurse to Maintain Work-Life Balance

Taking Care of Physical Health
- Taking care of physical health is very important.
- Mind–body connect
- Physical health helps in maintaining mental health.

Ensuring Adequate Physical Health
- Eat nutritious food and have your meals on time as much as you can.

- Stay hydrated.
- Maintain sleep hygiene—regular time to bed and rising.
- Avoid discussing work-related matters and other matters that are disturbing toward bedtime
- Exercise regularly (walk, yoga)
- Avoid excessive screen time, especially around bedtime.
- Medication and treatment adherence for comorbidities—ensure timely care.
- Consultation with your physician if you have comorbidities and difficulty in following the treatment

Tips to Develop a Better Work-Life Balance

- To ensure you make the best of your time at work and home, good ideas include new daily regime ensuring the main things remain the main things.
- Set a clear boundary between work and home. Ask your family to make you accountable to ensure you do not slip back into old habits.
- Allow yourself to focus on the parts of your life you really care about and give them 100% attention.
- Keeping a daily to-do list. Make sure you complete the important things and do not worry about the rest.

▌APPLYING SOFT SKILLS TO WORKPLACE AND SOCIETY

Presentation Skills

- Many clinical nurses are changing the way they deliver care for the benefit of their patients.
- To share ideas, knowledge, and opinions more widely, nurses need to either speak or write within the public arena.
- For all nurses, presentation skills are not just useful, they are essential, whether for sharing practice, influencing colleagues, or seeking a new job.
- Such skills can be learned, building on characteristics most nurses already possess.
- Effective presentations usually require learning to control nervousness and preparing properly.

Social Etiquette

Humans are social animals and it is important that they follow certain norms that facilitate interpersonal relationships. Social etiquette is exactly how it sounds, it refers to the behavior you resort to in social situations—interactions with your family, friends, coworkers, or strangers. We are expected to follow social norms to coexist and live in harmony.

Social etiquette influences how others perceive and treat you. It can help you create lasting impressions that establish trust and reliance. Practicing good social manners not only helps you build lifelong relationships, it also helps you create fruitful opportunities. Let's look at some real-life social etiquette examples to understand the concept better.

- Remembering people's names and making them feel good
- Saying "sorry" or "excuse me" immediately after sneezing
- Using "thank you" and "sorry" when a situation calls for it
- Saying "excuse me" while navigating your way through a crowd
- Holding the door for somebody standing in front of or behind you

Types of Social Etiquette

We practice different kinds of social etiquette depending on the situation we are in. For example, the way you behave at a family dinner is quite different from the way you behave at a business lunch. Let us look at the types of social etiquette we practice depending on different situations:

1. **Face-to-face etiquette:** Face-to-face interactions are not always easy. Here are a few etiquette practices to follow when you meet someone:

- Use your full name to introduce yourself and greet the other person. You can simply use "hello, nice to meet you" to break the ice. A smile and a firm handshake make it easier to build rapport.
- Pay attention to your body language so that you do not come off as rude or unprofessional. Good posture, eye contact, and a confident attitude can make a huge difference.
- One of the most important aspects of social etiquette is paying attention to people. Never interrupt anyone mid-sentence and always listen respectfully.

2. **Social media etiquette:** Social etiquette also extends to social media and online communication. Here are some ways to ensure proper conduct on social media platforms:
    - If someone does not accept your friendship or follow requests, leave them be. If it is important to connect with someone, message them and state your purpose.
    - Avoid posting insensitive content on your social media handles. If you make a mistake, own up and apologize.
    - Always get consent if you want to share someone else's information, photos, or content. Before tagging someone in a post or photograph, check if they are comfortable with it.

3. **Virtual meeting etiquette:** Work from home has become the new normal for most businesses today and virtual meetings have become a part of daily work routine. Here are a few tips to help you maintain proper social etiquette during online meetings:
    - Dress for success! Wearing appropriate attire can help you feel confident. It also shows that you pay attention to details and it will impress your audience.
    - Mute your microphone when you are not speaking. It ensures that there is no echo and you do not disrupt the flow of meetings.
    - It may be tempting to check your phone but try to stay present and active. Participate in discussions and show anyone who is speaking that you are respectfully listening to them.

4. **Telephone etiquette:** Implies the manners of using telephone communication including the way you represent your ideas and yourself:
    - Greeting the receiver, the tone of voice
    - The choice of words, listening skills, the closure to the call, etc.
    - In official calls do not use words like "any guess who I am."
    - Do not eat something when you are on call.
    - At the end of the conversation use pleasant words like take care, have a great day, feel grateful to talk with you.

Motivational Skills

❖ Maintaining our own motivation at work can be a challenge at times, let alone raising motivation of our team. Yet, the workplace is constantly changing and our ability to respond well to those changes depends on our own motivation and the motivation of our coworkers.
❖ The rewards of a motivated healthcare team are greater healthcare outcomes and greater efficiency in healthcare delivery.
❖ Developing your emotional intelligence will go a long way to improving your own and your staff's levels of motivation.
❖ We cannot expect to see motivation from our staff unless we exhibit it in our own attitude and behavior.

Nurses who maintain their motivation in the fast-paced world of the healthcare setting will be using one or all of the following techniques:

1. They are life-long learners. They feed their mind with knowledge. Maintaining a curiosity for knowledge goes a long way toward keeping motivated.
2. They choose their company. You become like the people you associate with, so

motivated people seek out like-minded colleagues.
3. They choose to see failure as feedback and not a setback. Positive people acknowledge their missteps and modify their behavior in pursuit of their desired outcome.
4. Maintaining motivation requires self-assessment. Seek feedback on your performance as a leader so that you can self-correct if necessary.

Teamwork

Today's healthcare organizations are filled with skilled, multigenerational, and culturally diverse interdisciplinary team members. Although each specialty has a specific focus, we all share a unified goal: We want both the patient care experience and our work environment to be positive. To ensure that patients are satisfied during their healthcare encounters, we must embrace a teamwork approach to care delivery.

Teamwork requires effective communication skills and collaborative care coordination. Team members should be encouraged to ask questions, share ideas or concerns, and discuss potential solutions. Each team member's strengths and skills must be utilized to achieve an optimal patient care experience and workplace satisfaction.

■ APPLICATION OF SOFT SKILLS IN NURSING

1. **Nurses develop emotional intelligence:** It takes all sorts of nurses to make up a class. While some nurses demonstrate a high level of emotional intelligence, some lack this ability.
2. **Nurture interpersonal relationship:** The classroom is the best platform that provides interaction between students. In this, they constantly engage in interaction during class hours or in the event of completing a group assignment and projects.
3. **Easily understanding of classroom teaching:** Student nurses come into a class with the main motive of the new learning of the subject matter. Soft skills make their learning more interesting and fruitful. Students can solve problems employing the principles of soft skills while staying inquisitive about their surroundings and their subject matter.
4. **Expose leadership qualities in students:** Some students are born with leadership qualities and for those who do not have these qualities soft skills come in as handy tools. Through soft skills, students will be able to motivate themselves to take on leadership roles so as to attract the attention of others.
5. **Uncover the hidden potential in students:** Soft-skilled students are now in a sweet spot to uncover the hidden potential that was lying dormant in them. Every student brings to the table a host of talents that amaze both the educators and their parents.

QUESTION BANK

MULTIPLE CHOICE QUESTIONS

1. **Soft skills are also known as:**
    a. Interpersonal skills
    b. Personal skills
    c. Student skills
    d. Learning skills

UNIT IX: Application of Soft Skills

2. Communication is a part of:
    a. Soft skills
    b. Hard skills
    c. Rough skills
    d. Short skills
3. The person who transmits the message:
    a. Receiver
    b. Feedback
    c. Sender
    d. Encode
4. _____ is the person who notices and decodes and attaches some meaning to a message.
    a. Receiver
    b. Driver
    c. Sender
    d. Cleaner
5. The response to a sender message is called:
    a. Decode
    b. Feedback
    c. Massage
    d. Encode
6. _____ refers to all these factors that disrupt communication.
    a. Nonsense
    b. Noise
    c. Nowhere
    d. Nobody
7. Environmental barriers are the same as _____ noise.
    a. Physiological
    b. Psychological
    c. Physical
    d. Sociological
8. Our dress code is an example of _____ communication.
    a. Verbal
    b. Nonverbal
    c. Written
    d. Spoken
9. _____ communication includes tone of voice, body language, facial expressions etc.
    a. Nonverbal
    b. Verbal
    c. Letter
    d. Noise
10. When there is similarity of background between the sender and the receiver such as age, language, nationality, religion, and gender then this is called _____ context.
    a. Social
    b. Cultural
    c. Physical
    d. Dynamic

ANSWER KEY
1. a   2. a   3. c   4. a   5. b   6. b   7. c   8. b
9. a   10. b

SHORT ANSWER TYPE QUESTIONS

1. Define communication.
2. Define time management.
3. What is resilience?
4. Enlist the methods of coping with stress.
5. Define work-life balance.

LONG ANSWER TYPE QUESTIONS

1. Define soft skills. What is the importance of soft skills in nursing?
2. What are the types of soft skills? Explain in detail the way of communication.
3. Explain how soft skills are beneficial for nursing in contrast to society.
4. Explain barriers in establishing interpersonal relationships and strategies to overcome barriers.

UNIT X

Self-empowerment

OUTLINE

- Meaning and Definition of Self-empowerment
- Dimensions of Self-empowerment
- Self-empowerment Development
- Women Empowerment
- Professional Etiquette and Personal Grooming
- Role of Nurse in Empowerment

■ SELF-EMPOWERMENT

Nowadays, depression or mental health issues are becoming severe. The World Health Organization (WHO) estimates that each year approximately one million people die from suicide. The reason behind it is that people do not have control of their own life.

In the age of remote control technology, people are losing control of life. In our day-to-day life, we have two options for every situation. But mainly, we chose the easiest one. That makes our life out of control.

But there is also a solution, which is "personal empowerment." It helps you to make positive decisions that make your life better. That gives positive energy within you.

■ PERSONAL EMPOWERMENT

Personal empowerment is the process of becoming more robust to take charge of your own life. It is a mixture of self-belief, self-awareness, and self-respect. To empower yourself, you need to understand the purpose of your life. And you also need to find out your weak points and strong points. Trying to overcome your weaknesses and making the right decisions in any situation is a base of personal empowerment. Personal empowerment gives you the right path to success. It is more than just feelings. It is a mindset that helps you improve yourself.

■ NURSING EMPOWERMENT

Nursing empowerment means the ability to effectively motivate and mobilize self and others to accomplish positive outcomes in nursing practice and work environment.

Definition of Self-empowerment

"Self-empowerment is seeking the solution rather than fixating on the problem."

—*Coach Bobbi*

Self-empowerment defines making a conscious decision to take charge of your destiny. It involves making positive choices, taking action to advance.

■ DIMENSIONS OF SELF-EMPOWERMENT

1. **Success:** When you start making yourself empowered, many things in your professional life start making it easier for you. Empowerment means a power given to change yourself. It also gives you a lot of self-confidence and also increases the

productivity and efficiency of your work. Because of all these things, you can set goals, make decisions faster, and do actions at your 100% efficiency. This helps you a lot to become successful.
2. **Health:** In this faster world, health becomes an essential thing for any person. Low self-confidence and poor self-care affect very hard on your physical as well as mental health. Personal empowerment gives you a lot of self-esteem. What motivates you to do things such as exercise, meditation, and others. It keeps your body fit both physically and mentally. Then you get a new version of yourself.
3. **Relationships:** When you are empowered, then you get control over your emotions. It shines your personality, which makes you a better person. You can easily give what your people want from you.

■ STEPS OF SELF-EMPOWERMENT DEVELOPMENT

It seems easy when we understand the meaning of self-empowerment. It is not a one-time thing but also a long process. When you start doing it, then may you realize it is hard to develop. Here are some steps that make this journey easier.

1. **Take a time and find inner peace:**
   - We are living in the 21st century; we are living in a race. So, we have no time for ourselves. But if you want to be empowered yourself, then it is a must to take time for yourself. Do whatever makes you calm. Meditation is a powerful way to get inner peace.
   - Stop, take some time in your daily race, go in peace and start thinking about what is going on in your life. Think deeper. You started getting answers to all your problems.
2. **Identify yourself:**
   - After getting answers to your problem, the second and most important step of empowering yourself is identifying yourself. Firstly identify your goal. Write it down where it will always be in front of your eyes so that you will never forget your goal.
   - Then find out your strengths and weaknesses. Ask yourself which things you can do better. Be honest with yourself. Think about your past achievements, what great things you did in the past. For example, you get good marks in 10th or 12th. Feel the power within yourself.
   - Then make a track for your goal. Decide action plan for it.
3. **Trust yourself:**
   - We live in this era, where Cristiano Ronaldo, Elon Musk exist. If they can, then you can also do.
   - If you decide to achieve it, then there is no limit to what you can earn.
   - You have a goal and a ready action plan. Now, you have to start believing in yourself. If you doubt your abilities, then you do not get success. Self-belief is the essential thing to get the win. Self-belief is a power that makes you stronger.
   - If you have a belief in yourself, then only the world starts to believe in you.
4. **Learn and develop yourself:**
   - To develop self-empowerment needs to improve your skills. Think about your goal and find what skills are required for achieving it. Then start learning these skills as much as possible. And the most important thing is to implement that learning. Learning is a sign of growing.
   - This gives you a lot of confidence to do things effectively.
5. **Start taking actions:**
   - Start taking actions that are essential for your development. Thinking about empowering yourself never makes you empowered. But doing things for that makes you empowered.
   - Remember, it is not only a one-time thing; it is a continuous process of making the right decisions for your development.

- Take small steps rather than significant steps. It helps to save you from the biggest failure.
6. **Share your experience:** Suppose you started feeling empowered or getting success. Then start sharing your knowledge of what you get from this journey. That helps you make an outstanding personality in the world and motivates you to achieve more goals.

TECHNIQUES TO BUILD PERSONAL EMPOWERMENT

- **Exercise:** Both mental and physical bodies are connected. If one of them is doing well, then the second will automatically do well. Doing daily exercise keeps your physical and mental health better. So, take some time in your daily schedule to go for a walk, gym, or swimming. It keeps you not only healthy but also happy.
- **Watch, listen and talk positive:** Empowering yourself is a long process. That needs a lot of time. To improve your thought process, you need to grasp positive things. There is a lot of negativity filled in today's world of social media and all over the internet. You need to focus on only positive things around you. Try to watch positive and knowledgeable content, listen to positive vibes. It helps in making your thought process positive in turn; you would talk positive. These all things make your mindset and atmosphere positive.
- **Visualization:** Take five minutes in your daily routine, close your eyes, and see yourself achieving your goal in future. That will inspire you a lot.
- **Affirmations:** Thinking positive statements which are helping you to complete your goals are affirmations. Like, "I will get success."

Writing these positive statements in a notebook is a powerful way to empower yourself. That helps a lot to make your mindset stronger.

EXAMPLE OF SELF-EMPOWERMENT

Everyone knows Cristiano Ronaldo. He is one of the best footballers in the world. A gardener's son becomes the most expensive athlete in the world. In all the world, people talk about their self-esteem, self-empowerment, mindset. Why? Cristiano has played football since his childhood. He was a very talented boy, that is why he was selected for his first club Andhorina at the age of 8.

When he was 11 years, older people appreciated his talent and said that he was very skinny. That one thing hurts Cristiano more. But small Cristiano knows he can change his body; he can develop his body. So, small Ronaldo decided to work harder than anyone else. He chooses to empower himself. When his teammates used to stop working, then Cristiano used to continue. He still follows this habit.

His new team Juventus medical report said that "Ronaldo's body is the same as a 20 years old player's body at the age of 32." He becomes a legendary footballer of all time because of his self-empowering mindset. Now you get the power of personal empowerment.

Therefore, personal empowerment is a compelling way to not only become successful but also live a great life. So, it is essential to take control of your own life. It is a long process, so you need some patience. Remember one thing: With the mindset of empowering yourself, you can achieve anything in your life.

WOMEN'S EMPOWERMENT

Women's empowerment can be defined as promoting women's sense of self-worth, their ability to determine their own choices, and their right to influence social change for themselves and others.

It is closely aligned with female empowerment—a fundamental human right that is also key to achieving a more peaceful, prosperous world. Women's empowerment and promoting women's rights have emerged as a part of a major global movement and are continuing to break new ground in recent years. Days such as International Women's Empowerment Day are also gaining momentum. But despite a great deal of progress, women and girls continue to face discrimination and violence in every part of the world.

Importance of Women Empowerment

In recent times, everyone is pointing to the empowerment of women. It is right to say that women's empowerment has become the necessity of the time. Women should possess liberty, faith, and self-worth to opt for their needs and demands. Discrimination based on gender is useless and is having zero worth by looking at the growth of women in the last few decades. Women are paid less and are treated as a cook and slave in families, and their real potential fails to get highlighted. Women empowerment in India is required to overcome situations of such types and to provide them with their independent role in Indian society. Empowering women is a necessary right of women. They should have proportional rights to contribute to society, economics, education, and politics. They are approved to gain higher education and receive a similar treatment as men are receiving.

1. **Ensures holistic development of society:** Women empowerment in India is one of the principal terms for society's overall development. There is nothing erroneous in participating in the development of society. In the whole world, women are playing numerous roles in meadows such as medical, engineering, and so on. Apart from taking part in the sphere of technology, they are energetically partaking in security services such as police, navy, military, etc. All these before-mentioned services are taking the community to another level.
2. **Determine their intelligence level:** Over the preceding decades, there has been a uniform increase in women's empowerment. Women must possess self-worth, confidence, and the freedom to choose their needs and requirements. Classifying people based on gender is unreasonable, and it has no worth. Still, women are paid less, expected to cook, and restricted by their family members. To overcome these situations and to have an independent role in society, women's empowerment is needed.

   Empowering women is the fundamental right of women. They can have equal rights to participate in education, society, economics, and politics. They are allowed to have higher education and treated in the way as men.
3. **Able to solve unemployment:** Unemployment is one of the common problems that can be seen in developing society. The research says that half of the population consists of women. The unemployment of women and unequal opportunities in the workplace can be eradicated with the help of women empowerment in India. Whenever women are facing unemployment, their true potential is left without any use. To make use of the strength and potential of the women, they must be provided with equal opportunities. You can motivate them by providing any special gifts. The best time to honor women is Women's Day. You can honor them with Women's Day gifts.
4. **Know about their intelligence:** It is unthinkable to understand and analyze the way of living of women by peeking at them. You can foresee their level of intelligence by way of moving toward the problems and in the solution-finding. In the contemporary era, women are nicely versed in technical troubles. Women's empowerment plays a vital role in these cases. Without women empowerment in India, you will not be able to determine and understand the intelligence of women. Therefore, making existence in work is particularly important and an advantageous one. You can present any gift to give recognition to their work.

5. **Capable enough to solve the issues of unemployment:** Unemployment is one of the widespread problems that can be glimpsed in societies in the developing stage. The study says that around half of the population comprises women. The unemployment of women and unbalanced opportunities in the working place can be eliminated with the assistance of women empowerment in India. Whenever women are confronting unemployment issues, their true capability is left without any intention. To make use of the courage and capacity of the women, they should be empowered with an equal number of opportunities.

PROFESSIONAL ETIQUETTE AND PERSONAL GROOMING

Etiquette is a code of good manners that a nurse should follow. The nurse is an important member of the healthcare team. All the health team members work corporately to achieve the patient health status at the desired level. Being a professional nurse you have to follow some essential manners.

1. You should be courteous to all. Be gentle and polite in your talk.
2. The nurse should greet their seniors, co-workers, patients, etc., with appropriate words and according to the time of the day, e.g., good morning, good evening.
3. The nurse should address the seniors with proper titles, e.g., sir, madam, sister, mister, miss, etc.
4. Stand up when people of higher rank enter your room.
5. Stand up when answering questions in the classroom.
6. Open the door for the seniors and stand aside for them to pass.
7. Excuse yourself when overtaking a senior person.
8. Stand aside and give way to seniors when you cross them on the ways, e.g., in the corridors, on the staircases, etc.
9. Maintain silence whenever and wherever necessary, e.g., classroom, library, study room, and dormitories.
10. Keep your dress neat and tidy.
11. While on duty never use any form of jewelry that may interfere with work.
12. Obey seniors without arguing.
13. Help the seniors to carry a heavy load if you find them on the way.
14. Say "Thank You" when someone is doing a favor for you, and also when someone corrects you.
15. Get prior permission from the sister in charge before you take any article from any department.
16. Do not delay the answers to the questions. Give the answer immediately and appropriately.
17. Always be punctual.
18. Avoid thumb sucking and nail-biting.
19. In an assembly, let the senior take the seat first.
20. Keep eye contact and sit face-to-face when listening to someone.
21. Say "Excuse me" even if you hurt others accidentally.
22. Never let others' secrets go out of you.
23. Always close the door after getting into a room or when you get out of the room if so desired.
24. Knock at the door and wait for the answer before you enter the other's room.
25. Excuse yourself before you interfere with others engaged in talking or doing some work.
26. The nurse should not give and receive any gifts or present especially from the patients and their relatives.

Importance of Etiquettes in Nursing Profession

1. **Introduce yourself:** Put out your hand for a handshake and say your name in a confident voice. Be ready to introduce colleagues to others as well. Mention the higher-ranking person in the organization

first. Give the name of the person you are making the introduction to first, then say the name of the person being introduced and say something about that person. Then say something about the first person.

2. **Have a confident handshake**: Many people judge others by the quality of their handshake, so make sure it is confident and firm (but not too firm—do not overdo it). Stand up, lean forward, make eye contact, and smile. However, take into consideration cultural preferences and sensitivities—for example, Hindu men do not shake hands with women.

3. **Keep conversations on track**: To avoid inadvertently offending someone, stay away from controversial topics such as religion and politics. When talking with a patient, remember that you are the caregiver. Do not unload your troubles on your patients. If you have trouble getting a conversation started, try using the acronym OAR to help: Make an **O**bservation. **A**sk questions. **R**eveal something about yourself, but avoid getting too personal.

4. **Watch your body language**: When making conversation, do not forget that the care you invest in your words can be undone by nonverbal communication. Stand tall with your shoulders back and your chin up; avoid slouching. Keep your hands out of your pockets, and do not put your hands on your hips or cross them over your chest. Use a sincere smile to convey warmth and friendliness. Look at the eyes of the person you are talking with to show your interest.

5. **Cultivate a positive work environment**: Be polite and courteous to your colleagues, no matter how stressful the situation. When you show respect for others and make others feel valued, you contribute to effective communication and team building.

6. **Dress for success**: If you dress too casually, patients may question your professionalism and attention to detail. Make sure your uniform, laboratory coat, scrubs, and shoes are clean and professional-looking. Clothes should not be too tight or skirts too short. If your hair is long, pull it up and out of your face. Make certain your name tag is visible and readable.

7. **Present a positive, professional image**: Recently, I went to a medical center across town for an audiology consult. When I checked in, I was given a form to fill out and was told to wait until someone called my name. A woman dressed in white called my name and put out her hand. Thinking it was for a handshake, I put my hand out. However, she indicated that she had put her hand out for the form I had filled out. She directed me to another room, sat down, and started asking me questions. Because she never introduced herself and her name tag was turned over, I had to ask her to identify herself and describe her role in the organization. Because she ignored my handshake, she missed an important opportunity to introduce herself and present a positive, professional image.

PERSONAL GROOMING

Grooming promotes the person's self-esteem and self-worth **(Fig. 1)**.

Characteristics of Personal Grooming

- Pleasing personality
- Good hygiene
- Mingle with everyone
- Extrovert character
- Good communication skills

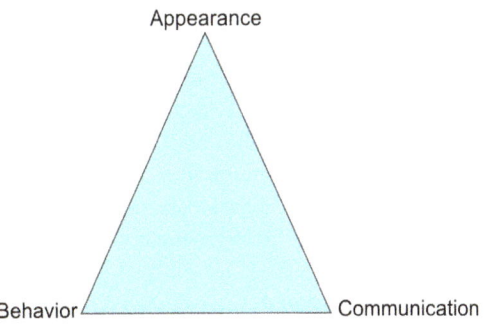

Fig. 1: Triangle for personal grooming.

- Compromise
- Willingness to contribute
- Taking responsibility for mistakes
- Positive attitude and self-esteem
- Time management
- Mutual respect for others and their contributions
- Punctuality
- Teamwork

Tips to Improve Personal Grooming

- **Uniform:** Your uniform tells a lot about your organization. Uniforms should be pressed, ID cards should be worn, and shoes should be clean and polished.
- **Hair:** It should be well-cleaned, natural looking, no bright colors, long hair tied properly at the back, avoid hair accessories.
- **Nails:** Nails should be cut short and nail art is not permitted.

ROLE OF NURSE IN EMPOWERING OTHERS

- As frontline care providers, nurses have the most direct knowledge of the practices that drive patient satisfaction and well-being.
- Because healthcare resources are limited and because there is waste in the system, the nurse must be good stewards of existing resources and capital equipment.
- The American Nurses Association (ANA)'s nursing code of ethics specifically states that nurses are responsible for continuously enhancing the quality and effectiveness of nursing practice.
- Nurses who are empowered feel supported which has a motivating effect, raises job satisfaction, creates an empowered team, and more.
- Empowerment helps nurse increase their job satisfaction overall.
- It offers a clear vision of the future. That helps leaders get buy-in and develop a strategy around their vision that can bring about change.
- Encourage nurses to become comfortable with change. Change is a certainty in the healthcare environment.
- Give nurses a voice. Leaders should hold a daily and weekly meeting where staff has the opportunity to share concerns.

QUESTION BANK

MULTIPLE CHOICE QUESTIONS

1. **Personal grooming refers to:**
   a. Maintaining personal hygiene for pleasing personality
   b. Brushing teeth
   c. Trimming nails
   d. None of these
2. **Personal grooming is best explained by**
   a. Appearance, behavior, communication
   b. Appearance, behavior, coordination
   c. Behavior, communication, skills
   d. Appearance, communication, etiquette
3. **Which among the following is not a dimension of self-empowerment?**
   a. Health
   b. Success
   c. Relationship
   d. Illness

4. **Domestic violence is:**
   a. Physical violence only
   b. Mental violence only
   c. Violence inside the house
   d. All of the above
5. **Empowerment is the opposite of:**
   a. Motivated
   b. Accomplishment
   c. Helplessness
   d. Goal
6. **Self-empowerment is important for:**
   a. Accomplishment
   b. Goal achievement
   c. Career success
   d. All of above
7. **Which strategies help women become more socially and economically empowered?**
   a. Women working together
   b. More income sources for women
   c. Improved access to education
   d. All of the above

ANSWER KEY
1. a   2. a   3. d   4. d   5. c   6. d   7. d

SHORT ANSWER TYPE QUESTIONS

1. Define self-empowerment.
2. Enlist the dimension of self-empowerment.
3. Why women empowerment is necessary?
4. Define professional etiquette.
5. Why personal grooming is important?

LONG ANSWER TYPE QUESTIONS

1. Define self-empowerment. Describe the importance of self-empowerment.
2. Explain the dimension of self-empowerment.
3. Enlist the steps of developing self-empowerment.
4. Explain professional etiquette and personal grooming.
5. Explain the role of the nurse in empowering others.

Bibliography

1. Amanpreet K. A Textbook of Psychology, 2nd edition: PV Publisher; 2022.
2. Babu S. Psychology for Nurses, 1st edition: Elsevier; 2014.
3. Baron RA, et al. Social Psychology, 12th edition: Person Education Publisher; 2009.
4. Bhatia and Craig's. Elements of Psychology and Mental Hygiene, 4th edition: University Press; 2019.
5. Clement I. Textbook on Psychology, 1st edition: Jaypee Brothers Medical Publishers; 2010.
6. en .wikipedia.org/wiki/Emotion
7. en .wikipedia.org/wiki/Psychology
8. Gowda K. Essential of Psychology. CBS Publisher; 2017.
9. https://openpress.usask.ca.
10. https://www.apa.org.
11. https://www.britannica.com.
12. https://www.cliffsnotes.com.
13. https://www.frontiersin.org.
14. https://www.homeobook.com.
15. https://www.Indeed.com.
16. https://www.Psychology.Fandom.com.
17. https://www.Publicservicedegree.org.
18. https://www.researchgate.net.
19. https://www.simplypsychology.org.
20. https://www.ukessays.com.
21. https://www.verywellmind.com.
22. https://www.yourdictionary.com
23. Jacob A. Psychology for Graduate Nurses, 4th edition: Jaypee Brothers Medical Publishers; 2007.
24. Mangal SK. Psychology for Nursing, 1st edition: Avichal Publisher; 2012.
25. Marks DF, Murray M, et al. Health Psychology, 3rd edition: Sage Publisher; 2011.
26. Morgan CT, King J RA, et al. Introduction to psychology. Tata McGraw-Hill Publisher; 1993.
27. Munn's. Introduction to Psychology, 5th edition: AITBS Publisher; 2001.
28. Prakash P. Textbook of Applied Sociology and Psychology, 1st edition: CBS Publishers; 2022.
29. Rajesh GK. Psychology for Graduate Nurses, 1st edition: Jaypee Brothers Medical Publishers; 2013.
30. Sharma H, Mann G. Psychology for Nurses, 5th edition: Lotus Publisher; 2013.
31. Snyder CR, Lopez SJ, Jennnifer T. Positive Psychology: The Scientific and Practical Explorations of Human Strengths, 2nd edition: Sage Publication; 2011.
32. Sreevani R. Applied Psychology for nurses, 4th edition: Jaypee Brothers Medical Publishers; 2022.

BSc Nursing 1st Year (Sample Paper)
Part B
Applied Psychology (Section B)

Total Marks: 38

Multiple Choice Questions (10 × 1 = 10)

1. Which of the following deals with the study of how a person's action, feelings or thoughts are influenced by others:
   a. Social psychology
   b. Clinical psychology
   c. Educational psychology
   d. Health psychology
2. Behavior includes which of the following activities:
   a. Motor
   b. Cognitive
   c. Affective
   d. All of the above
3. Which of the following is not a structure of the forebrain?
   a. Thalamus
   b. Substantia nigra
   c. Hippocampus
   d. Amygdala
4. Individual difference is influenced by following:
   a. Heredity
   b. Environment
   c. Personality
   d. Both a and c
5. A relatively consistent pattern of behavior in the individual is termed as:
   a. Traits
   b. Id
   c. Personality
   d. Ego
6. Which of the following test are used to measure the aptitude of individual?
   a. Personality test
   b. Mental ability
   c. Intelligence test
   d. Emotional test
7. Which of the following criteria of test determines the set of score of test?
   a. Reliability
   b. Norms
   c. Validity
   d. Practicality
8. What soft skill is mostly used by the patients for explaining treatment plan?
   a. Interpersonal skills
   b. Nonverbal
   c. Verbal
   d. Both a and b
9. The dimensions of self-empowerment includes:
   a. Developing self-confidence
   b. Skills and goals
   c. Values
   d. All of these
10. The professional etiquettes includes:
    a. Neat dressing
    b. Being assertive in appropriate manner
    c. Body language
    d. All of these

ANSWER KEY

1. a 2. d 3. b 4. d 5. a 6. b 7. b 8. d
9. d 10. d

Very Short Answer (Any Three) (3 × 2 = 6)
1. Biological motives
2. Reasoning
3. Meaning of perception
4. Defense mechanism
5. Mental health

Short Answer Questions (Any Three) (3 × 5 = 15)
1. Body-mind relationship
2. Branches of psychology
3. Characteristics of psychological test
4. Elaborate the effective of memorizing
5. Importance of guidance and counseling in mental health

Long Answer Questions (Any One) (1 × 7 = 7)
1. Significance of psychology in nursing
2. Explain concept and theories of motivation

Index

Page numbers followed by *b* refer to box, *f* refer to figure, *fc* refer to flowchart, and *t* refer to table.

A

Abductive reasoning 131
Acetylcholine 24, 26
Actual mental events 1
Adaptation 10
Adenohypophysis 29, 31
Adjustment at home 45
Adjustment at work 45
Adjustment in school 45
Adjustment in society 45
Adolescence 70
Adolescent, development stages of 72*t*
Adrenal glands 159
Adrenocorticotropic hormone 30, 31
Adulthood 70
   and old age 48
   development stages during 72*t*
Alcohol 27
Alderfer's ERG theory 151
Alopecia areata 213
Alpha/beta testing 190*f*
Altruism 53
Alzheimer's disease 11
American Nurses Association 226
American Psychological Association 208
Amnesia 129
Amphetamine 126
Amygdala 22, 158
Analogy and assimilation, law of 121
Anarchic theory 135
Anosmia 36
Anterior horn cells 23
Anthropology 7
Antidiuretic hormone 30
Anxiety 165
   disorders 165
Applied psychology, department of 2

Aptitude 139, 142, 188
   characteristic concept of 140
   for graphic art 142
   nursing implications of 142
   professional 141
   test 141, 192
      differential 192
      types of 141, 192
   types of 140
Army alpha and beta tests 188
Arousal reaction 158
Artistic aptitude 140
Ascending reticular activating system 158, 161
Assertiveness training
   purposes of 203
   techniques for 203
Asthma 19
Astigmatism 36
Attention 101, 104*f*
   and concentration, test of 193
   determinants of 102
   effect of 102*f*, 103*f*
   factors affecting 105
   nature of 101
   span of 105
   theories of 104
   types of 102, 102*fc*
Attitude 172
   ambivalent 76
   behavior process model 177, 177*fc*
   change, factor affecting 174
   components of 172
   formation of 173
      theories of 176
   functions of 172
   general appearance and 183
   in health and sickness, role of 178
   meaning of 172
   measurement of 177
   nature of 172
   negative 177

   rational 41
   testing 192
   types of 177
Attitudinal change 174
Auditory learners 113
Auditory sensation 35
Autistic withdrawal 51
Autonomy, sense of 41
Axon 24, 25

B

Balance theory 176
Bargaining 74
Basal ganglia 28
Basic desires theory 152
Behavior
   affective 15
   aggressive 76
   biological explanations of 16
   cognitive 15
   components of 2*f*
   connative 15
   constituents of 15*f*
   glandular controls of 29
   muscular control of 27
   patterns 85
Benton visual retention test 128
Benzodiazepines 18
BF skinner experiments 118*f*
Biochemistry 7
Biological amnesia 129
Biological and behavior 15
Biological psychology 17
Blood pressure 162
Body on mind, effect of 18
Body reaction 212
Body systems, wear and tear of 166
Body temperature, motive for regulation of 154
Body works 17
Brain 20, 86
   anatomy of 21*f*
   and behavior 19

Index

motor pathways in 29
parts of 21f
waves 162
Brainstem 28
  reticular formation 158
Broadbent's claim 104
Broadbent's filter theory 104, 104f
Build personal empowerment,
    techniques to 222
Build resilience, ways to 209

C

Cannabis 126
Cannon-Bard theory 158, 160f
Cardiovascular system 28
Cataract 36
Cathexis 92
Cattell and Horn's theory 136
Cattell's and Eysenck's
    theories 90
Cell
  body 23
  division 23
  kinds of 23
Central nervous system 17, 20, 20fc, 28
Central traits 90
Cerebellum 22, 28
Cerebral cortex 27, 28, 157, 160
Cerebrum 20
Child apperception test 156
Childhood 47
  psychology 3
Children apperception test 95, 96f
Chronic mental illnesses 97
Chronic stress 19
Clerical aptitude test 142
Clinical psychology 3
Cocaine 18, 126
Coginitive psychology 101
Cognition theory 136
Cognitive development 69, 71
Cognitive dissonance theory 176
Common health problems 69, 71, 72
Common illness, types of 77
Common mental
  health issues 79
  illness 38
Communication 175, 197, 199, 202
  advantages of 203
  and interpersonal
    relationships 206
  assertive 203, 204

aural 197
barriers of 205b
characteristics of 201
clear 57
controlling process 199
disadvantages of 204
elements of 200
formal 202
helps in socializing 199
importance of 199
informal network 202
mechanical 202
nonverbal 197, 202, 202f
one-way 175, 201
oral 202-204
physiological 202
principles of 201
process of 200, 200f
promotes motivation 199
psychic 202
source of 174
    information 199
strategies of 204
types of 197, 201
understanding 200
verbal 197, 202
visual 198, 202
written 197, 202-204
Community mental health 48
Comparative psychology 3
Comprehensive neuropsychiatric
    batteries 193
Concrete intelligence 135
Concrete operations 66
Conflict 58
  causes of 58
  resolution 58, 60
    facilitator of 62
  sources of 58f
  types of 55, 59
Congruity theory 176
Conscious
  consists of 85
  layer 91
Consultation services 49
Coping skill intervention 213
Coronary artery disease 19
Corpus callosum 20, 27
Cortex 20
  association of 27, 28f
Corticobulbar tract 23
Corticospinal tract 23
Counseling 10
  effective 11
Countershock phase 167

Crisis intervention 49
Crisis situations 48
Critical thinking skills 206
Cultivate compassion 210
Cultural factors 86
Cytoplasm 23

D

Deal with conflict, ways to 61f
Death and dying 74
Deductive reasoning 131
Defense mechanism 50, 91
  characteristics of 51f
  functions of 51
Delusion 133
  of grandeur 134
  of influence 133
  projection 51
Dendrites 24
Deoxyribonucleic acid 31
Depression 6, 25, 38, 74, 164
Deutsch-Norman
  model of selective attention 105f
  theory 104
Development, stages of 68t
Developmental disorders 11
Developmental psychology 65
Developmental theory 65
Diazepam 18
Diencephalon 22
Digestive system 162
Disability, developmental 75
Disabled, types of 75
Disfigurement 75
Displacement 52
  theory 129
Dissociation 53
Distortion 51
Distraction 105
  continuous 106
  discontinuous 106
  forms of 106
Dopamine 6, 24, 26
  activity 18
Droopy eyelids 154
Drug addictions 27
Dualistic theories 18
Dynamic organization 85

E

Early diagnosis and case finding 48
Early reference and follow-up services 49

Echoic memory 125
Eclectic theory 136
Edward L Thorndike's law 114*f*
Ego 91
　dealing with 55
　defense mechanism
　　classification of 51
　　implications of 54
　　functions of 55*f*
　　restores balance between id and superego 55*f*
Elements, pre-potency of 121
Eliminating distraction, methods of 106
Emotion 126, 156, 157, 160*f*, 161*fc*, 163
　activation theory of 161
　alteration in 164
　Arnold's theory of 162
　arousal 122
　biological basis of 157
　brain 22
　characteristics of 157
　conflicts 19
　development 69, 71, 72
　factors affecting 157
　in health and sickness 164
　insight 211
　intelligence 135, 156, 211
　measurement of 162
　physiological changes in 162
　stability 90
　theories of 159
　understand negative 163
　unpleasant 19
　verbal instruments to measure 163
Empathy, develop 164
Employee aide programs 213
Endocrine glands 29*f*
　functions of 29*f*
Ensuring adequate physical health 215
Environment 33
　factors 106
　frustration 56
　mastery 40
Erikson development stages 67*t*
Erikson's reasoning 66
Erikson's theory 66
Etiquettes, importance of 224
Exercise 126, 222
　law of 120
　mindfulness 209
Expectancy theory 151

Experimental method 156
Extrapyramidal system 23
Extrapyramidal tract 23
Extrinsic motivation 148

F

Face-to-face etiquette 216
Factors affecting attitude 173
　change 174*fc*
Family members, impact on 78
Fantasy 52
Farsightedness 36
Female gamete 68
Figure ground perception 109*f*
First psychology laboratory 2
Fluid intelligence 136
Focused attention 104
Folstein test 193
Forebrain 20
Forensic psychiatric test 192
Forgetting, causes of 128
Formal psychology, birth of 1
Free movement, sensation of 36
Freud's iceberg of mind 17*f*
Frontal lobe 21
　association cortex 27
Frustration 76
　and conflict 55
　conflict leading to 56
　dealing with 57
　in students, causes of 56
　process of 56*f*
　sources of 56
　symptoms of 56

G

Galen's theory 89*f*
Galvanic skin response 162
Gamma-Aminobutyric acid 19, 26
General adaptation syndrome 167, 168*f*
General aptitude battery test 192
Generativity 67
Genes 31
　strands of 31
　transmission of 32*f*
　types of 31
Genetic 34
　and behavior 31
　disorders 34
　diversity 33
　variability 33
Genital stage 92
Gestalt principles 108, 109*f*

Gestalt psychology 4
Goal-oriented behavior 148
Gonadotropic hormone 30, 31
Good learning, symbols of 119
Gordon Allport's trait theory 89
Group
　development of 81
　　stages of 81*f*
　nonverbal tests 138
　psychological issues in 81
　types of 80, 80*fc*
　verbal tests 138
Group tests
　advantages of 138
　disadvantages of 138
Growth hormone 30

H

Habit
　formation of 121, 122
　types of 122
Hallucination 110*t*
Harmonious development 44
Health
　problems, types of 123
　professionals, training of 49
Hearing
　abnormalities related to 36
　sense of 35
Heartbeat 162
Hereditary 41
Heredity 33
　and environment 33
　product of 85
Herzberg's two factor theory 151
Hindbrain 20, 22
Homeostasis 153
Hormonal changes 162
Hormone 29, 30*t*, 159
Hot lines service link 49
Human behavior 15, 16
Human beings, behavior of 7
Human memory 125*fc*
Human mind, Freud's view of 91*f*
Human Y chromosome 31
Humanistic approach 5
Humanistic psychology 5
Humor 54, 87
Hunger pangs 153
Hygiene factors 151
Hyperopia 36
Hypertension 19, 123
Hypochondriacal delusions 133
Hypothalamus 22, 158

I

Iconic memory 125
Idealization 52
Identity *vs* confusion 67
Illness on sick individuals, effects of 78*f*
Illusion 110, 110*t*
  personal 110
  universal 110
Improve personal grooming 226
Impulse transmission, mechanism of 25
Inattention 103, 104*f*
Incentive theory 152
Individual across life span, development of 68
Individual and family therapy 50
Individual performance test 137
Individual verbal test 137
Inductive reasoning 131
Industrial psychology 3
Industry *vs* inferiority 66
Infancy 47
Infant development
  scales, types of 189*t*
  stages of 68*t*
Information
  gathering exercise 203
  novelty of 175
  transfer 24
Infundibulum 29
Inkblot test 95
Insight learning, theory of 115, 115*f*
Instrumental conditioning 117
Integrity *vs* despair 67
Intellectualization 53
Intelligence 134, 142, 188
  abstract 135
  characteristics of 134
  crystallized 136
  information processing theory of 136
  level 223
  measurement of 137
  test 137*fc*, 188, 192
    evolution of 188
    limitations of 139
    uses of 139, 190
  theories of 135
  types of 134, 135
Intensity on attention, effect of 102*f*
Interactional skill training 50
Interactionism theorized 18
Interference theory 129
Internal factors 106
Interpersonal relationship 206, 206*f*
  at workplace 208
  factors enhancing 207
  phases of 206
  role of nurse in improving 207
Interpersonal relationships 12
Intimacy *vs* isolation 67
Intrinsic motivation 148, 152
Introjection 54
Isolation 53

J

James-Lange theory 159, 160*f*
Janani Suraksha Yojna 79
Jean Piaget theory 65, 66*t*, 93
Jensen's theory 137
Journal writing 57
Jung's classification 88

K

Kinesthetic learners 113
Kinesthetic sensations 35
Korsakoff's syndrome 127, 129
Kretschmer types of physique 87
Kubler-Ross grief cycle 74*f*

L

Lactic acid 154
Lazarus theory 161
Learning 111, 112
  by conditioning 115
  by observation 115
  conceptual 112
  factors influencing 112
  factors operating after 128
  humanistic theories of 119, 119*f*
  in sickness and health, role of 123
  laws of 120
  material, nature of 113
  method of 128
    nature of 113
  motor 112
  nature of 112
  paired-associate 112
  primary laws of 120
  problem-solving 112
  process 113
  Roger's theory of 119
  secondary laws of 120
  serial 112
  speed of 128
  styles, types of 113
  subordinate laws of 121
  theories of 114
  transfer of 121
  trial and error theory of 114
  types of 112, 119
  verbal 112
Life, positive philosophy of 40
Limbic system 21, 22, 158
  parts of 22
Local adaptation syndrome 168
Loci, method of 126
Lorazepam 18
Luria-Nebraska-neuropsychological battery 193

M

Marijuana 126
Maslow's hierarchy 150*f*
Maslow's theory of Hierarchy 150
Maternal drive 154
Mature and responsible 40
Maturity 93
Mechanical aptitude 140
  test 141
Medulla 23, 159
  oblongata 22
Melanocyte-stimulating hormone 30
Memory 124
  and forgetting 124
  disorders of 183
  explicit 125
  factors influencing 126
  immediate 125
  implicit 126
  long-term 125
  methods to improve 126
  nature of 124
  process 124, 124*f*
  short-term 124, 125
  test for 127, 193
  types of 125
Mental age and intelligence quotient 139
Mental agility 210
  develop 210
Mental alertness and retention, test for 193
Mental and physical health 113
Mental development 68
Mental disorders 38, 42

Index

Mental functioning 137
Mental health 38, 39, 43, 44, 99
   and mental hygiene 38
   concept of 38
   dimensions of 39, 39f
   education 49
   factors affecting 41, 41t
   illness continuum 42f
   promotion of 43
   services 50t
      preventive 46
      promotive 46
Mental hospital, programs in 49
Mental hygiene 43, 44
   concept of 38
   functions of 44
   history of 44
   limitations of 45
   movement 45
   objectives of 44
   principles of 45
Mental iceberg 91f
Mental ill health 41
Mental illness 42
   prevention of 43
   types of 38
Mental process 17
   understanding 11
Mental representation 17
Mental status examination 182
Mentally challenge 75, 76
Mentally disturbed patients 11
Mentally healthy 38
   characteristics of
      individual 40
      person 40b
Mesencephalon 22
Midbrain 20, 22
   parts of 22
Middle adulthood 93
Mind 17
   on body, effect of 19
   topography of 5
Mind-body
   concept of 16
   interaction 16f, 18
   interventions 19
   relationship 11, 16
      history of 16
      theories of 17, 18t
Mini-mental state examination 184, 193
   interpretation of 185
Mini-mental status examination 183

Monarchic theory 135
Monistic theories 17
Moral anxiety 91
Moral character 85
Motivated forgetting 129
Motivation 146, 147, 147f
   and emotional processes 146
   concept of 146
   cycle 153
   expectancy theory of 151f
   nature of 148, 148f
   process of 153fc
   skills 217
   theories of 150
   types of 148, 149f
Motivator-hygiene theory 151
Motive 147f
   achievement 149, 155
   acquisitive 155
   affiliation 150, 155
   aggressive 155
   biological 153
   classification of 149
   curiosity 155
   general 149
   hunger 153
   love and hope 156
   measurement of 156
   physiological 153
   power 155
   primary 149
   secondary 149
   self-esteem 155
   sex 154
   social 154
   stimulus and exploration 155
   thirst 153
Motor activity, disorder of 183
Motor development 68
Motor sensations 35
Multifactor theory 135
Multiple responses, law of 121
Muscle
   tissue 27
   tremors 154
Musical aptitude tests 142
Myelin sheath 24
Myopia 36

N

Nature *vs* nurture 33
Near-sightedness 36
Negative attitude, characteristics of 177t

Nerve cells 24
   communicate 24
Nerve impulse 25f
   conduction 24
Nervous system 20
Nervous tension 38
Neurohypophysis 29, 31
Neurological disorders, types of 11
Neurologically handicapped 75
Neuron 6, 23, 25
   parts of 23
   structure of 23f
   terminal of 24
Neuropsychological assessment 193
Neurotic anxiety 91
Neuroticism 90
Neurotransmitter 24
   disease variability 27
   types of 26t
Nicotine 18
Nihilistic delusions 133
Nodes of Ranvier 24
Noradrenaline 26
Norepinephrine 24, 159
Nucleus 23
Nurse with good personality, qualities of 98
Nurse-patient relationship, therapeutic 206
Nursing
   empowerment 220
   implication in 82
Nurture interpersonal relationship 218

O

Occipital lobe 22
Occupational training 50
Older adult, development changes in 73t
Olfaction, abnormalities related to 36
Olfactory sensation 35
Operant conditioning
   application of 119
   principles of 117
Optimum health, reduce 166
Oral sensory 92
Original learning, strength of 128
Orthopedically handicapped 75
Osgood and Tannenbaum congruity theory 176f
Oxygen, need for 154
Oxytocin 30

Index

P

Pain, avoidance of 154
Parapsychology 4
Parietal lobe 21
   association cortex 27
Parkinson's disease 6, 11
Passive aggression 52
Pavlov's experiments 116f
Peplau's theory 206f
Peptic ulcers 19
Perception 106
   abnormalities in 110
   alterations in 111
   determinants influencing 107
   disorder of 183
   factors influencing 110
   laws of 108
   principles of 108
   process of 107, 107f
   types of 108
Perceptual disorder 111
Performance intelligence test 190
Performance testing 192
Perinatal period 47
Persecutory delusions 133
Person's behavior 15
Personal affairs, management of 196
Personal empowerment 220
Personal frustration 56
Personal grooming 224, 225
   characteristics of 225
   triangle for 225f
Personality 84
   alterations in 97
   and behavior 10
   assessment, techniques of 94
   characteristics of 85
   classification of 87
   constituents of 84
   determinants 86fc
      affecting 86
   determine 87
   development, psychosocial stages of 92
   disorder 98, 123
      categories of 98t
   disturbed 76
   Eysenck's three dimensions of 90
   five-factor theory of 90
   Freudian components of 90f
   functions 86
   improvement in altered 99
   inventories 94
   measurement and evaluation of 94
   nature of 85
   symptoms of alterations in 97
   testing 191
      methods of 191
   theories of 87
   traits of 89f
Phenylketonuria 34
Philosophy and psychology 6
Physical factors 86
Physical growth 68-72
Physical health, taking care of 215
Physics and psychology 7
Physiologic reactions 163
Physiological development 69-72
Physiology and psychology 7
Piaget's stages 93
Picture arrangement 190f
Pituitary gland 29
Pons varolii 22
Poor mental health, warning signs of 42
Poor reputation 214
Poor time management, implications of 214
Positive attitude 177
   characteristics of 177t
   toward self 39
Positive motivation 148
Postsynaptic membrane 24, 25
Potassium ions 24
Preconscious layer 91
Prenatal period 47
Preschooler, development stages of 70t
Presynaptic membrane 24, 25, 26
Proactive inhibition 129
Problem-solving strategies 57
Professional aptitudes, tests of 142
Professional education 12
Professional etiquette 224
Projected techniques 94
Projection 52
Prolactin 30, 31
Promote positive feeling 163
Psychiatry and psychology 7
Psychic energy 91
Psychoanalysis 5
Psychoanalytical model 41
Psychoanalytical theory 90
Psychodynamic approach 5
Psychological amnesia 130
Psychological assessment 182
Psychological distress 79
Psychological needs 71
Psychological problems 78
Psychological syndrome 42
Psychological test 2, 182, 185, 186
   characteristics of 187
   principles of 187
   types of 188
   uses of 187
Psychological well-being, techniques to help with 170
Psychology 1, 6, 7, 11, 12
   abnormal 3, 7
   applications of 11
   areas of 2
   behavioral 6
   biological 6
   clinical method 9
   cognitive approach 5
   contemporary approaches to 5
   correlation method 9
   development of 3, 8
   educational 3
   evolutionary approach 5
   experimental 3
   general 2
   humanistic approach 5
   in nursing profession 11
   interview method 9
      types of 10
   introspection method 7
   meaning of 1
   methods of 7
   natural observation 8
   nature of 1
   observation method 8
   of challenged 75
   of elderly people 77
   of groups 80
   of sensation 34
   of sick individuals 77
   of vulnerable groups 75
   of women 79
   positive 6
   principles of 11
   psychodynamic approach 5
   schools of thought in 4, 4f
   scientific method 8
   scope of 2, 3f
   sociocultural approach 5
   subfields of 2
   subject matter of 1
   to nursing, relevance of 10

Psychometric assessment 182
  advantages of 194
  disadvantages of 194
Psychomotor activity 15
Psychoneuroimmunology 19
  concept of 19*f*
Psychosis 133
Psychosocial assessment,
    methods for 182
Psychosocial development 66, 69,
    70, 72
Psychosomatic illness, prevent
    164
Psychosomatic medicine 18
Psychotherapy 7
Psychotic denial 51
Pulse rate 162
Punishment 117

R

Raven's progressive matrices 191*f*
Reaction
  expressive 163
  formation 53
  to frustration 56*f*
Realistic goal settings 57
Reasoning 131
Regression 52
Rehabilitation 50
Reinforcement
  negative 118*f*
  positive 118*f*
  types of 6
Relaxation techniques 57, 168
Repression 53
  theory 129
Reproductive and child health 79
Research 10
  studies, types of 8
Resent sympathy 76
Resilience 208
  in workplace 209
Resilient nurse, qualities of 209*f*
Respiratory rate 162
Reticular formation 158
Revised Stanford-Binet scales
    189*f*
Roger classifies 119
Role of nurse 76, 79
  dealing with frustration 57
  empowering 226
  good communication 205
  identification of individual
    personality 98

maintain work-life balance
    215
  primary prevention 47
  psychological testing 194
  secondary prevention 48
  tertiary prevention 49
Rorschach inkblot test 96*f*, 156
Rorschach interpretation 96
Rorschach's test 95
  goals of 96

S

Schachter-Singer theory 160,
    161*fc*
Scholastic aptitude 141
  tests of 142
School children 70
  development stages of 71*t*
Screening programs 48
Selecting appropriate tests 186
Self-actualized persons,
    characteristics of 151
Self-consciousness 85
Self-empowerment 220, 222
  development, steps of 221
  dimensions of 220
Semantic memory 126
Semiconscious, consists of 85
Sensation 34
  attributes of 34
  types of 35
Sensorimotor stage 65
Sensory 125
  aptitude 140
  development 69
  input 124
Serial communication 202
Serotonin 6, 24, 26
Set attitude, law of 121
Sex cell 68
Sexual development 65, 68-72
Sharing views 57
Sheldon theory 87
  classification to 88*t*
Shock phase 167
Sick individual, hospitalization
    of 78
Sickness, forgetting during 129
Sight, sense of 35
Sin and guilt, delusions of 133
Situational factors 86
Situational judgement test 193
Skills training 214
Skinner's view 6

Sleep
  need for 154
  problems 69
Slender cellular structure 25
Smell, sense of 35
Social etiquette 216
  types of 216
Social factors 86
Social intelligence 135
Social isolation, feeling of 76
Social media etiquette 217
Social psychology 4
Socially challenged 76
Sociology and psychology 6
Soft skill 196, 204
  application of 196, 218
  develop 198
  types of 197, 197*f*, 197*t*
Spearman's two-factor theory 136
Speech
  and hearing handicapped 75
  disorder of 183
Spinal cord 28
Spiritual conditions 212
Spiritual development 69, 71, 72
Spirituality 211
Staff development program 213
Stagnation 67
Stanford-Binet test 188
Stress 165, 212
  acute 167
  and adaptation 165, 167
  chronic 167
  cycle 165, 166*f*
  diary 171
  effect of 166, 213
    emotional response 166
    physical response 166
    psychological response
      166
  episodic acute 167
  in nursing 171
  in relation to sickness 171
  management 168, 211
  strategies 213
  reaction to 166
  types of 167, 213
  workplace 212
Stressors 165
  day-to-day 165
  types of 212
Stress-stressors, sources of 165
Sublimation 53
Superego 91

Index

Suppression 54
Symbolic communication 202
Sympathetic nervous system 159
Synapse 24
Synaptic cleft 25

T

Tachistoscope 105
Tactile sensations 35
Taste
  buds 35
  sensation 35
  sense of 35
Teacher's role 57, 119
Tectum and tegmentum 22
Telephone etiquette 217
Telodendria 24
Temper tantrums 69
Temperament theory 87
Temporal lobe 21
  association cortex 27
Tertiary prevention, components of 49f
Test development, history of 186
Thalamus 22
Thematic apperception test 94, 95f, 156
Theories, types of 87
Therapeutic modalities 12
Thinking 130
  abstract 130
  alterations in 133
  conceptual 130
  concrete 130
  convergent 132
  creative 130
  divergent 132
  levels of 132
  logical 131
  perceptual 130
  types of 130
Thorndike's law 122
Thought
  disorder of 183
    content of 183
    form of 183
  negative 19
Thumb sucking 69
Thurston's group factor theory 136
Thurstone attitude scale 192
Thyroid-stimulating hormone 30, 31
Toddler, development stages of 69t
Touch, sense of 35
Trait
  secondary 90
  theories 89
Transfer, types of 121
Treisman's attenuation model 104, 105f
Two factor theory 160

U

Unconscious
  consists of 85
  layer 91
Unemployment, issues of 224
Unitary theory 135

V

Verbal learning 112
Verbal *vs* nonverbal test 138
Virtual meeting etiquette 217
Visual agnosia 111
Visual discrimination 111
Visual learners 113
Visual memory 126
Visual processing 111
Visual sensation 35
Visually handicapped 75

W

Walk-in clinics 49
Waste, elimination of 154
Wechsler intelligence
  scale 137, 190f
  test 189
Wechsler IQ test classification 139t
Wechsler memory scale 127
Wechsler-Bellevue intelligence test 137, 138
White blood corpuscles 162
Women's empowerment 222, 223
Word association test 96
Working memory 125
Work-life balance 215

Y

Yoga, practice 27

EU GSPR Authorised Reprsentative
Logos Europe, 9 rue Nicolas Poussin
1700, La Rochelle, France
Phone: +33 (0) 6 67 93 73 78
E-mail: contact@logoseurope.eu

www.ingramcontent.com/pod-product-compliance
Ingram Content Group UK Ltd.
Pitfield, Milton Keynes, MK11 3LW, UK
UKHW050429150426
5217IPUK00019B/1302